theclinics.com

# MEDICAL CLINICS OF NORTH AMERICA

## Colon Cancer Screening, Surveillance, Prevention, and Treatment: Conventional and Novel Technologies

GUEST EDITOR

Mitchell S. Cappell, MD, PhD, FACG

January 2005 • Volume 89 • Number 1

SAUNDERS

An Imprint of Elsevier, Inc.

PHILADELPHIA LONDON TORONTO MONTREAL SYDNEY TOKYO

**W.B. SAUNDERS COMPANY**
*A Division of Elsevier Inc.*

The Curtis Center • Independence Square West • Philadelphia, Pennsylvania 19106

http://www.theclinics.com

**THE MEDICAL CLINICS OF NORTH AMERICA**
**January 2005**
Editor: Heather Cullen

**Volume 89, Number 1**
**ISSN 0025-7125**



*The Medical Clinics of North America* (ISSN 0025-7125) is published bimonthly by Elsevier. Corporate and editorial offices: 170 S Independence Mall W 300 E, Philadelphia, PA 19106-3399. Accounting and circulation offices: 6277 Sea Harbor Drive, Orlando, FL 32887-4800. Periodicals postage paid at Orlando, FL 32862, and additional mailing offices. Subscription prices are USD 140 per year for US individuals, USD 244 per year for US institution, USD 70 per year for US students, USD 180 per year for Canadian individuals, USD 311 per year for Canadian institutions, USD 205 per year for international individuals, USD 311 per year for international institutions and USD 103 per year for Canadian and foreign students/residents. To receive student/resident rate, orders must be accompanied by name of affiliated institution, date of term, and the *signature* of program/residency coordinator on institution letterhead. Orders will be billed at individual rate until proof of status is received. Foreign air speed delivery is included in all *Clinics* subscription prices. All prices are subject to change without notice. POSTMASTER: Send address changes to *The Medical Clinics of North America,* W.B. Saunders Company, Periodicals Fulfillment, Orlando, FL 32887-4800. **Customer Service: 1-800-654-2452 (US). From outside of the US, call 1-407-345-1000. E-mail: hhspcs@harcourt.com.**

*Reprints.* For copies of 100 or more, of articles in this publication, please contact the Commercial Reprints Department, Elsevier Inc., 360 Park Avenue South, New York, New York 10010-1710. Tel.: (212) 633-3813; Fax: (212) 633-3820; E-mail: reprints@elsevier.com.

*The Medical Clinics of North America* is also published in Greek by Althayia S. A., Athens, Greece; in Spanish by McGraw-Hill Interamericana Editores S. A., P.O. Box 5-237, 06500 Mexico, D.F., Mexico; and in Portuguese by Reichmann and Affonso Editors, Rio de Janeiro, Brazil.

*The Medical Clinics of North America* is covered in *Index Medicus, Current Contents, ASCA, Excerpta Medica, Science Citation Index,* and *ISI/BIOMED.*

Printed in the United States of America.

## GOAL STATEMENT

The goal of *Medical Clinics of North America* is to keep practicing physicians up to date with current clinical practice by providing timely articles reviewing the state of the art in patient care.

## ACCREDITATION

The *Medical Clinics of North America* is planned and implemented in accordance with the Essential Areas and Policies of the Accreditation Council for Continuing Medical Education (ACCME) through the joint sponsorship of the University of Virginia School of Medicine and W. B. Saunders Company. The University Of Virginia School of Medicine is accredited by the ACCME to provide continuing medical education for physicians.

The University of Virginia School of Medicine designates this educational activity for a maximum of 90 category 1 credits per year, 15 category 1 credits per issue, toward the AMA Physician's Recognition Award. Each physician should claim only those credits that he/she actually spent in the activity.

The American Medical Association has determined that physicians not licensed in the US who participate in this CME activity are eligible for AMA PRA category 1 credit.

Category 1 credit can be earned by reading the text material, taking the CME examination online at ***http://www.theclinics.com/home/cme***, and completing the evaluation. Each test question must be answered correctly; you will have the opportunity to retake any questions answered incorrectly. Following successful completion of the test and the evaluation, you may print your certificate.

## FACULTY DISCLOSURE

As a provider accredited by the Accreditation Council for Continuing Medical Education (ACCME), the Office of Continuing Medical Education of the University of Virginia School of Medicine must ensure balance, independence, objectivity, and scientific rigor in all its individually sponsored or jointly sponsored educational activities. All authors/editors participating in a sponsored activity are expected to disclose to the readers any significant financial interest or other relationship (1) with the manufacturer(s) of any commercial product(s) and/or provider(s) of commercial services discussed in an educational presentation and (2) with any commercial supporters of the activity (significant financial interest or other relationship can include such things as grants or research support, employee, consultant, stock holder, member of speakers bureau, etc.). The intent of this disclosure is not to prevent authors/editors with a significant financial or other relationship from writing an article, but rather to provide readers with information on which they can make their own judgments. It remains for the readers to determine whether the author's/editor's interest or relationships may influence the article with regard to exposition or conclusion.

***The authors/editors listed below have identified no professional or financial affiliations related to their presentation:*** Prathap Bandipalliam, MD; Manoop S. Bhutani, MD, FACG, FACP; C. Richard Boland, MD; Mitchell S. Cappell, MD, PhD, FACG; J. Heather Cullen; Gregory B. Haber, MD, FRCPC; Kareem Hamdy, MD; Ernest T. Hawk, MD, MPH; Atsushi Irisawa, MD, PhD; Zvi Lefkovitz, MD; Gregory J. Monkewich, MD, FRCPC, ABIM; Ellen Richmond, MSN, RN; Robert Shapiro, MD; Sapna Syngal, MD, MPH; Radha Tamerisa, MD; Jose E. Torres, MD; George Tsoulfas, MD; Asad Umar, PhD, DVM; and, Jaye L. Viner, MD, MPH.

***The authors/editors listed below have identified the following professional or financial affiliations related to his presentation:*** **Jack S. Mandel, MD, PhD** has disclosed that he serves as a member of a scientific advisory committee for Enterix, the manufacturer of an immunochemical screening test.

***Disclosure of discussion of non-FDA approved uses for pharmaceutical products and/or medical devices:*** The University of Virginia School of Medicine, as an ACCME provider, requires that all authors/editors identify and disclose any "off label" uses for pharmaceutical products and/or for medical devices. The University of Virginia School of Medicine recommends that each reader fully review all the available data on new products or procedures prior to instituting them with patients.

***All authors/editors who provided disclosures will not be discussing any off-label uses except:*** **Ernest T. Hawk, MD, MPH, Ellen Richmond, MSN, RN; Asad Umar, PhD, DVM**; and, **Jaye L. Viner, MD, MPH** will be discussing the off-label use of ASA, Selenium, Calcium, Eflornithine, Celecox B, Folate, and Antioxidants for Cancer Prevention.

***The authors/editors listed below have not provided disclosure or off-label information:*** Stephen Koch, MD; and, Carol E. H. Scott-Conner, MD, PhD.

## TO ENROLL

To enroll in the Medical Clinics of North America Continuing Medical Education program, call customer service at 1-800-654-2452 or sign up online at ***http://www.theclinics.com/home/cme***. The CME program is available to subscribers for an additional annual fee of $195.00.

## FORTHCOMING ISSUES

March 2005

**Screening, Prevention, and Treatment of Esophageal, Gastric, and Hepatic Malignancies**
Mitchell S. Cappell, MD, PhD, FACG,
*Guest Editor*

May 2005

**Renal Disease**
Ajay K. Singh, MB, MRCP, *Guest Editor*

July 2005

**Minority Health Issues, Part I**
Charles R. Thomas, Jr., MD, and
Eddie L. Greene, MD, *Guest Editors*

## RECENT ISSUES

November 2004

**Treating Tobacco Dependence**
Virginia Cullen Reichert, NP, Arunabh Talwar, MD, FCCP, Alan M. Fein, MD, FACP, FCCP, FCCM
*Guest Editors*

September 2004

**Primary Prevention of Heart Failure**
Jagat Narula, MD, PhD, Clyde W. Yancy, MD, and James B. Young, MD, *Guest Editors*

July 2004

**Type 2 Diabetes Mellitus**
Alan J. Garber, *Guest Editor*

# GUEST EDITOR

**MITCHELL S. CAPPELL, MD, PhD, FACG,** Director, Gastroenterology Fellowship Training Program, Division of Gastroenterology, Albert Einstein Medical Center, Philadelphia, Pennsylvania

# CONTRIBUTORS

**PRATHAP BANDIPALLIAM, MD,** Research Fellow, Dana-Farber Cancer Institute, Boston, Massachusetts

**MANOOP S. BHUTANI, MD, FACG, FACP,** Professor, Department of Medicine; Co-Director, Center for Endoscopic Research, Training and Innovation (CERTAIN); and Director, Center for Endoscopic Ultrasound, University of Texas Medical Branch, Galveston, Texas

**C. RICHARD BOLAND, MD,** Chief, Division of Gastroenterology, Baylor University Medical Center, Dallas, Texas

**MITCHELL S. CAPPELL, MD, PhD, FACG,** Director, Gastroenterology Fellowship Training Program, Division of Gastroenterology, Albert Einstein Medical Center, Philadelphia, Pennsylvania

**GREGORY B. HABER, MD, FRCPC,** Director, Division of Gastroenterology, Lenox Hill Hospital, New York, New York

**KAREEM HAMDY, MD,** House Staff, Department of Surgery, Roy J. and Lucille C. Carver College of Medicine, University of Iowa, Iowa City, Iowa

**ERNEST T. HAWK, MD, MPH,** Chief, Gastrointestinal and Other Cancers Research Group, Division of Cancer Prevention, National Cancer Institute, Bethesda, Maryland

**ATSUSHI IRISAWA, MD, PhD,** Lecturer, Fukushima University School of Medicine, Fukushima, Japan

**STEPHEN KOCH, MD,** Clinical Instructor, Department of Radiology, Mount Sinai School of Medicine, Mount Sinai Medical Center, New York, New York

**ZVI LEFKOVITZ, MD,** Clinical Associate Professor and Vice-Chairman, Department of Radiology, Mount Sinai School of Medicine, Mount Sinai Medical Center, New York, New York

**JACK S. MANDEL, PhD, MPH,** Rollins Professor of Epidemiology and Chairman, Department of Epidemiology, Rollins School of Public Health, Emory University, Atlanta, Georgia

**GREGORY J. MONKEWICH, MD, FRCPC,** Gastroenterology and Therapeutic Endoscopy, Vancouver, British Columbia, Canada

**ELLEN RICHMOND, RN, MS,** Program Director, Gastrointestinal and Other Cancers Research Group, Division of Cancer Prevention, National Cancer Institute, Bethesda, Maryland

**CAROL E.H. SCOTT-CONNER, MD, PhD,** Professor, Department of Surgery, Roy J. and Lucille C. Carver College of Medicine, University of Iowa, Iowa City, Iowa

**ROBERT SHAPIRO, MD,** Section Head, Body Imaging; and Clinical Associate Professor, Department of Radiology, Mount Sinai School of Medicine, Mount Sinai Medical Center, New York, New York

**SAPNA SYNGAL, MD, MPH,** Associate Physician, Division of Gastroenterology, Brigham and Women's Hospital; Staff Physician, Population Sciences Division, Dana-Farber Cancer Institute; and Assistant Professor, Medicine, Harvard Medical School, Boston, Massachusetts

**RADHA TAMERISA, MD,** Senior Gastroenterology Fellow, Department of Medicine, University of Texas Medical Branch, Galveston, Texas

**JOSE E. TORRES, MD,** House Staff, Department of Surgery, Roy J. and Lucille C. Carver College of Medicine, University of Iowa, Iowa City, Iowa

**GEORGE TSOULFAS, MD,** Department of Surgery, Roy J. and Lucille C. Carver College of Medicine, University of Iowa, Iowa City, Iowa

**ASAD UMAR, PhD, DVM,** Program Director, Gastrointestinal and Other Cancers Research Group, Division of Cancer Prevention, National Cancer Institute, Bethesda, Maryland

**JAYE L. VINER, MD, MPH,** Program Director, Gastrointestinal and Other Cancers Research Group, Division of Cancer Prevention, National Cancer Institute, Bethesda, Maryland

# CONTENTS



A review of the pathophysiology, clinical presentation, and diagnosis of colon cancer and colonic polyps is important and timely. This field is rapidly changing because of breakthroughs in the molecular basis of carcinogenesis and in the technology for colon cancer detection and treatment. This article reviews colon cancer and colonic polyps, with a focus on recent dramatic advances, to help the primary care physician and internist appropriately refer patients for screening colonoscopy and intelligently evaluate colonoscopic findings to reduce the mortality from this cancer.



Both the incidence and the mortality from colorectal cancer can be substantially reduced by primary and secondary prevention. There are many screening tests for colorectal cancer, and any test should result in a reduction in colorectal cancer incidence and mortality. If the age-eligible population undergoes these screening tests, the burden of colorectal cancer should be substantially reduced. The scientific evidence related to secondary prevention, specifically screening of individuals at average risk for colorectal cancer, is presently reviewed.



Colorectal cancer (CRC) mortality may be greatly reduced by clinically feasible screening programs. The benefits of surveillance of

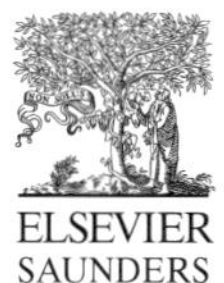

ELSEVIER
SAUNDERS

THE MEDICAL
CLINICS
OF NORTH AMERICA

Med Clin N Am 89 (2005) xi–xiii

Preface

# Colon Cancer Screening, Surveillance, Prevention, and Treatment: Conventional and Novel Technologies

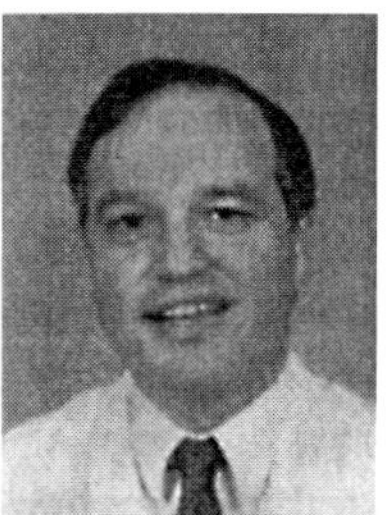

Mitchell S. Cappell, MD, PhD, FACG
*Guest Editor*

During the past year about 55,000 Americans succumbed to colon cancer [1]. This number is about 55 times the number of American fatalities up to now in the current Iraqi conflict and is about the same number of American fatalities during one decade of war in Vietnam. Indeed, during the approximately 15 minutes it takes to read this preface another American will succumb to colon cancer. These deaths are largely preventable. Unfortunately, the major recent advances in colon cancer pathogenesis, screening, and prevention have been inadequately translated and ineffectively implemented for patient care and public benefit.

The American public needs further awareness and education about the importance of colon cancer screening, prevention, and therapy. You, the internists and general practitioners, have the direct and nearly universal patient access to educate the American public about this cancer and to refer them one-at-a-time for appropriate screening and surveillance. Colon cancer is the most dramatic example of the importance of educating the internist, and through him or her the general public about cancer, because this cancer is so ubiquitous and so preventable. This issue of the *Medical Clinics of North America* is dedicated to you, the internist: to educate you to educate your patients, to instruct you to refer your patients for screening and surveillance, and to inform you of novel diagnostic tests and therapies to offer your patients.

The gastroenterologist and the gastrointestinal surgeon, radiologist, and oncologist will also refer to this issue for a critical review of new and

0025-7125/05/$ - see front matter 
doi:10.1016/j.mcna.2004.09.002

important developments in colon cancer. Educating the physician should benefit the patient by access to better and more modern therapies. By emphasizing recent developments and future directions in this issue, it is hoped to stimulate basic and clinical research to help reduce the cancer incidence and mortality, until some day soon—through an integrated strategy of cancer prevention, screening, and therapy of premalignant lesions—colon cancer shall become as extinct as scourges of the past.

I provide a comprehensive overview of this subject with an emphasis on colonic adenomas, the major precurson lesion, and on screening and surveillance for cancer prevention. This article introduces the next article on screening of patients at average risk for colon cancer. In Dr. Mandel's excellent historical approach to this subject, the seminal clinical trials are critically reviewed. This is a highly important clinical area for the internist and gastroenterologist, as evidenced by the recent explosive growth of screening colonoscopy. Dr. Syngal and colleagues present a concise but thorough review of high-risk groups for colon cancer, their surveillance protocols, and the surveillance techniques. This work provides a user-friendly reference for the general clinician and practicing gastroenterologist. Chemoprevention of colon cancer is a pioneering field with immense clinical potential, as demonstrated by the limited, but established, efficacy of nonsteroidal anti-inflammatory agents. Ernest Hawk and colleagues review all the promising chemopreventive agents, as well as the rapidly changing chemotherapeutic armamentarium for advanced colon cancer.

Novel technologies are increasingly being applied to diagnose and treat colon cancer as well as other gastrointestinal cancers. Applications of these novel technologies are reviewed with respect to colon cancer as well as other gastrointestinal cancers. Virtual colonoscopy is a rapidly evolving and highly clinically relevant technology. The literature on this subject is growing exponentially with widely divergent results between studies [2,3]. This field is critically and comprehensively reviewed by Dr. Lefkovitz and colleagues, including reviews of very recent clinical studies. Endoscopic ultrasound is becoming increasingly important in the staging of upper gastrointestinal and rectal cancers. Proper staging permits more precise therapy. For example, detection of clinically unsuspected metastases by endoscopic ultrasound can help prevent unnecessary cancer surgery. Drs. Tamerisa, Irisawa, and Bhutani thoroughly review this subject, and new techniques of endoscopic ultrasound–guided ablative, chemotherapeutic, and radiation therapy. Although already established in Japan and Europe, endoscopic mucosal resection and endoscopic ablation are being increasingly applied in America to treat precancerous or early cancerous lesions. The excellent review by Drs. Monkewich and Haber should be of great interest to gastrointestinal endoscopists, but should also provide useful information to internists and other generalists about these rapidly evolving therapeutic options for their patients with gastrointestinal cancers. With the recent explosion of laparoscopic surgery, surgeons have increasingly applied this technology to treat precancerous and cancerous gastrointestinal neoplasms because of the reduced perioperative morbidity and mortality with this minimally invasive technique. Dr. Torres and colleagues review in detail the principles, technique, results, and controversies of laparoscopic surgery for cancer. Although laparoscopic surgeons will find this review of particular interest, all physicians treating gastrointestinal malignancies should find this article informative and important.

I want to thank my family for enduring too many days of work on this issue and too few with my family; my wife for her patience and understanding; and my children Adina, David, Miriam, and Daniel for their support. I want to thank J. Heather Cullen, the Publishing Manager of the *Medical Clinics of North America*, for her cheerful assistance and support during a collaboration of nearly 10 years. I thank the librarians at Maimonides Medical Center, Lydia Friedman, Richard Patrimonio, and James Verlander, for bibliographic assistance during my writing of several articles in the issue.

If clinicians apply the currently available knowledge, techniques, and modalities as herein presented, for more aggressive screening, surveillance, prevention, and early intervention of colon cancer, tens of thousands of lives shall be saved. Reading and comprehension are the prerequisite; application is the essence.

Mitchell S. Cappell, MD, PhD, FACG
*Director*
*Gastroenterology Training Program*
*Division of Gastroenterology*
*Albert Einstein Medical Center*
*5501 Old York Road*
*Philadelphia, PA 19141-3098, USA*

*E-mail address:* mscappell@yahoo.com

## References

[1] Jemal A, Tiwari RC, Murray T, Ghafoor A, Samuels A, Ward E, et al. Cancer statistics, 2004. CA Cancer J Clin 2004;54:8–29.
[2] Cotton PB, Durkalski VL, Pineau BC, Palesch YY, Mauldin PD, Hoffman B, et al. Computed tomographic colonography (virtual colonoscopy): a multicenter comparison with standard colonoscopy for detection of colorectal neoplasia. JAMA 2004;291:1713–9.
[3] Pickhardt PJ, Choi JR, Hwang I, Butler JA, Puckett ML, Hildebrandt HA, et al. Computed tomographic virtual colonoscopy to screen for colorectal neoplasia in asymptomatic adults. N Engl J Med 2003;349:2191–200.

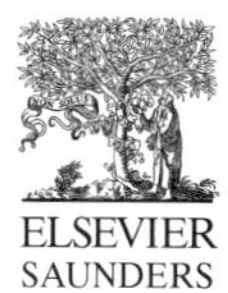

ELSEVIER
SAUNDERS

Med Clin N Am 89 (2005) 1–42

THE MEDICAL CLINICS OF NORTH AMERICA

# The pathophysiology, clinical presentation, and diagnosis of colon cancer and adenomatous polyps

Mitchell S. Cappell, MD, PhD, FACG

*Division of Gastroenterology, Department of Medicine, Albert Einstein Medical Center, 5501 Old York Road, Philadelphia, PA 19141-3098, USA*

Colon cancer afflicts more than 135,000 patients per year in America. It kills more than 55,000 patients per year [1] and many more patients suffer morbidity from curative colon cancer surgery or chemotherapy. Recently promulgated screening and surveillance colonoscopy regimens, as recommended by medical professional societies (including the American Gastroenterological Association [2], the American Society for Gastrointestinal Endoscopy [3], the American College of Gastroenterology [4], and the American Cancer Society [5,6]), and as approved by Medicare [7] and most private medical insurance companies [8] for reimbursement, can largely avoid this morbidity by colonoscopic removal of premalignant polyps [9], and can largely prevent this mortality by early detection of colon cancer at a curable stage [9–11].

Yet only about one quarter of eligible patients currently undergo any form of colon cancer screening [12]. This failure tragically results in tens of thousands of preventable deaths and even greater morbidity per annum in America. Aside from patient reluctance to undergo colonoscopy because of the invasiveness, risks, and discomfort of the test [13], a major factor in this breakdown is the failure by primary care physicians and internists to educate their patients and refer them for screening colonoscopy [14]. Contrariwise, primary care physicians and internists occasionally refer patients who are inappropriate candidates for screening colonoscopy because of age less than 50 years, a negative screening colonoscopy within the past decade, or severe medical comorbidity and a poor prognosis. Education of primary care physicians and internists, who can in turn educate their patients, should

*E-mail address:* mscappell@yahoo.com


doi:10.1016/j.mcna.2004.08.011

eliminate these barriers to mass screening and optimize referral for colonoscopy [14].

A review of the pathophysiology, clinical presentation, and diagnosis of colon cancer and colonic polyps is important and timely for the internist and primary care physician. This field is rapidly changing because of breakthroughs in the molecular basis of carcinogenesis and in the technology for colon cancer detection and treatment. This article reviews colon cancer and colonic polyps, with a focus on recent dramatic advances, to help the primary care physician and internist appropriately refer patients for screening colonoscopy and intelligently evaluate colonoscopic findings to reduce the mortality from this cancer. Companion articles elsewhere in this issue focus on screening for colon cancer in average-risk patients, surveillance of colon cancer in high-risk patients, and chemoprevention and therapy for colon cancer.

## Pathophysiology

### *Histopathogenesis*

Colon cancer arises from mucosal colonic polyps. The critical parameter of polyps in terms of natural history, particularly malignant potential, is histology. The two most common histologic types are hyperplastic and adenomatous. Histologically, hyperplastic polyps contain an increased number of glandular cells with decreased cytoplasmic mucus, but lack nuclear hyperchromatism, stratification, or atypia [15]. Adenomatous nuclei are usually hyperchromatic, enlarged, cigar-shaped, and crowded together in a palisade pattern [16]. Adenomas are classified as tubular or villous. Histologically, tubular adenomas are composed of branched tubules, whereas villous adenomas contain digitiform villi arranged in a frond. Tubulovillous adenomas contain both elements.

Virtually all colon cancers arise from adenomas as demonstrated by multiple epidemiologic, clinical, and pathologic findings. First, about one third of operative specimens containing colon cancer contain one or more synchronous adenomas, a significantly higher rate than in age-matched controls without colon cancer [17]. Second, the risk of colon cancer markedly increases with increasing number of adenomatous polyps [18]. Third, adenomatous tissue is frequently found contiguous to frank carcinoma [19]. Fourth, patients with familial adenomatous polyposis (FAP), who have hundreds or thousands of adenomatous colonic polyps, inevitably develop colon cancer if colectomy is not performed [20]. Fifth, patients who refuse polypectomy for adenomas develop colon cancer at a rate of about 4% after 5 years and 14% after 10 years [21]. This adenoma-to-cancer sequence is supported by recent findings about the molecular basis of colon cancer, as described later.

A relationship between hyperplastic polyps and colon cancer is controversial. Hyperplastic polyps may increase slightly the risk of colon cancer, but the effect is small [22,23]. Risk factors for malignancy in hyperplastic polyps include large polyp size (> 1 cm diameter); location in the right colon; a focus of adenoma within the polyp (mixed hyperplastic-adenomatous polyp); occurrence of more than 20 hyperplastic polyps in the colon; a family history of hyperplastic polyposis; and a family history of colon cancer [24]. Serrated polyps sometimes previously classified as a type of hyperplastic polyp may, like adenomas, be a significant risk factor for colon cancer [25]. Serrated polyps, unlike ordinary hyperplastic polyps, tend to be large and to occur in the right colon [26]. The colonocytes in these polyps frequently have BRAF genetic mutations and DNA methylation [27].

## *Molecular pathogenesis*

### *History of recent molecular advances*

Colon cancer is probably the best understood complex (multistep) cancer in terms of molecular genetics. A brief history helps summarize and place in perspective the recent, revolutionary advances in the molecular basis of colon cancer. Investigation of the pathogenesis of two uncommon familial colon cancer syndromes, FAP and hereditary nonpolyposis colon cancer (HNPCC), led to dramatic breakthroughs in understanding the molecular basis of the more common sporadic (nonsyndromic) form of colon cancer. The clinical genetics and clinical phenotype of FAP was described during the last two centuries: patients with FAP develop hundreds or thousands of adenomatous polyps throughout the colon beginning after puberty and inevitably develop colon cancer (Table 1) [20,28–37]. This syndrome is inherited as a classic mendelian autosomal-dominant single gene. During the past two decades FAP was shown to be caused by germline mutation of the adenomatous polyposis coli (*APC*) gene located on chromosome 5q. A patient with FAP carries this germline mutation in one allele in all somatic cells, including colonocytes (Table 2) [38–44]. This mutation underlies the development of hundreds of adenomatous polyps throughout the colon; colonic adenomas form when the second APC allele is damaged or lost in a colonocyte.

The clinical genetics and clinical phenotype of HNPCC were characterized during the twentieth century (Table 3) [45–53]. In HNPCC multiple cases of colon cancer, without gastrointestinal polyposis, occur within a family. Colon cancer typically occurs in the right colon beginning as sessile polyps in middle age. The Amsterdam Criteria, as recently modified by the Amsterdam II Criteria, are used clinically to diagnose HNPCC. These criteria include all the following: three or more relations with colon cancer, one of whom is a first-degree relative of the other two; colon cancer involving at least two generations in the family; and at least one colon cancer diagnosed before age 50 years [54]. During the past 15 years, HNPCC was shown to be caused by mutations of one of the mismatch repair genes, including hMSH2,

Table 1
Milestones in the clinical genetics of familial adenomatous polyposis

| Author, year of discovery [Ref.] | Discovery and finding |
|---|---|
| Menzelio, 1721 [28] | Report of a patient with many colonic polyps of undetermined histology |
| Corvisart, 1847 [29] | Possible first case report of FAP |
| Chargelaigue, 1859 [30] | Possible second case report of FAP |
| Cripps, 1882 [31] | First confirmed case report of FAP; noted syndrome was possibly familial |
| Bickersteth, 1890 [32] | Confirmed familial nature of the syndrome |
| Smith, 1887 [33] | Described colon cancer arising in the polyps of FAP |
| Handford, 1890 [34] | Second report of colon cancer arising in polyps of FAP |
| Lockhart-Mummery, 1925 and 1934 [35] | Reported numerous cases of FAP |
| Dukes, 1930 [36] | Recognized clinical variability in the expression of adenomatous polyps, and developed clinical diagnostic criteria for FAP |
| Gardner and Richards, 1953 [37] | Described extracolonic tumors and other abnormalities associated with FAP (Gardner's syndrome) |
| Bussey, 1975 [20] | Described the natural history of FAP in a large clinical series |

hMSH6, hMLH1, hMLH3, hPMSI, and hPMS2 [55]. Germline mutations of the hMLH1 and hMSH2 genes account for most of the cases. Mismatch repair enzymes, encoded for by mismatch repair genes, normally recognize errors in nucleotide matching of complementary chromosome strands and initiate segmental excision of the newly synthesized strand to ensure faithful strand replication [56]. Cells with mismatch repair gene mutations cannot repair spontaneous DNA errors and progressively accumulate mutations throughout the genome with succeeding DNA replications. This progressive

Table 2
Milestones in the molecular genetics of familial adenomatous polyposis

| Author, year of discovery [Ref.] | Discovery and finding |
|---|---|
| Veale, 1965 [38] | Determined by pedigree analysis that FAP is caused by a single dominant mutation |
| Cockyne, 1967 [39] | Confirmed Veale's discovery |
| Herrera et al, 1986 [40] | Reported a de novo *APC* mutation associated with a large deletion in chromosome 5 |
| Bodmer et al, 1987 [41] | Applied restriction length polymorphism to localize the *APC* mutation to the long arm of chromosome 5 |
| Leppert et al, 1990 [42] | Confirmed Bodmer's findings |
| Kinzler et al, 1991 [43] | Identified the *APC* gene on chromosome 5 by positional cloning |
| Olschwang et al, 1993 [44] | Confirmed the identification of the *APC* gene |

Table 3
Milestones in the clinical and molecular genetic basis of hereditary nonpolyposis colon cancer

| Author, year of discovery [Ref.] | Discovery and finding |
|---|---|
| *Clinical genetics* | |
| Broca, 1869 [45] | Described transmission of breast cancer and intestinal cancer through several generations in one pedigree |
| Warthin, 1913 [46] | Reported high incidence of intestinal cancer in one family (family G) through multiple generations |
| Lynch and Lynch, 1982 [47] | Refined Warthin's findings by describing clinical presentation of Lynch types I and II family cancer syndromes (now called HNPCC) |
| *Molecular genetics* | |
| Peltomaki et al, 1993 [48] | Described microsatellite instability in HNPCC |
| Fishel et al, 1993 [49] | Identified and cloned the first human mismatch repair gene *hMSH2* (*hMLH2*) |
| Leach et al, 1993 [50] | Confirmed Fishel's discovery 2 weeks after the publication of Fishel's study |
| Bronner et al, 1994 [51] and Papopoulos et al, 1994 [52] | Identified the second mismatch repair gene, *hMLH1*, and localized it to chromosome 3p |
| Kolodner et al, 1994 [53] | Showed patients with Muir-Torre syndrome (HNPCC associated with sebaceous gland and skin tumors) have hMSH2 mutations or other mutations that cause microsatellite instability |

accumulation leads to genetic hypermutability and chaos; mutations accumulate in oncogenes and tumor suppressor genes that can result in colon cancer [57]. Mismatch repair gene mutation is detected as microsatellite instability, in which errors occur in simple DNA repetitive sequences, such as in poly-A or CA-tandem repeating sequences [56]. The molecular genetics of variants of FAP and HNPCC are described in Table 4. The molecular genetics of other intestinal polyposis syndromes are described in Table 5 [58–63].

### *Molecular biology*

These breakthroughs provided not only the molecular basis of syndromic hereditary colon cancer but also of sporadic colon cancer. Colon cancer is believed caused by a cascade of genetic mutations leading to progressively disordered local DNA replication and accelerated colonocyte replication. The progressive accumulation of multiple genetic mutations results in the transition from normal mucosa to benign adenoma to severe dysplasia to frank carcinoma (Table 6). Mutations of the mismatch repair genes are believed to account for about 15% of sporadic colon cancers [64]. APC mutation is believed to account for about 80% of sporadic colon cancers [64]. Spontaneous somatic APC mutation in colonocytes is believed to underlie

Table 4
Molecular genetics of syndromic colon cancer

| Gene mutation | Clinical syndromes | Manifestations |
|---|---|---|
| *APC* | Familial adenomatous polyposis | Development of hundreds of colonic adenomas and inevitably of colon cancer without colon resection |
| | Attenuated familial adenomatous polyposis | Mutations at specific sites (both terminals or exon 9) of *APC* gene can cause attenuated familial polyposis syndrome with development of dozens of colonic adenomas |
| | Gardner's syndrome | Variant of familial adenomatous polyposis with prominent extracolonic growths, such as osteomas |
| | Turcot's syndrome | Variant of familial adenomatous polyposis with typical colonic manifestations and medulloblastomas or other tumors of CNS often caused by mutations of the *APC* gene |
| Mismatch repair | HNPCC | Develop several adenomatous colonic neoplasms, primarily in the right colon, with rapid malignant transformation |
| | Turcot's syndrome | Variant of HNPCC with typical colonic findings of few colonic neoplasms and glioblastoma multiforme tumors of CNS sometimes caused by mutations of mismatch repair genes |

*Abbreviation:* CNS, central nervous system.

the development of sporadic adenomatous polyps. *APC* gene mutations occur early in adenoma development and are often found in aberrant crypt foci, the earliest identifiable dysplastic crypts [65]. APC mutations are found in about 50% of sporadic adenomas [66]. Adenomas usually remain benign. Malignant transformation requires further genetic alterations.

The *DCC* (deleted in colon cancer) gene encodes for a neural cell adhesion molecule receptor and normally promotes apoptosis and suppresses tumors. Loss of the normal *DCC* gene is believed to be important in the transition from an intermediate to a late adenoma. Its role in this transition is supported by its frequent allelic deletion during this transformation [67].

The normal *p53* gene product arrests the cell cycle following DNA injury to permit either DNA repair if the damage is correctable, or apoptosis if the damage is too severe. The wild-type p53 protein product is up-regulated after cell stress from radiation exposure, DNA injury, or other noxious events to prevent new DNA synthesis and halt cell division. Loss of p53

Table 5
History of molecular genetics of other intestinal polyposis syndromes

| Author, year of discovery [Ref.] | Discovery and finding |
|---|---|
| Zigman et al, 1997 [58] | Showed the Ruvalcaba-Myhre-Smith syndrome (hamartomatous, lipomatous hemangiomatous, and lymphangiomatous gastrointestinal polyps) is caused by an autosomal-dominant mutation of the *PTEN* gene on chromosome 10q |
| Nelen et al, 1996 [59] and 1997 [60] | Showed Cowden's disease (gastric and colonic hamartomatous polyps) is caused by an autosomal-dominant mutation of the *PTEN* gene on chromosome 10q |
| Houlston et al, 1998 [61]; Howe et al, 1998 [62] | Showed familial juvenile polyposis (more than 10 juvenile intestinal polyps) is caused by an autosomal-dominant mutation in the *SMAD4 (DRC4)* gene on chromosome 10q |
| Jenne et al, 1998 [63] | Showed Peutz-Jeghers syndrome (small number of intestinal polyps associated with mucocutaneous pigmentation) is caused by an autosomal-dominant mutation in the *STK11* gene on chromosome 19p |

function can promote genomic instability as genetic errors are replicated without check, resulting in loss of heterozygosity. Mutation of the *p53* gene is believed to be important in the transition from late adenoma to frank carcinoma. About 50% of lesions with high-grade dysplasia and about 75% of frank cancers exhibit loss of normal *p53* function, usually from a missense point mutation of one allele and deletion of the other, wild-type, allele [56,68].

The K-*ras* gene encodes for a protein involved in signal transduction from the cell membrane to the nucleus [69]. Specific mutations of this gene result in constitutive activation of this signal pathway and increased colonocyte replication. These mutations are associated with exophytic growth of adenomas in the transition to carcinoma [70]. About 50% of colon cancers have K-*ras* mutations [67].

The accumulation of genetic mutations leads to genetic instability, manifested by loss of heterozygosity [71]. Loss of heterozygosity accelerates carcinogenesis. Cells with loss of heterozygosity have one, instead of the normal two, alleles of some genes because of loss of individual chromosomes during mitosis. A tumor suppressor gene is more likely to lose normal function when only one allele is present after loss of heterozygosity. Only one, rather than two, allelic mutations are then required for loss of its function.

DNA methylation at the promotor region can terminate and silence gene expression without DNA mutation [72]. In particular, DNA methylation can inactivate suppressor genes, thereby promoting cancer [73]. Colon cancer is sometimes associated with methylation and inactivation of p14,

Table 6
Molecular genetics of sporadic colon cancer

| Gene | Chromosome location | Normal physiologic function of encoded protein | Clinical manifestations of mutation |
|---|---|---|---|
| *APC* | 5q | Regulates cell growth and apoptosis | Homozygous somatic mutation associated with colonic adenomas |
| K-*ras* family | Various chromosomes | Encodes a small GTP binding protein on cell membrane involved in transduction of mitogenic signals across cell membrane | Mutated in about one half of colon cancers; may act in an intermediate stage of carcinogenesis; mutation common in hyperplastic polyps |
| *p53* | 17p | Regulates G1 cell cycle and apoptosis | Critical in transition from late adenoma to early cancer |
| *DCC* | 18q | Encodes a neural cell adhesion molecule, facilitates apoptosis, tumor suppressor | Believed to promote progression to frank carcinoma |
| Mismatch repair genes | Located on several chromosomes | Recognize errors in nucleotide matching of complementary chromosome strand and initiate excision of erroneous strand | Progressive accumulation of mutations throughout the genome in affected cells leading to hypermutability and genetic chaos; mutations of oncogenes or tumor suppressor genes can lead to colon cancer |

normally an upstream inducer of the *p53* tumor suppressor pathway. This occurs in about 25% of colon cancers [74]. The inactivation produces the same cancer phenotype as mutation of the tumor suppressor gene *p53* [72]. Methylation of the tumor suppressor gene *p16*, designated *CDKN2A*, occurs in about 35% of colon cancers [75].

## Pathology

### *Histology*

Colon cancers are classified as well-differentiated, moderately well differentiated, or poorly differentiated on the degree of preservation of normal glandular architecture and cytologic features. Progressively more poor differentiation is presumably a histologic marker of further underlying genetic mutations, but the mutations associated with poor differentiation are currently unknown. About 20% of cancers are poorly differentiated. They have a poor prognosis [76]. About 15% of colon cancers are classified as mucinous or colloid because of prominent intracellular accumulation of mucin. These cancers are more aggressive [77].

### *Gross pathology*

About 65% of colon cancers are distal to the splenic flexure and potentially detectable by sigmoidoscopy [78]. Contrariwise, about 35% of colon cancers are proximal to the sigmoid and not detectable by flexible sigmoidoscopy. Colon cancer can occur in a pedunculated polyp, sessile polyp, mass, or stricture. Small polyps rarely contain cancer. Only about 1% of diminutive polyps contain cancer [79]. Cancer in a sessile polyp may metastasize faster than cancer in a pedunculated polyp because of the closer proximity of the lymphatic drainage [80].

### *Stage*

Carcinoma in situ, or high-grade dysplasia, is histologically cancer but is pathologically confined to the mucosa without penetration of the muscularis mucosa. Invasive colon cancer is most commonly staged from A through D according to the Dukes classification, with stage A penetrating beyond the colonic muscularis mucosa into the submucosa. Stage B1 extends beyond the submucosa into the muscularis propria; stage B2 extends through the muscularis propria into the serosa. Stage C has regional lymph node metastases, and stage D has distant metastases.

Colon cancer is recently staged according to the tumor–node–metastases (TNM) classification by mural depth of the primary tumor (T), by presence of local lymph node metastases (N), and by presence of distant metastases (M) [81]. This classification is particularly helpful in endosonographic staging of colon cancer [82]. In the TNM classification, invasive colon cancer is classified from stage I to IV. Stage I in the TNM classification corresponds to Dukes A or B1 lesions, stage II corresponds to a Dukes B2 lesion, stage III corresponds to a Dukes C lesion, and stage IV corresponds to a Dukes D lesion. Pathologic stage, as classified by either scheme, is highly correlated with cancer prognosis [83]. Diagnostic delays result in a more advanced pathologic stage at diagnosis.

*Metastases*

About 20% to 25% of patients initially present with Dukes D colon cancer with identifiable metastases [84]. Perhaps another 30% of patients have no detectable metastases preoperatively or intraoperatively but eventually succumb to colon cancer after apparently curative surgery because of gross cancer recurrence presumably from initially undetected micrometastases. The most common sites of gross metastases are the regional lymph nodes and liver [85]. The lungs, peritoneum, pelvis, and adrenals are less common sites [85]. These sites typically become involved only after hepatic or lymphatic metastases occur.

## Epidemiology

Colon cancer is the second most common cause of mortality from cancer [1]. The lifetime risk of colon cancer is about 1 in 17 [1]. Colon cancer incidence declined by about 2% per annum in America from 1985 through 1995, but has increased recently [86]. This probably reflects increased (earlier) detection through screening programs [10,86]. If so, the incidence should begin to decline again in several years as the benefits of aggressive screening colonoscopy become manifest. Colon cancer has numerous environmental and demographic risk factors (Table 7) [1,37,62,87–117]. Environmental factors play a major etiologic role in colon cancer despite the importance of genetic mutations in colon cancer pathogenesis. Environmental factors presumably modulate the risk of the genetic mutations responsible for colon cancer, although the precise molecular mechanisms are currently unknown.

The incidence of colon cancer exhibits a striking geographic variation: the age-adjusted incidence varies by up to 15-fold among different countries [118]. Industrialized nations, except Japan, have the highest incidence, whereas South American countries and China have a relatively low incidence [1]. The wide variation in incidence is largely attributed to national differences in diet and other environmental factors [119]. In contrast to native Japanese, descendants of Japanese immigrants to America have, like other Americans, a high incidence of colon cancer attributed to dietary and other environmental adaptations [120]. Indeed, the incidence of colon cancer has recently increased in native Japanese attributed to their adopting a Westernized diet and other environmental changes with industrialization [119].

American blacks have an increased risk of colon cancer compared with whites, but the difference is small [121]. Native American Indians have a significantly lower risk [122]. The incidence is slightly higher in American men than women [123]. The incidence of colon cancer rises sharply with age, beginning at age 50 years [124]. This phenomenon is attributed to accumulation of chance somatic mutations with age.

## Clinical presentation of colon cancer

### *Symptoms*

Symptoms are common and prominent late in colon cancer when the prognosis is poor but are less common and less obvious early in the disease. Common symptoms include abdominal pain, rectal bleeding, altered bowel habits, and involuntary weight loss [125]. Although colon cancer can present with either diarrhea or constipation, a recent change in bowel habits is much more likely to be from colon cancer than chronically abnormal bowel habits. Less common symptoms include nausea and vomiting, malaise, anorexia, and abdominal distention [10].

Symptoms depend on cancer location, cancer size, and presence of metastases. Left colonic cancers are more likely than right colon cancers to cause partial or complete intestinal obstruction because the left colonic lumen is narrower and the stool in the left colon tends to be better formed because of reabsorption of water in the proximal colon [126]. Large exophytic cancers are also more likely to obstruct the colonic lumen. Partial obstruction produces constipation, nausea, abdominal distention, and abdominal pain. Partial obstruction occasionally paradoxically produces intermittent diarrhea as stool moves beyond the obstruction.

Distal cancers sometimes cause gross rectal bleeding, but proximal cancers rarely produce this symptom because the blood becomes mixed with stool and chemically degraded during colonic transit [127]. Bleeding from proximal cancers tends to be occult, and the patient may present with iron deficiency anemia without gross rectal bleeding [128]. The anemia may produce weakness, fatigue, dyspnea, or palpitations. Advanced cancer, particularly with metastasis, can cause cancer cachexia [129], characterized by a symptomatic tetrad of involuntary weight loss, anorexia, muscle weakness, and a feeling of poor health.

### *Signs*

Just as with symptoms, colon cancer tends not to produce signs until advanced [10]. Anemia from gastrointestinal bleeding may produce pallor. Iron deficiency anemia can cause koilonychia manifested by brittle, longitudinally furrowed, and spooned nails; glossitis manifested by lingual erythema and papillae loss; and cheilitis manifested by scaling or fissuring of the lips [130]. Hypoalbuminemia may clinically manifest as peripheral edema, ascites, or anasarca. Hypoactive or high-pitched bowel sounds suggest

Table 7
Risk factors for colon cancer

| Parameters | Proposed mechanism | References |
|---|---|---|
| *Epidemiology* | | |
| Old age | Acquired colonocyte mutations accumulate with age | [87] |
| Living in United States and other highly industrialized nations, possibly excluding Japan | Dietary and environmental carcinogens | [1] |
| Physical inactivity? | Physical activity may stimulate immunosurveillance, and stimulate intestinal peristalsis to decrease mucosal contact with fecal carcinogens | [88] |
| *Diet* | | |
| High fat? | Various theories (eg, increased bile secretion) | [89] |
| Low fruit and vegetable consumption | Anticarcinogenic substances in fruits and vegetables (eg, folic acid) | [90,91] |
| Low calcium? | Calcium binds to bile acids that are otherwise potentially colonotoxic | [92] |
| High red meat? | Animal fat in red meat or carcinogens (eg, nitrosamines) in cooked meat | [93] |
| Low selenium? | Selenium can help neutralize toxic free radicals because of antioxidant effects | [94] |
| Low folate? | Folate needed for DNA synthesis and repair | [95] |
| Low carotenoid diet? | Carotenoids can help neutralize free radicals because of antioxidant effects | [96] |
| Low-fiber diet? | Dilution of carcinogens in stool cause by increased stool bulk and stool water with a high-fiber diet | [89,97] |
| Obesity | Carcinogens in an unhealthy diet, or role of abnormal insulin levels in carcinogenesis? | [98,99] |
| *Social habits* | | |
| Smoking cigarettes | Carcinogens present in tobacco | [100] |
| Alcohol | May promote cell proliferation and inhibit DNA repair | [101] |
| *Genetics and family history* | | |
| FAP | Develops hundreds of adenomatous colonic polyps. Inevitably develops colon cancer because of small but significant risk of malignant transformation in each adenoma | See text |

Table 7 (*continued*)

| Parameters | Proposed mechanism | References |
|---|---|---|
| Gardner's syndrome | Variant of FAP | [37] |
| HNPCC (Lynch syndrome) | Mutant mismatch repair gene leads to accumulation of genetic mutations, including mutations of tumor suppressor genes | See text |
| Peutz-Jeghers syndrome | Syndromic hamartomatous polyps may occasionally transform to adenomas | [102] |
| Juvenile polyposis | Syndromic juvenile polyps can transform to adenomas and then cancers over time | [62] |
| Family history of nonsyndromic colon cancer | Postulated shared genetic factors leading to mild susceptibility to colon cancer and possibly shared environmental factors | [103] |
| Hyperplastic polyposis | Genetic mutation in hyperplastic polyposis may predispose to cancer | [104] |
| *Inflammatory bowel disease* | | |
| Chronic ulcerative colitis | Dysplasia and genetic mutations associated with mucosal injury and repair | [105] |
| Chronic Crohn's colitis | Dysplasia and genetic mutations associated with cell injury and repair | [106] |
| *History of prior neoplasia* | | |
| Colonic adenomatous polyps | Precursor lesions to colon cancer | [107] |
| Prior colon cancer | Genetic predisposition or environmental factors | [108] |
| Breast cancer? | Shared reproductive hormonal or environmental factors | [109] |
| *Other* | | |
| Pelvic radiation | Carcinogenic effects caused by radiation-induced mutations | [110] |
| Diabetes mellitus? | Insulin may modulate colonocyte proliferation | [111] |
| *Streptococcus bovis* bacteremia | May promote colonocyte proliferation | [112,113] |
| Ureterosigmoidostomy | Carcinogens excreted in urine or colonic mucosal proliferation during repair after urine-induced mucosal injury | [114] |
| Acromegaly | Growth hormone promotes proliferation of pre-existing colonic adenomas and cancers | [115,116] |
| Prior cholecystectomy? | Continuous colonic exposure to potentially carcinogenic bile acids after cholecystectomy | [117] |

*Abbreviation:* ?, questionable, controversial, or weak risk factor for colon cancer.

gastrointestinal obstruction. A palpable abdominal mass is a rare finding that suggests advanced disease. Rectal examination, including fecal occult blood testing (FOBT), is important in the evaluation of possible colon cancer, as discussed later in the section on colon cancer screening. Rectal cancer may be palpable by digital rectal examination. Other physical findings, although rare, should be systematically searched for, including peripheral lymphadenopathy, especially a Virchow's node in the left supraclavicular space; hepatomegaly from hepatic metastases; and temporal or intercostal muscle wasting from cancer cachexia. Very rare findings with colon cancer include a Sister Mary Joseph node caused by metastases to a periumbilical node, and a Blumer's shelf caused by perirectal extension of the primary tumor [127].

### *Laboratory abnormalities*

Patients with suspected colon cancer should have routine blood tests including a hemogram with platelet count determination, serum electrolytes and glucose determination, evaluation of routine serum biochemical parameters of liver function, and a routine coagulation profile. About half of patients with colon cancer are anemic [10]. Anemia, however, is very common, so that only a small minority of patients with anemia have colon cancer. Iron deficiency anemia of undetermined etiology, however, warrants evaluation for colon cancer, particularly in the elderly [131]. Hypoalbuminemia is uncommon, but not rare, in colon cancer. It usually indicates poor nutritional status from advanced cancer [132].

Routine serum biochemical parameters of liver function are usually within normal limits in patients with colon cancer. Abnormalities, particularly elevation of the alkaline phosphatase level, often indicate hepatic metastases [133]. The serum lactate dehydrogenase level may increase with colon cancer. Diarrhea associated with colon cancer can rarely produce electrolyte derangements or dehydration. Nausea and vomiting from colon cancer can rarely produce metabolic derangements of hypovolemia, hypokalemia, or alkalosis.

The serum carcinoembryonic antigen level is not useful to screen for colon cancer [134]. It is only moderately sensitive. Although patients with very advanced cancer tend to have highly elevated levels, patients with early and highly curable colon cancer tend to have only minimally elevated levels, with considerable overlap with the levels of patients without colon cancer [135]. It is poorly specific. Other colonic diseases or systemic disorders can cause a carcinoembryonic antigen elevation. Preoperative testing is, however, useful to determine cancer prognosis and to provide a baseline for comparison with postoperative levels. An elevated serum level preoperatively is a poor prognostic indicator: the higher the serum level the more likely the cancer is extensive and will recur postoperatively [135]. After apparently complete colon cancer resection the serum level almost always normalizes; failure to normalize postoperatively suggests incomplete resection [136]. A sustained and progressive rise after postoperative normalization strongly suggests cancer recurrence [137]. Patients with this finding require prompt surveillance colonoscopy to exclude colonic recurrence and abdominal imaging to exclude metastases.

### *Unusual clinical syndromes caused by colon cancer*

Colon cancer can cause acute colonic obstruction, most commonly from exophytic intraluminal growth, and most uncommonly from intussusception or volvulus. Obstruction typically occurs in the sigmoid colon because of the narrow lumen and hard stool in this region. Patients present with abdominal pain, nausea and vomiting, obstipation, abdominal tenderness, abdominal distention, and hypoactive bowel sounds. Colon cancer can rarely perforate acutely through the colonic wall and cause acute generalized peritonitis, and can rarely perforate slowly to form a walled-off inflammatory mass or abscess with localized peritoneal signs. Factors promoting colonic perforation include disruption of mucosal integrity because of transmural malignant extension or colonic ischemia, and increased intraluminal pressure because of colonic obstruction. Presentation with colonic obstruction or perforation indicates a poor prognosis. Colon cancer rarely causes ischemic colitis because of colonic dilatation proximal to malignant obstruction or malignant infiltration of blood vessels [138]. Colon cancer occasionally causes gross rectal bleeding because of cancerous mucosal ulceration.

## Clinical presentation of colonic adenomas

Adenomatous polyps are most commonly asymptomatic. In a review of 800 patients with colorectal polyps about two thirds were asymptomatic [139]. Moreover, these symptoms are often coincidental and not caused by the polyps. For example, rectal bleeding in a patient with a small colonic polyp is more often caused by other conditions, particularly hemorrhoids. Hemorrhoidal bleeding characteristically is postdefecatory, coats the stools, and produces very bright red blood [140]. Polyps more than 1 cm in diameter are more likely to produce symptoms, and polyps less than 0.5 cm rarely produce symptoms [141,142]. The most common symptoms attributable to polyps are rectal bleeding, abdominal pain, and change in bowel habits. A rectal polyp can rarely cause rectal prolapse. A large polyp rarely forms the leading edge of a colonic intussusception [143]. Large villous adenomas, especially in the distal colon, can rarely cause profuse watery diarrhea [144].

Physical findings and laboratory abnormalities are uncommon with adenomatous colonic polyps. A rectal polyp may be palpable by digital rectal examination. Only about half of adenomas cause fecal occult blood [145]. Large adenomas are more likely to cause occult bleeding and small adenomas rarely cause occult bleeding [141,142]. A benign colonic polyp rarely causes iron deficiency anemia; iron deficiency anemia is much more common with a malignant polyp because of quantitatively greater chronic blood loss.

Symptoms and signs are common when colon cancer is advanced and likely to be incurable, are less common when colon cancer is early and highly curable, and are relatively uncommon with adenomatous polyps. This phenomenon renders adenomas or early cancer difficult to detect by clinical presentation and provides the rationale for mass screening of the general asymptomatic population for early detection and prevention of colon cancer.

## Screening and diagnostic tests for colonic lesions

### *Screening of average-risk patients*

#### *Fecal occult blood testing*

FOBT was the traditional mainstay of screening for colon cancer and colonic polyps. It is most commonly tested by a colorimetric assay of a reaction on guaiac catalyzed by the pseudoperoxidase present in blood. It has advantages as a screening test of low cost, test simplicity, noninvasiveness, and safety. It has a disadvantage as a screening test because of low specificity. FOBT is based on increased microscopic rectal bleeding in patients with colon cancer compared with patients without colonic disease. Patients with and without colon cancer, however, have a wide range of microscopic bleeding with considerable overlap [145]. This overlap results in low test specificity [146]. Specificity is increased by avoiding ingestion of broccoli, cauliflower, or red meats and by avoiding therapy with aspirin for 3 days before the test. Whether iron causes a false-positive FOBT is controversial [147], but withholding iron therapy for several days before the test is prudent because of possible test interference. Even in ideal research studies, only 5% to 10% of patients with fecal occult blood have colon cancer, and another 20% to 30% have colonic adenomatous polyps [148–150]. Although true-positive tests can lead to early colon cancer detection and cure, false-positive FOBT results in a large number of expensive and nondiagnostic colonoscopies.

FOBT is, moreover, only moderately sensitive. Sensitivity is improved by performing stool tests on three different occasions because colon cancer typically only intermittently bleeds, and by avoiding ascorbic acid for several days before the test because ascorbic acid inhibits the guaiac reaction [151]. Test sensitivity is also improved by performing the test on fresh stool or by rehydrating the stool specimen, but rehydration decreases the test specificity. Nevertheless, the sensitivity of FOBT for colon cancer using ideal techniques under the ideal circumstances of a research study is only about 85% [152]. The sensitivity for detecting adenomas is considerably lower because colonic adenomas bleed less frequently than colon cancer. The sensitivity for adenomas is only about 50% [145]. The sensitivity is particularly low for adenomas that are small or located in the proximal colon [145].

Despite these flaws, FOBT is an important element in the armamentarium of colon cancer screening because of test safety and convenience. Mandel et al [153] demonstrated in a large, prospective, randomized, controlled study that annual screening by FOBT results in reduced mortality from colon cancer. Unexplained fecal occult blood mandates further evaluation of the colon to exclude colon cancer or polyps in any patient more than 40 years old [154].

*Barium enema*

Barium enema was touted as a cheaper, less invasive, and safer alternative to colonoscopy. Barium enema entails a risk of colonic perforation of only about 1 per 25,000 examinations [155]. Patients are exposed to about 0.03 Gy of radiation during a barium examination. Indeed, Medicare approved barium enema for reimbursement for screening for colon cancer. Barium enema, however, is only moderately sensitive at detecting colon cancer. For example, in a review of 2193 consecutive colorectal cancers, barium enema was much less sensitive (82.9% sensitivity) than colonoscopy (95% sensitivity) in detecting colon cancer [156]. Barium enema is even less sensitive at detecting colonic polyps. For example, in a study of 580 patients undergoing both barium enema and colonoscopy, barium enema detected only 32% of colonic polyps less than 6 mm in diameter, 53% of colonic polyps between 6 and 10 mm, and 48% of polyps larger than 10 mm [157]. Diverticulosis, colonic spasm, poor colonic preparation, and redundant overlapping colonic loops interfere with barium enema interpretation and accuracy. Rectal lesions may be missed because of interference by the intrarectal occluding balloon. Barium enema does not permit histologic characterization of an identified lesion because of an inability to perform biopsies, and does not permit therapeutic removal of polyps. Detection of a polyp at barium enema necessitates colonoscopy as a second examination for biopsy or polypectomy.

*Flexible sigmoidoscopy*

Flexible sigmoidoscopy every 3 to 5 years has been recommended in conjunction with annual FOBT for screening for colon cancer [5,158,159]. Sigmoidoscopy decreases mortality from rectosigmoid colon cancer. For example, Selby et al [160] reported a 59% reduction of rectosigmoid cancer in patients undergoing one or more rigid sigmoidoscopies in the prior decade compared with unscreened controls matched for age and sex.

The role of flexible sigmoidoscopy is becoming increasingly limited in the screening and diagnosis of colon cancer. Sigmoidoscopy is relatively insensitive at colon cancer or colon polyp detection because the proximal half of the colon is not endoscopically visualized. From one third to one half of lesions are proximal to the sigmoid colon [161,162]. This effect has become quantitatively larger with the recent shift of colonic polyps and cancers to the right side of the colon [163]. Even a screening strategy that calls for colonoscopy when a patient has a distal colonic polyp detected by sigmoidoscopy misses most proximal lesions because most proximal lesions do not have synchronous distal lesions [164,165]. Sigmoidoscopy is also an inadequate test for patients with distal colon cancer. About 3% to 5% of patients with an index colon cancer have a synchronous cancer [166,167]. The presence of proximal synchronous lesions affects distal cancer management. If a synchronous proximal lesion is malignant, the patient requires larger colonic resection to extirpate both lesions. If the proximal lesion is a benign adenoma, the patient should undergo colonoscopic polypectomy before undergoing sigmoid colectomy. Finding an adenomatous polyp or cancer at sigmoidoscopy mandates a full colonoscopy to diagnose synchronous lesions.

*Diagnostic colonoscopy*

Colonoscopy is recommended for screening of patients more than 50 years old at average risk for colon cancer or colonic polyps [5,159]. Colonoscopy is highly sensitive at detecting large ( > 1 cm) colonic polyps, with a miss rate of only 6%, and is moderately sensitive at detecting diminutive (<0.6 cm) polyps with a miss rate of about 27% [168]. Colonic polyps may be missed around sharp turns, especially the hepatic and sigmoid flexures; at areas of colonic spasm, especially in the sigmoid or with severe diverticulosis; and areas covered by stool because of poor colonic preparation. Colon cancers are rarely missed at colonoscopy because they tend to be larger than adenomatous polyps. Colonoscopy is a highly specific test. At colonoscopy polyps are removed and masses biopsied for a pathologic diagnosis.

Colonoscopy, however, has disadvantages as a screening test because it is resource intensive; expensive; somewhat invasive; uncomfortable; and entails a small, but significant, risk of serious complications. It requires a team including a technician, nurse, and highly trained colonoscopist. Colonoscopy is not readily available with long waiting times because of a shortage of highly trained colonoscopists [169,170]. The test requires patient preparation for 24 hours before the procedure. The test is uncomfortable and generally requires sedation and analgesia. The patient requires postprocedure monitoring until the effects of the sedatives and analgesics wear off. The complication rate of diagnostic colonoscopy is about 0.4% [171,172]. The most common major complications are gastrointestinal bleeding and colonic perforation. Most colonic perforations require colonic surgery, but conservative management with parenteral fluids, antibiotics, and surgical back-up occasionally suffices [173].

At colonoscopy, polyps are characterized according to size; color; number; segmental location; intramural location (mucosal versus submucosal); presence or absence of a stalk (pedunculated versus sessile); and superficial appearance. Polyp characteristics at colonoscopy provide important clues concerning polyp histology and malignant potential, which can influence the colonoscopic management. Hyperplastic polyps are usually small, pale, unilobular, and located in the rectum [174]. Adenomas are larger, redder, more multilobular, and distributed throughout the colon. Villous adenomas tend to be large, bulky, sessile, shaggy, soft, velvety, and friable [140]. Colonoscopic appearance is, however, only moderately correlated with polyp histology. Pathologic examination of a colonoscopic biopsy provides an indication of polyp histology, but is subject to sampling error. A polyp is definitively classified by pathologic examination of the entire polyp after polypectomy. Colonoscopic polypectomy is diagnostic and therapeutic for noncancerous adenomatous polyps.

Flat adenomas tend to be small, discoid, and erythematous plaques. Flat adenomas are important because of a significant risk of high-grade dysplasia and occasionally of cancer. Flat adenomas are difficult to detect and are often missed at colonoscopy. These lesions are identified by chromoendoscopy with colonoscopic instillation of methylene blue or indigo carmine [175,176].

The differential diagnosis of numerous polypoid colonic masses detected at colonoscopy includes FAP, attenuated FAP, hyperplastic polyposis, juvenile polyposis, Peutz-Jeghers syndrome, pseudopolyposis, diffuse colonic hemangiomatosis, and pneumatosis coli. These conditions are differentiated by clinical, radiologic, colonoscopic, and histologic findings. In patients with FAP, the colonic mucosa is carpeted by hundreds or thousands of adenomatous polyps. In patients with attenuated FAP, only about 30 adenomatous polyps are present. These polyps are usually located in the proximal colon and tend to be flat growths because of intramural, rather than intraluminal, growth [42]. Classic and attenuated FAP are both caused by APC mutations. In attenuated FAP, APC mutations occur at certain sites, particularly the extreme proximal or distal ends of the *APC* gene [177]. Patients with FAP must undergo prophylactic colectomy after puberty to prevent colon cancer [178]. Hyperplastic polyposis is characterized by 20 or more polyps in the colon, a predominantly right colonic polyp distribution, and a positive family history [104]. Juvenile polyposis is characterized by a family history of juvenile polyposis, more than five juvenile polyps in the colon, multiple juvenile polyps throughout the rest of the gastrointestinal tract, and polyp development at a young age [179]. In Peutz-Jeghers syndrome multiple hamartomatous polyps, which characteristically contain abundant branching smooth muscle, occur throughout the gastrointestinal tract. Patients characteristically have perioral and oral hyperpigmentation because of melanin deposition [180]. Pseudopolyps represent islands of variably inflamed residual mucosa surrounded by a background of previously sloughed off mucosa. It is most commonly associated with ulcerative colitis. Other colonoscopic findings of ulcerative colitis, including mucosal erythema, granularity, blunting of the normal vascular pattern, friability, mucopus, mucosal hemorrhage, and superficial ulcerations, may be present. At colonoscopy, hemangiomas often appear as multiple violet-blue, sessile, polypoid lesions [181]. They are associated with characteristic dermatologic lesions in the blue rubber bleb nevus syndrome. In pneumatosis coli multiple air-filled cysts are present in the colonic submucosa. Colonoscopy reveals multiple, pale, cystic, round polypoid masses with overlying intact mucosa [182].

Early colon cancer may occur in an adenomatous polyp and may be difficult to distinguish by colonoscopy from a nonmalignant adenomatous polyp. For example, a 2-cm-wide villous adenoma has an approximately 40% chance of harboring cancer [183]. Polyp risk factors for malignancy include villous rather than tubular histology, large size, sessile morphology, and increasing number of colonic polyps [17]. Advanced colon cancer typically appears as a large, exophytic mass because of intraluminal growth, or as a colonic stricture because of circumferential growth. A colonic stricture may, however, be benign. Malignancy is suggested when a colonic stricture is ulcerated, indurated, asymmetric, and friable, and has irregular or overhanging margins. The colonoscopic appearance is not definitive. Pathologic examination of multiple colonic biopsies and cytologic analysis of stricture brushings are usually diagnostic.

### *Surveillance of high-risk patients and diagnostic testing of patients with strong clinical indications*

Patients at average risk for colonic adenomatous polyps or cancer undergo screening colonoscopy every 10 years, or alternative screening tests at periodic intervals, as outlined previously and described in detail elsewhere in this issue. Patients who are members of high-risk groups, as listed in Box 1,

**Box 1. Indications for colonoscopic surveillance for colon cancer**

*Personal history*

- Prior colonic adenomatous polyps
- Prior colon cancer
- Peutz-Jeghers syndrome
- HNPCC (Lynch syndrome)
- Juvenile polyposis syndrome
- Chronic ulcerative colitis
- Chronic Crohn's colitis

*Family history*

- Colon cancer
- Colonic adenomatous polyps
- HNPCC (Lynch syndrome)
- Familial adenomatous polyposis

undergo periodic surveillance more frequently. In these high-risk groups colonoscopy is the recommended test. The age of beginning surveillance and the frequency of surveillance depends on the age of onset of the increased cancer risk and the quantitative risk of cancer. These indications are discussed elsewhere in this issue. Aside from periodic screening or surveillance, patients require colonoscopy to exclude colon cancer, adenomatous polyps, or other colonic diseases for specific acute indications, as listed in Box 2.

## Testing for intramural penetration and extracolonic spread of colon cancer

### *CT*

CT has been the standard modality to image the abdomen in patients with colorectal cancer. CT is relatively highly accurate at detecting liver metastases. For example, CT was 85% accurate in a multicenter study [184]. CT is much more sensitive at detecting large than small hepatic lesions [185]. CT is only moderately accurate at T staging. For example, the accuracy for T staging was only 74% in a large multicenter study [184]. CT errors typically occur from underestimating the T stage. CT is only about 50% to 70% accurate in N staging of rectal cancer [184].

**Box 2. Acute indications for colonoscopy to exclude colonic adenomas, colon cancer, or other colonic diseases**

- Fecal occult blood
- Iron deficiency anemia
- Hematochezia
- Melena with a nondiagnostic esophagogastroduodenoscopy
- *Streptococcus bovis* bacteremia
- After finding colonic polyps at sigmoidoscopy
- Adenocarcinoma metastatic to the liver with an unknown primary
- Change in bowel habits in the elderly
- Follow-up after colonoscopic removal of a large sessile proximal colonic polyp
- Abnormal radiologic study (barium enema, virtual colonoscopy) suggestive of colon cancer
- Colonic stricture
- Dye injection to label a malignant polyp for subsequent surgical removal
- Intraoperative colonoscopy to localize a lesion for surgical removal

### *MRI*

MRI seems to be superior to CT in detecting focal liver metastases from colon cancer. It is more sensitive than CT, particularly for small metastases, because of the typically sharp contrast between metastatic lesions and normal liver on MRI [186]. Administration of contrast agents, such as superparamagnetic iron oxide, further improves the sensitivity of MRI [187]. MRI is also more specific for hepatic metastases than CT. Hepatic metastases have a much shorter T2 sequence than hepatic hemangiomas or cysts [188]. Hepatic metastases typically demonstrate rapid and strong enhancement with intravascular contrast because of enhanced vascularity, but may enhance inhomogeneously because of nonperfused or hypovascular areas within metastases [189]. Although MRI has advantages over CT for detecting hepatic metastases, CT has been the standard test because of lower cost, greater machine availability, and more widely available expertise in image interpretation [190]. MRI is traditionally reserved for characterizing ambiguous hepatic lesions detected by abdominal ultrasound or CT.

### *Transrectal and colonic ultrasonography*

The relative inaccuracy of CT for T and N staging of rectal cancer has led to application of endoscopic ultrasound for this purpose. Preoperative evaluation of the T stage (depth of mural invasion) and the N stage (nodal involvement) greatly impacts the therapy for rectal cancer. Patients with superficial cancer (T1N0) can be treated by local endoscopic or transanal resection without wide excision. Patients with T2N0 lesions are treated surgically without preoperative adjuvant therapy. Patients with deep intramural involvement (T3 or T4) or with nodal involvement (N1 or N2) should receive preoperative radiation and possibly chemotherapy. Patients without rectal sphincter involvement may avoid a colostomy.

Endoscopic ultrasound is more accurate than CT for T staging. For example, in a study of 80 patients with rectal cancer undergoing both CT and rectal ultrasonography, the accuracy of T staging by endosonography was 91% compared with 71% for CT [191]. This difference was statistically significant ($P = .02$). Other studies report that rectal endosonography has about 85% accuracy for T staging [192–194]. Tumors generally appear at endosonography as homogeneous hypoechoic masses that disrupt the normal five-layer ultrasound structure of the rectal wall [195]. Errors in endosonographic T staging may be caused by distortion of the ultrasound image by inflammation in tissue just beneath cancer [196]. Endosonography is more accurate for staging T1, T3, and T4 lesions than T2 lesions because of difficulty in assessing cancer invasion through the muscularis propria [82]. Endosonography has about 80% accuracy for N staging [82,191]. At endosonography malignant lymph nodes tend to be large ($> 1$ cm); hypoechoic; have sharply demarcated borders; and a round, rather than an ovoid or flat, shape [195].

Rectal ultrasound has become the standard preoperative imaging modality for local T and N staging of rectal cancer because of relatively high accuracy. It has not yet, however, been proved to prolong survival [197]. The rectum is easily accessible to an ultrasound probe, using either a rigid probe inserted blindly or an echoendoscope inserted under endoscopic guidance. The procedure is very safe. Endoscopic ultrasound findings frequently change the treatment plan. For example, in a study of 80 patients, endoscopic ultrasound findings resulted in the addition of preoperative neoadjuvant therapy in 25 patients [191]. The accuracy of endoscopic ultrasound is operator dependent. Other factors affecting the accuracy of tumor staging include the ultrasound frequency, with higher frequency improving the resolution but decreasing the depth of penetration; the location of the tumor, with reduced accuracy for tumors low in the rectum; and prior radiotherapy caused by an increase in wall echogenicity after radiation [198].

There are scant data on the impact of endoscopic ultrasound–guided fine-needle aspiration in rectal cancer staging [82,199]. In one study of 41 patients, endoscopic ultrasound–guided fine-needle aspiration of a lymph node upgraded the N stage in one patient and downgraded the N stage in eight patients [191]. Unfortunately, these changes were incorrect in three of the nine cases. Although a fine-needle aspiration diagnosis of cancer in a lymph node is secure, a finding of benignity may be erroneous because of sampling error. The current data are insufficient to recommend standard use of fine-needle aspiration in N staging of rectal cancer [82].

Locally recurrent rectal cancer is potentially important to detect early so that patients can undergo salvage surgery for possible cure. Endoscopic ultrasound is currently the most reliable imaging study for detecting postoperative rectal cancer recurrence. It is superior to CT. In a study of 62 patients undergoing surveillance after rectal cancer surgery, endoscopic ultrasound detected all 11 cancer recurrences [200]. An array of other studies, including serial serum carcinoembryonic antigen levels, digital rectal examination, colonoscopy, and pelvic CT, failed to detect two of these cancer recurrences. The clinical benefit of early detection of rectal cancer recurrence is limited, however, by the low cure rate of salvage surgery [201].

The data on endosonography for colon cancer are much more limited than that for rectal cancer. Most patients with colon cancer without distant metastases undergo colonic resection, regardless of T or N stage. Colonic endosonography is also technically more demanding and time consuming than rectal endosonography. In a study of 50 small colon cancers, endosonography was 91.8% accurate in T staging, compared with 63.3% for magnifying colonoscopy [202]. This difference was statistically significant. Endosonography was, however, only 24.1% accurate for N staging in this study. In a study of 86 patients with colon cancer, endosonography using a balloon-sheathed miniprobe inserted during colonoscopy was 85% accurate for T staging and 73% accurate for N staging [203].

## Prevention of colon cancer

### *Dietary modifications*

Dietary fiber may reduce the risk of colon cancer. Proposed mechanisms include decreased mucosal exposure to intraluminal carcinogens caused by stimulated intestinal transit, decreased concentration of carcinogens in stool caused by increased stool bulk, increased concentrations of anticarcinogenic short-chain fatty acids, and stabilization of insulin levels caused by delayed starch absorption that might otherwise promote colonic carcinogenesis [86]. The effect of dietary fiber is controversial with numerous studies suggesting a large protective effect [97], and several studies suggesting no effect [93]. Regardless of the effect on colon cancer, a high-fiber diet is recommended because of other health benefits. Patient obesity and a diet rich in animal fat and red meat have been proposed as risk factors for colon cancer. The evidence for this is insufficient to recommend avoidance of these factors to reduce the incidence of colon cancer, but avoidance of these factors is recommended because of other, primarily cardiovascular, health benefits. The known effects of dietary factors on colon cancer prevention are summarized in Table 7. These effects are reviewed in detail elsewhere in this issue and in several other recent reviews [123,204].

### *Chemoprevention with aspirin and other nonsteroidal anti-inflammatory drugs*

Nonsteroidal anti-inflammatory drugs (NSAIDs) reduce cellular proliferation, slow cell cycle progression, and stimulate apoptosis [86]. Experimental data suggest that NSAIDs may prevent colonic adenomas or cancer. For example, various NSAIDs prevent carcinogen-induced colon cancer in rodents [205]. Several NSAIDs inhibit adenoma formation in the Min-mouse model of human FAP [123,206]. Case-control and cohort epidemiologic studies also provide evidence of decreased adenoma incidence or decreased colon cancer mortality with regular chronic NSAID use, particularly of aspirin [207]. The Cancer Prevention Study II prospectively analyzed the effect of aspirin on colon cancer mortality during a 6-year period in more than 600,000 adults who provided information on their aspirin use at their enrollment in the trial. The relative mortality from colon cancer was about 0.6 in men and 0.58 in women who used aspirin 16 or more times per month compared with nonusers of the same sex [208]. The relative risk was unchanged when adjusted for dietary factors, physical activity, family history, or diseases that might affect colon cancer mortality or aspirin use. In the Nurses Health Study, the relation between chronic aspirin use and the incidence of colorectal cancer from 1984 through 1992 was analyzed. Women who took aspirin for at least 20 years had a relative risk of 0.56 for developing colon cancer compared with nonusers [209]. Other NSAIDs seem to cause similar reductions in colon cancer incidence, although the effects are less well analyzed [210].

Waddell et al [211] first demonstrated that open-labeled treatment with sulindac, an NSAID, caused regression of colonic adenomas in patients with FAP. They reported disappearance of most rectal polyps in seven patients with a rectal stump status post–subtotal colectomy and of most colorectal polyps in another four patients with FAP with intact colons [211]. Subsequent trials have confirmed that sulindac causes regression of existing adenomas and suppression of new adenomas in patients with FAP [123].

NSAIDs are believed to reduce adenoma formation and inhibit colon cancer development by inhibiting the cyclooxygenase (COX) enzymes required for the synthesis of prostaglandin $E_2$; prostaglandin $E_2$ promotes cell proliferation and tumor growth [212]. NSAIDs may also retard carcinogenesis by effects on cell adhesion and apoptosis [204]. Cyclooxygenase has two isoforms, COX-1 and COX-2. Although nonselective NSAIDs inhibit both isoforms, several COX-2 selective inhibitors have been recently developed. COX-2 inhibitors are used clinically to avoid, or at least reduce, the gastrointestinal toxicity of nonselective NSAIDs [213]. COX-2 is believed to mediate cell proliferation and tumor growth. Hence, selective COX-2 inhibitors may block adenoma formation and cancer development.

Celecoxib, a selective COX-2 inhibitor, was effective in preventing and treating adenomas in the Min-mouse model of FAP [214]. Celecoxib has shown some promise in causing regression of colonic adenomas in patients with FAP. In a study of 77 patients with FAP, patients receiving celecoxib, 400 mg twice daily, had a 28% reduction in the mean number of rectal polyps as compared with a 4.5% reduction in the placebo-treated group [215].

Several trials have examined the effect of NSAIDs on sporadic adenomas. The effects are generally less dramatic [123]. If the benefit of NSAIDs in patients with sporadic adenomas is less clinically significant than in patients with FAP, the toxicity of NSAIDs becomes a more important issue in these patients. Although data support that NSAIDs inhibit colonic carcinogenesis, the optimum specific NSAID, dosage, and duration of treatment are unknown. The role of COX-2 selective inhibitors versus nonselective COX inhibitors needs to be better analyzed and defined.

### *Colonoscopic polypectomy*

Colonic polyps less than 0.8 cm in diameter are usually removed by hot biopsy, especially when sessile, whereas polyps that are larger than 0.8 cm in diameter are usually removed by snare polypectomy, especially when pedunculated [216]. Hot biopsy is performed cautiously in the cecum using a low amplitude and brief duration of current because the colonic wall is thinnest and most vulnerable to transmural necrosis in this region [217]. Diminutive polyps, less than 6 mm in diameter and sessile, may be removed by cold snare polypectomy, wherein the polyp is snared and transected in guillotine fashion without electrocautery. Cold snare polypectomy avoids diathermy artifact in the resected specimen, but entails a theoretical risk of incomplete removal of neoplastic tissue. Electrocautery, in contrast, destroys residual neoplastic tissue in the unremoved stump. Cold snare polypectomy is safe, with a low risk of postpolypectomy hemorrhage [218]. Ultradiminutive (<4 mm) polyps may be removed by repeated cold biopsies without electrocautery.

Large polyps that are likely or obviously malignant should be extensively sampled by multiple biopsies to increase the diagnostic yield, but not removed in toto by polypectomy to avoid the extra risks of polypectomy when cancer surgery is likely to be subsequently required [219]. Sessile polyps between 2 and 3 cm in diameter may be removed by snare polypectomy after creating a pseudopedicle by injecting normal saline or another solution into the polyp base, as described next under endomucosectomy [218]. Sessile polyps more than 3 cm in diameter may be unamenable to conventional snare polypectomy, but may be removed by sequential piecewise polypectomy during several colonoscopic sessions [220]. Pedunculated polyps more than 5 cm in diameter or occluding the lumen may be unamenable to conventional colonoscopic polypectomy because of the technical difficulty of looping a snare around these polyps. These polyps may require surgical resection even when benign.

The complication rate of therapeutic colonoscopy is about 1.4% [171,172]. The most common major postpolypectomy complications are gastrointestinal bleeding, colonic perforation, and the postpolypectomy syndrome. In the postpolypectomy syndrome, a patient develops abdominal pain, pyrexia, leukocytosis, and localized peritoneal irritation from an almost transmural burn from polypectomy. This occurs in up to 1% of polypectomies [221]. This syndrome is usually managed medically, with cessation of oral intake, intravenous hydration, and antibiotic administration [222].

The pathophysiology of the adenoma-to-carcinoma sequence and the molecular pathophysiology of colon carcinogenesis strongly suggest that polypectomy of adenomas should substantially prevent colon cancer. This is strongly supported by clinical trials. For example, in the National Polyp Study 699 patients underwent surveillance colonoscopy at 1, 3, and every 2 subsequent years after detecting at least one adenomatous polyp at an index colonoscopy [223]. The 699 patients had only five colorectal cancers detected during a mean surveillance period of 5.9 years. This represented a 76% to 90% decline in the incidence of colon cancer compared with three historical reference groups. All the cancers were detected early.

### *Endomucosectomy*

Endomucosectomy, or endoscopic mucosal resection, adapts the classic principles of conventional snare polypectomy combined with submucosal injection to remove more deeply affected mucosa or submucosa by resecting through the middle or deep submucosa. Endomucosectomy provides an alternative to surgery for deeper superficial lesions without evident penetration of the deep muscle layer, regional lymph nodes, or distant metastases. Sessile villous adenomas, adenomas with carcinoma in situ (T0 lesions), and some early cancers invading the submucosa (T1N0M0) lesions are candidates for endomucosectomy in suitable patients. Usually the tumor is characterized by endoscopy, sampled by endoscopic biopsy, and locally staged by endosonography before considering endomucosectomy. Patients are evaluated for the suitability of endomucosectomy based on tumor size; endoscopic appearance; pathology of the initial endoscopic biopsy; and the estimated depth of tumor penetration (T stage). Endomucosectomy is usually applied to polypoid (protruding) lesions, but can be applied to flat or even minimally depressed lesions provided the previously mentioned criteria are satisfied. Endomucosectomy has an advantage over endoscopic ablative therapy (using laser, argon plasma coagulation, or photodynamic therapy) because the entire treated specimen is removed and available for histologic analysis and pathologic staging. Endomucosectomy has an advantage over the alternative of surgical resection of less procedure morbidity and minimal mortality.

The basic technique of endomucosectomy is deep submucosal injection of normal saline or another solution to thicken the colonic wall at the polypectomy site to permit deep resection of the submucosa without incurring a risk of a transmural burn or frank colonic perforation. This injection also tamponades the feeding artery to reduce postpolypectomy bleeding, promotes vasospasm, and increases tissue liquidity and electrical conductivity at the polyp base to facilitate electrocautery. The effects of the submucosal injection are carefully evaluated during endoscopy. A lesion that lifts during submucosal injection is amenable to endomucosectomy; a lesion that partly lifts may be amenable to endomucosectomy after due consideration; and a lesion that fails to lift (nonlift sign) is not amenable to endomucosectomy because of a high risk of invasive carcinoma [224,225]. Deep carcinomatous invasion is the major cause of adherence of submucosa to deep muscle and the nonlift sign [225]. Failure to lift also increases the risk of endomucosectomy because of poorly defined tissue planes for endoscopic resection.

The tumor may then be resected by conventional snare polypectomy to resect subcutaneous tissue. Adjunctive techniques used to increase the depth of endoscopic resection include the following. (1) The use of a special shark tooth snare with small hooks along the wire loop. The hooks dig into the lesion to prevent slippage of the lesion during snare closure. (2) The use of a transparent cap inserted at the tip of the endoscope. The cap contains an internal rim at the tip in which an open snare is prepositioned. After the lesion is sucked into the cap using endoscopic suction, the snare is closed on the suctioned tissue (neopolyp) and electrocautery is applied to remove deeper tissue. (3) The use of a double-channel endoscope with a biopsy forceps and a snare advanced through separate channels and with the snare loop opened around the biopsy forceps. The lesion is grasped and lifted by the biopsy forceps and the snare is then closed around the lifted submucosal tissue.

Endomucosectomy has been frequently used by Japanese and European endoscopists, but is increasingly being used by American investigators. It is most commonly applied to remove early gastric cancers or esophageal lesions but is being increasingly used to remove colorectal lesions, particularly large adenomas.

Complications of endomucosectomy include abdominal pain, bleeding, perforation, and stricture formation. The risks of bleeding vary from 1.5% to 24%, depending on the size and type of the lesion and the definition of bleeding [224]. Endoscopic hemostasis is frequently required during endomucosectomy because of transection of submucosal vessels. The endoscopist must be experienced and highly competent at endoscopic hemostasis to address the problem promptly. The simplest technique of hemostasis is endoscopic clipping.

The major problem of endomucosectomy is that it is insufficient therapy for locally extensive or metastatic disease. This occurs much more frequently for lesions staged as T1 than T0 by endosonography. About 10% of apparently T1 lesions turn out to be more deeply invasive cancers, including about 5% with residual cancer in the bowel wall and about 5% with undetected nodal metastases [226,227]. Such patients usually require cancer surgery for cure following endomucosectomy. Endomucosectomy is described in greater detail elsewhere in this issue.

## New and evolving developments

Colon cancer incidence and survival has improved only slightly in the United States during the past decade despite the apparent efficacy of colonoscopic polypectomy at cancer prevention [228]. This failure is caused by insufficient implementation of colonoscopy screening partly because of the expense, invasiveness, discomfort, and risks of colonoscopy. New simpler, less invasive, and safer tests are being designed to overcome these barriers to universal screening for colon cancer.

### *Stool genetic markers*

DNA from colon cancer is shed into the fecal stream in greater quantities than DNA from normal colonic mucosa. Cancerous DNA is not degraded with time or by contiguity with stool during colonic passage [229]. Much as minute quantities of blood in stool are detected by guaiac testing, minute quantities of DNA in stool can be assayed by polymerase chain-reaction amplification. This technique has shown clinical promise in preliminary clinical studies for noninvasive detection of cancerous DNA in stool specimens. For example, a multiarray assay for common mutations in colon cancer, including *APC*, *p53*, K-*ras*, and *BAT-26* (a marker for microsatellite instability) mutations had a sensitivity of 91% and specificity of 100% for detection of colon cancer in a study of 22 patients with colon cancer and 28 patients with endoscopically normal colons [230,231]. In another study, an assay for genetic mutations in *TP53*, *BAT-26*, and K-*ras* detected mutations in 36 (71%) of 51 patients with colon cancer [232]. Most of the detected cases, however, had histologically advanced and clinically symptomatic colon cancer; an ideal screening test should also detect early asymptomatic and potentially curable colon cancer [233]. Genetic stool screening has the potential test advantages of noninvasiveness and user friendliness, but needs further refinement in technique and testing in large clinical trials [229,231]. Incorporation of additional molecular markers may further improve test sensitivity and specificity.

Colorectal cancer can also be detected in the serum, but the clinical studies are so far preliminary and small. The studies have shown low test sensitivity [234,235]. With further technical refinements, these molecular and noninvasive approaches could become highly useful for screening for colon cancer.

## *Virtual colonoscopy*

Vining introduced virtual colonoscopy in 1994 to maintain the desirable features of colonoscopy of ease of lesion detection while avoiding the undesirable features of colonoscopy of test invasiveness, patient discomfort, need for sedation and analgesia, and test risks [236]. In virtual colonoscopy CT images are obtained in the prone and supine positions during a prolonged breathhold. The CT images are reformatted into two-dimensional images in the three orthogonal (axial, sagittal, and coronal) planes, or reconstructed into three-dimensional endoluminal (virtual colonoscopy) images that simulate the conventional colonoscopic view. Like colonoscopy, virtual colonoscopy generally requires colonic preparation with oral laxatives. Application of digital stool subtraction technology with administration of oral contrast may, however, obviate the need for colonic preparation [237]. Unlike colonoscopy, sedation and analgesia are not required. CT colonography is extremely safe with rarely reported significant complications [238,239]. Unlike colonoscopy, virtual colonoscopy can visualize extracolonic intra-abdominal organs. It can provide cancer staging simultaneous with colon cancer detection, and can visualize intra-abdominal abnormalities, such as extracolonic malignancies and aneurysms [240].

Virtual colonoscopy is currently under intense analysis. The accuracy is controversial, with conflicting data. For example, Pickhardt et al [239] reported in 2003 that CT colonography had a sensitivity of 93.8% for polyps at least 10 mm in diameter, 93.9% for polyps at least 8 mm in diameter, and 88.7% for polyps at least 6 mm in diameter. In this study CT colonography was an excellent screening test for colonic polyps with a very high sensitivity and specificity. Contrariwise, Cotton et al [241] reported in 2004 in a study of 600 patients undergoing both CT colonography and colonoscopy that the sensitivity of CT colonography was only 39% for lesions less than 6 mm in diameter, and only 55% for lesions sized more than 10 mm in diameter. In this study CT colonography was so poorly sensitive and specific as not to be useful as a screening test [242]. The wide discrepancy between the various studies may be caused by different CT technology, especially use of 4- versus 16-slice scanners, use of supine versus supine and prone views, different computerized software for colonic fly-through endoluminal views, different levels of radiologist training and expertise, and administration of dual oral contrast versus single oral contrast versus no oral contrast for tagging stool [242]. In all studies the accuracy of virtual colonoscopy is a function of polyp size. It is much more accurate for lesions larger than 10 mm than for lesions less than 5 mm [239,243,244]. It is consequently more accurate at detecting cancers than adenomas because cancers tend to be larger [244,245]. The most important disadvantage of virtual colonoscopy is the inability to remove polyps for histologic analysis and definitive therapy; the inability to biopsy masses for histologic classification; and the inability to apply other therapies, such as injection or ablation, which are available by colonoscopy. Detection of a polyp or mass at virtual colonoscopy currently requires colonoscopy as a second test for polypectomy or biopsy. Virtual colonoscopy is reviewed in detail elsewhere in this issue.

### *Videocapsule endoscopy*

The videocapsule is delivered perorally to the small intestine by peristalsis to provide wireless endoscopy by radiofrequency transmission [246]. The videocapsule contains a miniaturized image-capturing system, battery, light source, and transmitter, all of which are contained within an 11-by-30 mm capsule.

Videocapsule endoscopy has developed a niche in the evaluation of jejunoileal bleeding [247,248]. Although chronic blood loss is usually caused by an upper or lower gastrointestinal lesion, the bleeding occasionally arises from the jejunoileum. The jejunoileum is poorly accessible by traditional tube endoscopy. Only the distal 20 to 30 cm of the ileum is potentially accessible during colonoscopy [249]. Likewise traditional tube esophagogastroduodenoscopy can be extended by push enteroscopy into, but not beyond, the proximal jejunum because of instrumental looping [250]. The videocapsule has shown significant potential for jejunoileal evaluation.

Videocapsule endoscopy might potentially provide effective screening examination of the colon in the average-risk patient if the technology becomes reasonably priced [251]. Videocapsule endoscopy is theoretically attractive as a screening test because of examination simplicity, noninvasiveness, minimal patient discomfort, and an apparently high safety profile.

The test has serious practical disadvantages for colonic examination because of the high cost of the technology and poor sensitivity in the presence of stool; the instrument is unable to wash away, aspirate, or navigate around stool. Stool is a greater problem for colonic than small intestinal examination. The videocapsule lacks biopsy capability. It lacks therapeutic capabilities of injection, decompression, ablation, and polypectomy. The videocapsule moves passively from proximal to distal by gastrointestinal peristalsis. The videocapsule cannot rotate to view different sides of mucosa and to inspect lesions from different angles. The videocapsule currently provides telecommunications for only 6 hours; this is insufficient to examine the entire colon. Peristalsis is relatively slow in the colon and the videocapsule travels slowly through the colon. The weak illumination provided by the videocapsule, while adequate for the small-caliber small intestine, is inadequate for the large-caliber large intestine. At colonoscopy, the colon is insufflated to distend and display the colonic wall. The videocapsule lacks air insufflation capabilities and collapsed portions of the colon may be poorly visualized. Ideally, if these deficiencies are corrected, videocapsule endoscopy could provide an initial screening examination of the colon; a lesion detected by this examination would prompt colonoscopy, for direct colonoscopic confirmation, for a histologic diagnosis by colonoscopic biopsy, and for possible colonoscopic polypectomy.

## Summary

Epidemiologists, basic researchers, clinicians, and public health administrators unite! Develop and implement a simple, safe, and effective preventive and screening test for colon cancer. The public will willingly and enthusiastically accept such a test. Many thousands of lives are at stake every year.

## References

[1] Jemal A, Tiwari RC, Murray T, Ghafoor A, Samuels A, Ward E, et al. Cancer statistics, 2004. CA Cancer J Clin 2004;54:8–29.

[2] Winawer SJ, Fletcher RH, Miller L, Godlee F, Stolar MH, Mulrow CD, et al. Colorectal cancer screening: clinical guidelines and rationale. Gastroenterology 1997;112:594–642.

[3] American Society for Gastrointestinal Endoscopy. Guidelines for colorectal screening and surveillance. Gastrointest Endosc 2000;51:777–82.

[4] Bond JH. Polyp guidelines: diagnosis, treatment, and surveillance for patients with colorectal polyps. Practice Parameters Committee of the American College of Gastroenterology. Am J Gastroenterol 2000;95:3053–63.

[5] Smith R, Cokkinides V, Eyre H. American Cancer Society guidelines for the early detection of cancer. CA Cancer J Clin 2003;53:27–43.

[6] Smith RA, von Eschenbach AC, Wender R, Levin B, Byers T, Rothenberger D, et al. American Cancer Society guidelines for the early detection of cancer: update of early detection guidelines for prostate, colorectal, and endometrial cancers. Also: update 2001 – testing for early lung cancer detection. CA Cancer J Clin 2001;51:38–75.

[7] Prajapati DN, Saeian K, Binion DG, Staff DM, Kim JP, Massey BT, et al. Volume and yield of screening colonoscopy at a tertiary medical center after change in Medicare reimbursement. Am J Gastroenterol 2003;98:194–9.
[8] Harewood GC, Lieberman DA. Colonoscopy practice patterns since the introduction of Medicare coverage for average risk screening. Clin Gastroenterol Hepatol 2004;2:72–7.
[9] Pignone M, Rich M, Teutsch SM, Berg AO, Lohr KN. Screening for colorectal cancer in adults at average risk: a summary of the evidence for the US Preventive Services Task Force. Ann Intern Med 2002;137:132–41.
[10] Cappell MS, Goldberg ES. The relationship between the clinical presentation and spread of colon cancer in 315 consecutive patients: a significant trend of earlier cancer detection from 1982 through 1988 at a university hospital. J Clin Gastroenterol 1992;14:227–35.
[11] Trowbridge B, Burt RW. Colorectal cancer screening. Surg Clin North Am 2002;82:943–57.
[12] Nelson DE, Bolen J, Marcus S, Wells HE, Meissner H. Cancer screening estimates for US metropolitan areas. Am J Prev Med 2003;24:301–9.
[13] Harewood GC, Wiersma MJ, Melton LJ III. A prospective, controlled assessment of factors influencing acceptance of screening colonoscopy. Am J Gastroenterol 2002;97:3186–94.
[14] Taylor ML, Anderson R. Colorectal cancer screening: physician attitudes and practices. World Med J 2002;101:39–43.
[15] Tsai CJ, Lu DK. Small colorectal polyps: histopathology and clinical significance. Am J Gastroenterol 1995;90:988–94.
[16] Rubin CE, Bronner MP. Endoscopic mucosal biopsy: a memorial to Rodger C. Haggitt, M.D. In: Yamada T, Alpers D, Kaplowitz N, et al, editors. Textbook of gastroenterology. 4th edition. Philadelphia: Lippincott Williams & Wilkins; 2003. p. 2893–946.
[17] Morson BC, Dawson IMP. Gastrointestinal pathology. Oxford: Blackwell Scientific; 1972.
[18] Heald RJ, Bussey HJR. Clinical experiences at St. Mark's Hospital with multiple synchronous cancers of the colon and rectum. Dis Colon Rectum 1975;18:6–10.
[19] Day DW, Morson BC. The adenoma-carcinoma sequence. In: Morson BC, editor. The pathogenesis of colorectal cancer. Philadelphia: WB Saunders; 1978. p. 58–71.
[20] Bussey HJR. Familial polyposis coli: family studies, histopathology, differential diagnosis and results of treatment. Baltimore: Johns Hopkins University Press; 1975.
[21] Stryker SJ, Wolff BG, Culp CE, Libbe SD, Ilstrup DM, MacCarty RL. Natural history of untreated colonic polyps. Gastroenterology 1987;93:1009–13.
[22] Cappell MS, Forde KA. Spatial clustering of multiple hyperplastic, adenomatous, and malignant colonic polyps in individual patients. Dis Colon Rectum 1989;32:641–52.
[23] Blue MG, Sivak MV Jr, Achkar E, Matzen R, Stahl RR. Hyperplastic polyps seen at sigmoidoscopy are markers for additional adenomas seen at colonoscopy. Gastroenterology 1991;100:564–6.
[24] Jass JR. Hyperplastic polyps of the colorectum: innocent or guilty? Dis Colon Rectum 2001;44:163–6.
[25] Higuchi T, Jass JR. My approach to serrated polyps of the colorectum. J Clin Pathol 2004; 57:682–6.
[26] Montgomery E. Serrated colorectal polyps: emerging evidence suggests the need for a reappraisal. Adv Anat Pathol 2004;11:143–9.
[27] Wynter CV, Walsh MD, Higuchi T, Leggett BA, Young J, Jass JR. Methylation patterns define two types of hyperplastic polyps associated with colorectal cancer. Gut 2004;53: 573–80.
[28] Menzelio D. De excescentals verrucosa cristosis in intestinins crassis dysentarium passi observatis. Acta Med Berolinensium 1721;4:68–71.
[29] Corvisart L. Hypertrophie partielle de la muqueuse intestinale [Partial hypertrophy of the intestinal mucosa]. Bull Soc Anat 1847;22:400 [in French].
[30] Chargelaigue A. Des polypes du rectum [Polyps of the rectum]. Paris: Thesis; 1859 [in French].

[31] Cripps WH. Two cases of disseminated polyps of the rectum. Trans Pathol Soc London 1882;33:165–8.
[32] Bickersteth RA. Multiple polypi of the rectum occurring in a mother and child. St. Bartholomew's Hosp Rep 1890;26:299–301.
[33] Smith T. Three cases of multiple polypi of the lower bowel occurring in one family. St. Baretholomew's Hosp Rep 1887;23:225–9.
[34] Handford H. Disseminated polypi of the large intestine becoming malignant. Trans Pathol Soc London 1890;41:133–4.
[35] Lockhart-Mummery JP. Cancer and heredity. Lancet 1925;I:427–9.
[36] Dukes CF. The hereditary factors in polyposis intestini or multiple adenomata. Cancer Rev 1930;5:241–56.
[37] Gardner EJ, Richards RC. Multiple cutaneous and subcutaneous lesions occurring simultaneously with hereditary polyposis and osteomatosis. Am J Hum Genet 1953;5:139–47.
[38] Veale AMO. Intestinal polyposis. Eugenis Laboratory Memoirs Series 40. New York: Cambridge University Press; 1965.
[39] Cockyne EA. Hereditary in relation to cancer. Cancer Rev 1967;2:337–47.
[40] Herrera L, Kataki S, Gibas L, Pietrzak E, Sandberg AA. Gardner syndrome in a man with an interstitial deletion of 5q. Am J Med Genet 1986;25:473–6.
[41] Bodmer WF, Bailey CJ, Bodmer J, Bussey HJ, Ellis A, Gorman P, et al. Localization of the gene for familial adenomatous polyposis on chromosome 5. Nature 1987;328:614–6.
[42] Leppert M, Burt R, Hughes JP, Samowitz W, Nakamura Y, Woodward S, et al. Genetic analysis of an inherited predisposition to colon cancer in a family with a variable number of adenomatous polyps. N Engl J Med 1990;322:904–8.
[43] Kinzler KW, Nilbert MC, Su LK, Vogelstein B, Bryan TM, Levy DB, et al. Identification of FAP locus genes from chromosome 5q21. Science 1991;253:661–5.
[44] Olschwang S, Laurent-Puig P, Groden J, White R, Thomas G. Germ-line mutations in the first 14 exons of the adenomatous polyposis coli (APC) gene. Am J Hum Genet 1993;52:273–9.
[45] Broca PP. Traite des tumeurs [Treatise on tumors], vols. I and II. Paris: Asselin; 1866 and 1869 [in French].
[46] Warthin AS. Heredity with reference to carcinoma as shown by the study of the cases examined in the pathological laboratory of the University of Michigan, 1895–1913. Arch Intern Med 1913;12:546–55.
[47] Lynch HT, Lynch PM. What is hereditary colon cancer? In: Ingall JRF, Mastromarino AJ. Prevention of hereditary large bowel cancer: proceedings of a conference held in Troy, Michigan, June 3–4, 1982. New York: Alan R. Liss; 1982. p. 3–38.
[48] Peltomaki P, Aaltonen LA, Sistonen P, Pylkkanen L, Mecklin JP, Jarvinen H, et al. Genetic mapping of a locus predisposing to human colorectal cancer. Science 1993;260:810–2.
[49] Fishel R, Lescoe MK, Rao MRS, Copeland NG, Jenkins NA, Garber J, et al. The human mutator gene homolog MSH2 and its association with hereditary nonpolyposis colon cancer. Cell 1993;75:1027–38.
[50] Leach FS, Nicolaides NC, Papadopoulos N, Liu B, Jen J, Parsons R, et al. Mutations of mutS homolog in hereditary nonpolyposis colorectal cancer. Cell 1993;75:1215–25.
[51] Bronner CE, Baker SM, Morrison PT, Warren G, Smith LG, Lescoe MK, et al. Mutation in the DNA mismatch repair gene homolgue hMLH1 is associated with hereditary nonpolyposis colon cancer. Nature 1994;368:258–61.
[52] Papadopoulos N, Nicolaides NC, Wei YF, Ruben SM, Carter KC, Rosen CA, et al. Mutation of a mutL homolog in hereditary colon cancer. Science 1994;263:1625–9.
[53] Kolodner RD, Hall NR, Lipford J, Kane MF, Rao MRS, Morrison P, et al. Structure of the human MSH2 locus and analysis of the two Muir-Torre kindreds for MSH2 mutations. Genomics 1994;24:516–26.

[54] Vasen HF, Mecklin JP, Khan PM, Lynch HT. The International Collaborative Group on Hereditary Non-Polyposis Colorectal Cancer (ICG-HNPCC). Dis Colon Rectum 1991;34: 424–5.
[55] Ivanovich JL, Read TE, Ciske DJ, Kodner IJ, Whelan AJ. A practical approach to familial and hereditary colon cancer. Am J Med 1999;107:68–77.
[56] Robbins DH, Itzkowitz SH. The molecular and genetic basis of colon cancer. Med Clin North Am 2002;86:1467–95.
[57] Chung DC, Rustgi AK. DNA mismatch repair and cancer. Gastroenterology 1995;109: 1685–99.
[58] Zigman AF, Lavine JE, Jones MC, Boland CR, Carethers JM. Localization of the Bannayan-Riley-Ruvalcaba syndrome to chromosome 10q23. Gastroenterology 1997;113: 1433–7.
[59] Nelen MR, Padberg GW, Peeters EA, Lin AY, van den Helm B, Frants RR, et al. Localization of the gene for Cowden disease to chromosome 10q22–23. Nat Genet 1996;13:114–6.
[60] Nelen MR, van Staveren WC, Peeters EA, Hassel MB, Gorlin RJ, Hamm H, et al. Germline mutations in the PTEN/MMAC1 gene in patients with Cowden disease. Hum Mol Genet 1997;6:1383–7.
[61] Houlston R, Bevan S, Williams A, Young J, Dunlop M, Rozen P, et al. Mutations in DPC4 (SMAD4) cause juvenile polyposis syndrome, but only account for a minority of cases. Hum Mol Genet 1998;12:1907–12.
[62] Howe JR, Roth S, Ringold JC, Summers RW, Jarvinen HJ, Sistonen P, et al. Mutations in the SMAD4/DPC4 gene in juvenile polyposis. Science 1998;280:1086–8.
[63] Jenne DE, Reimann H, Nezu J, Friedel W, Loff S, Jeschke R, et al. Peutz-Jeghers syndrome is caused by mutations in a novel serine threonine kinase. Nat Genet 1998;18:38–43.
[64] Suraweera N, Duval A, Reperant M, Vaury C, Furlan D, Leroy K, et al. Evaluation of tumor microsatellite instability using five quasimonomorphic repeats and pentaplex PCR. Gastroenterology 2002;123:1804–11.
[65] Jen J, Powell SM, Papadopoulos N, Smith KJ, Hamilton SR, Vogelstein B, et al. Molecular determinants of dysplasia in colorectal lesions. Cancer Res 1994;54:5523–6.
[66] Miyaki M, Konishi M, Kikuchi-Yanoshita R, Enomoto M, Igari T, Tanaka K, et al. Characteristics of somatic mutation of the adenomatous polyposis coli gene in colorectal tumors. Cancer Res 1994;54:3011–20.
[67] Vogelstein B, Fearon ER, Hamilton SR, Kern SE, Preisinger AC, Leppert M, et al. Genetic alterations during colorectal-tumor development. N Engl J Med 1988;319:525–32.
[68] Baker SJ, Fearon ER, Nigro JM, Hamilton SR, Preisinger AC, Jessup JM, et al. Chromosome 17 deletions and p53 gene mutations in colorectal carcinomas. Science 1989; 244:217–21.
[69] Slebos RJ, Rodenhuis S. The ras gene family in human non-small-cell lung cancer. J Natl Cancer Inst Monogr 1992;13:23–9.
[70] Yashiro M, Carethers JM, Laghi L, Saito K, Slezak P, Jaramillo E, et al. Genetic pathways in the evolution of morphologically distinct colorectal neoplasms. Cancer Res 2001;61: 2676–83.
[71] Kern SE, Fearon ER, Tersmette KW, Enterline JP, Leppert M, Nakamura Y, et al. Clinical and pathological associations with allelic loss in colorectal carcinoma. JAMA 1989;261: 3099–103.
[72] Brenner DA and editors, Gastroenterology. Gastrointestinal basic science 2002–2003: the year in review. Clin Gastroenterol Hepatol 2004;2:9–13.
[73] Myohanen SK, Baylin SB, Herman JG. Hypermethylation can selectively silence individual p16ink4A alleles in neoplasia. Cancer Res 1998;58:591–3.
[74] Burri N, Shaw P, Bouzourene H, Sordat I, Sordat B, Gillet M, et al. Methylation silencing and mutations of the p14ARF and p16NK4A genes in colon cancer. Cancer Lab Invest 2001;81:217–29.

[75] Shannon BA, Iacopetta BJ. Methylation of the hMLH1, p16, and MDR1 genes in colorectal carcinoma: associations with clinicopathological features. Cancer Lett 2001;167:91–7.
[76] Deans GT, Patterson CC, Parks TG, Spence RA, Heatley M, Moorehead RJ, et al. Colorectal carcinoma: importance of clinical and pathological factors in survival. Ann R Coll Surg Engl 1994;76:59–64.
[77] Kanazawa T, Watanabe T, Kazama S, Tada T, Koketsu S, Nagawa H. Poorly differentiated adenocarcinoma and mucinous carcinoma of the colon and rectum show higher rates of loss of heterozygosity and loss of E-cadherin expression due to methylation of promoter region. Int J Cancer 2002;102:225–9.
[78] McCallion K, Mitchell RM, Wilson RH, Kee F, Wastson RG, Collins JS, et al. Flexible sigmoidoscopy and the changing distribution of colorectal cancer: implications for screening. Gut 2001;48:522–5.
[79] Church JM. Clinical significance of small colorectal polyps. Dis Colon Rectum 2004;47: 481–5.
[80] Nivatvongs S. Surgical management of malignant colorectal polyps. Surg Clin North Am 2002;82:959–66.
[81] Cooper HS, Slemmer JR. Surgical pathology of carcinoma of the colon and rectum. Semin Oncol 1991;18:367–80.
[82] Sandhu IS, Bhutani MS. Gastrointestinal endoscopic ultrasonography. Med Clin North Am 2002;86:1289–317.
[83] Fisher ER, Sass R, Palekar A, Fisher B, Wolmark N. Dukes' classification revisited: findings from the national surgical adjuvant breast and bowel projects (protocol R-01). Cancer 1989;64:2354–60.
[84] Boland CR. Malignant tumors of the colon. In: Yamada T, Alpers D, Kaplowitz N, et al, editors. Textbook of gastroenterology. 4th edition. Philadelphia: Lippincott Williams & Wilkins; 2003. p. 1940–90.
[85] Welch JP, Donaldson GA. The clinical correlation of an autopsy study of recurrent colorectal cancer. Ann Surg 1979;189:496–502.
[86] Hawk ET, Limburg PJ, Viner JL. Epidemiology and prevention of colorectal cancer. Surg Clin North Am 2002;82:905–41.
[87] Fleshner P, Slater G, Aufses AH Jr. Age and sex distribution of patients with colorectal cancer. Cancer Detect Prev 2001;25:55–61.
[88] Giovannucci E, Ascherio A, Rimm EB, Colditz GA, Stampfer MJ, Willett WC. Physical activity, obesity and risk of colon cancer and adenoma in men. Ann Intern Med 1995;122: 327–34.
[89] Willett WC, Stampfer MJ, Colditz GA, Rosner BA, Speizer FE. Relation of meat, fat, and fiber intake to the risk of colon cancer in a prospective study among women. N Engl J Med 1990;323:1664–72.
[90] Thun MJ, Calle EE, Namboodiri MM, Flanders WD, Coates RJ, Byers T, et al. Risk factors for fatal colon cancer in a large prospective study. J Natl Cancer Inst 1992;84: 1491–500.
[91] Kampman E, Verhoeven D, Sloots L, van't Veer P. Vegetable and animal products as determinants of colon cancer in Dutch men and women. Cancer Causes Control 1996;6: 225–34.
[92] Bergsma-Kadijk JA, van't Veer P, Kampman E, Burema J. Calcium does not protect against colorectal neoplasia. Epidemiology 1996;7:590–7.
[93] Fuchs CS, Giovannucci EL, Colditz GA, Hunter DJ, Stampfer MJ, Rosner B, et al. Dietary fiber and the risk of colorectal cancer and adenoma in women. N Engl J Med 1999;340: 169–76.
[94] Ghadirian P, Maisonneuve P, Perret C, Kennedy G, Boyle P, Krewski D, et al. A case-control study of toenail selenium and cancer of the breast, colon, and prostate. Cancer Detect Prev 2000;24:305–13.

[95] Baron JA, Sandler RS, Haile RW, Mandel JS, Mott LA, Greenberg ER. Folate intake, alcohol consumption, cigarette smoking, and risk of colorectal adenomas. J Natl Cancer Inst 1998;90:57–62.
[96] Modan B, Cuckle H, Lubin F. A note on the role of dietary retinol and carotene in human gastrointestinal cancer. Int J Cancer 1981;28:421–4.
[97] Howe GR, Benito E, Castelleto R, Cornee J, Esteve J, Gallagher RP, et al. Dietary intake of fiber and decreased risk of cancers of the colon and rectum: evidence from the combined analysis of 13 case-control studies. J Natl Cancer Inst 1992;84:1887–96.
[98] Betes M, Munoz-Navas MA, Duque JM, Angos R, Macias E, Subtil JC, et al. Use of colonoscopy as a primary screening test for colorectal cancer in average risk people. Am J Gastroenterol 2003;98:2648–54.
[99] Schindler AE. Obesity and risk of cancer in the woman. Zentralbl Gynakol 1998;120: 235–40.
[100] Anderson JC, Attam R, Alpern Z, Messina CR, Hubbard P, Grimson R, et al. Prevalence of colorectal neoplasia in smokers. Am J Gastroenterol 2003;98:2777–83.
[101] Goldbohm RA, van den Brandt PA, van't Veer P, Dorant E, Sturmans F, Hermus RJ. Prospective study on alcohol consumption and the risk of cancer of the colon and rectum in the Netherlands. Cancer Causes Control 1994;5:95–104.
[102] Spigelman AD, Arese P, Phillips RK. Polyposis: the Peutz-Jeghers syndrome. Br J Surg 1995;82:1311–4.
[103] Fuchs CS, Giovannucci EL, Colditz GA, Hunter DJ, Speizer FE, Willett WC. A prospective study of family history and the risk of colorectal cancer. N Engl J Med 1994;331:1669–74.
[104] Jeevaratnam P, Cottier DS, Browett PJ, van de Water NS, Pokos V, Jass JR. Familial giant hyperplastic polyposis predisposing to colon cancer: a new hereditary bowel cancer syndrome. J Pathol 1996;179:20–5.
[105] Eaden JA, Abrams KR, Mayberry JF. The risk of colorectal cancer in ulcerative colitis: a meta-analysis. Gut 2001;48:526–35.
[106] Hamilton SR. Colorectal carcinoma in patients with Crohn's disease. Gastroenterology 1985;89:398–407.
[107] Morson BC. The evolution of cancer of the colon and rectum. Cancer 1975;36:2251–70.
[108] Lockhart-Mummery HE, Heald RJ. Metachronous cancer of the large intestine. Dis Colon Rectum 1972;15:261–4.
[109] Neugut AI, Murray TI, Lee WC, Robinson E. The association of breast cancer and colorectal cancer in men: an analysis of surveillance, epidemiology, and end results program data. Cancer 1991;68:2069–73.
[110] Sandler RS, Sandler DP. Radiation-induced cancers of the colon and rectum: assessing the risk. Gastroenterology 1983;84:51–7.
[111] Will JC, Galuska DA, Vinicor F, Calle EE. Colorectal cancer: another complication of diabetes mellitus? Am J Epidemiol 1998;147:816–25.
[112] Klein RS, Catalano MT, Edberg SC, Casey JI, Steigbigel NH. *Streptococcus bovis* septicemia and carcinoma of the colon. Ann Intern Med 1979;91:560–2.
[113] Ellmerich S, Scholler M, Duranton B, Gosse F, Galluser M, Klein JP, et al. Promotion of intestinal carcinogenesis by *Streptococcus bovis*. Carcinogenesis 2000;21:753–6.
[114] Azimuddin K, Khubchandani IT, Stasik JJ, Rosen L, Riether D. Neoplasia after ureterosigmoidostomy. Dis Colon Rectum 1999;42:1632–8.
[115] Ron E, Gridley G, Hrubec Z, Page W, Arora S, Fraumeni JF Jr. Acromegaly and gastrointestinal cancer. Cancer 1991;68:1673–7.
[116] Webb SM, Casanueva F, Wass JA. Oncological complications of excess GH in acromegaly. Pituitary 2002;5:21–5.
[117] Ekbom A, Yuen J, Adami HO, McLaughlin JK, Chow WH, Persson I, et al. Cholecystectomy and colorectal cancer. Gastroenterology 1993;105:142–7.

[118] Ziegler RG, Devesa SS, Fraumeni JF. Epidemiologic patterns of colorectal cancer. In: De Vita VT Jr, Hellman S, Rosenberg SA, editors. Important advances in oncology, 1986. Philadelphia: JB Lippincott; 1986. p. 209–31.
[119] Tamura K, Ishiguro S, Munakata A, Yoshida Y, Nakaji S, Suguwara K. Annual changes in colorectal carcinoma incidence in Japan: analysis of survey data on incidence in Aomori Prefecture. Cancer 1996;78:1187–94.
[120] Haenszel W, Kurihara M. Studies of Japanese immigrants: I. Mortality from cancer and other diseases among Japanese in the United States. J Natl Cancer Inst 1968;40:43–68.
[121] Satia-Abouta J, Galanko JA, Martin CF, Ammerman A, Sandler RS. Food groups and colon cancer risk in African-Americans and Caucasians. Int J Cancer 2004;109:728–36.
[122] Ries LAG, Eisner MP, Kosary CL, et al. SEER cancer statistics review, 1973–1998. Bethesda: National Cancer Institute; 2001.
[123] Gatof D, Ahnen D. Primary prevention of colorectal cancer: diet and drugs. Hematol Oncol Clin North Am 2003;17:575–610.
[124] Miller AB. Trends in cancer mortality and epidemiology. Cancer 1983;51:2413–8.
[125] Falterman KW, Hill CB, Markey JC, Fox JW, Cohn I Jr. Cancer of the colon, rectum, and anus: a review of 2313 cases. Cancer 1974;34:951–9.
[126] Posner MC, Steele GD Jr, Mayer RJ. Adenocarcinoma of the colon and rectum. In: Zuidema GD, editor. Shackelford's surgery of the alimentary tract. 5th edition. Philadelphia: WB Saunders; 2002. p. 219–36.
[127] Cappell MS. Colon cancer during pregnancy: the gastroenterologist's perspective. Gastroenterol Clin North Am 1998;27:225–56.
[128] Harewood GC, Ahlquist DA. Fecal occult blood testing for iron deficiency: a reappraisal. Dig Dis 2000;18:75–82.
[129] Theologides A. Cancer cachexia. Cancer 1979;43:2004–12.
[130] Anderson NP. Syndrome of spoon nails, anemia, cheilitis, and dysphagia. Arch Dermatol 1938;37:816.
[131] Ioannou GN, Rockey DC, Bryson CL, Weiss NS. Iron deficiency and gastrointestinal malignancy: a population-based cohort study. Am J Med 2002;113:276–80.
[132] Spratt JS, Spjut HJ. Prevalence and prognosis of individual clinical and pathologic variables associated with colorectal carcinoma. Cancer 1967;20:1976–85.
[133] Jonsson PE, Bengtsson G, Carlsson G, Jonson G, Tryding N. Value of serum 5-nucleotidase, alkaline phosphatase and gamma-glutamyl transferase for prediction of liver metastases preoperatively in colorectal cancer. Acta Chir Scand 1984;150:419–23.
[134] Moertel CG, O'Fallon JR, Go VLW, O'Connell MJ, Thynne GS. The preoperative carcinoembryonic antigen test in the diagnosis, staging, and prognosis of colorectal cancer. Cancer 1986;58:603–10.
[135] Fletcher RH. Carcinoembryonic antigen. Ann Intern Med 1986;104:66–73.
[136] Arnaud JP, Koehl C, Adloff M. Carcinoembryonic antigen (CEA) in diagnosis and prognosis of colorectal carcinoma. Dis Colon Rectum 1980;23:141–4.
[137] Koch M, Washer G, Gaedke H, McPherson TA. Carcinoembryonic antigen: Usefullness as a postsurgical method in the detection of recurrence in Dukes stages B2 and C colorectal cancers. J Natl Cancer Inst 1982;69:813–5.
[138] Brandt LJ, Boley SJ, Mitsudo S. Clinical characteristics and natural history of colitis in the elderly. Am J Gastroenterol 1982;77:382–6.
[139] Rex DK. Colonoscopy: a review of its yield for cancers and adenomas by indication. Am J Gastroenterol 1995;90:353–65.
[140] Cappell MS, Friedel D. The role of sigmoidoscopy and colonoscopy in the diagnosis and management of lower gastrointestinal disorders: endoscopic findings, therapy, and complications. Med Clin North Am 2002;86:1253–88.
[141] Lieberman D. Rectal bleeding and diminutive colon polyps. Gastroenterology 2004;126: 1167–74.

[142] Ransohoff DF, Lang CA. Small adenomas detected during fecal occult blood test screening for colorectal cancer: the impact of serendipity. JAMA 1990;264:76–8.
[143] Arthur AL, Garvey R, Vaness DG. Colocolonic intussusception in a three-year-old child caused by a colonic polyp. Conn Med 1990;54:492–4.
[144] Steven K, Lange P, Bukhave K, Rask-Madsen J. Prostaglandin E2-mediated secretory diarrhea in villous adenoma of rectum: effect of treatment with indomethacin. Gastroenterology 1981;80:1562–6.
[145] Macrae FA, St. John DJ. Relationship between patterns of bleeding and Hemoccult sensitivity in patients with colorectal cancers or adenomas. Gastroenterology 1982;82:891–8.
[146] Helm JF, Sandler RS. Colorectal cancer screening. Med Clin North Am 1999;83:39–44.
[147] McDonnell WM, Ryan JA, Seeger DM, Elta GH. Effect of iron on the guaiac reaction. Gastroenterology 1989;96:74–8.
[148] Hardcastle JD, Armitage NC, Chamberlain J, Amar SS, James PD, Balfour TW. Fecal occult blood screening for colorectal cancer in the general population: results of a controlled trial. Cancer 1986;58:397–403.
[149] Simon JB. Fecal occult blood testing: clinical value and limitations. Gastroenterologist 1998;6:66–78.
[150] Winchester DP, Shull JH, Scanlon EF, Murrell JV, Smeltzer C, Vrba P, et al. A mass screening program for colorectal cancer using chemical testing for occult blood in the stool. Cancer 1980;45:2955–8.
[151] Jaffe RM, Kasten B, Young DS, Maclowry JD. False negative stool occult blood tests caused by ingestion of ascorbic acid (vitamin C). Ann Intern Med 1975;83:824–6.
[152] Church TR, Ederer F, Mandel JS. Fecal occult blood screening in the Minnesota Study: sensitivity of the screening test. J Natl Cancer Inst 1997;89:1440–8.
[153] Mandel JS, Bond JH, Church TR, Snover DC, Bradley GM, Schuman LM, et al. Reducing mortality from colorectal cancer by screening for fecal occult blood. Minnesota Colon Cancer Control Study. N Engl J Med 1993;328:1365–71.
[154] Goulston KJ, Cook I, Dent OF. How important is rectal bleeding in the diagnosis of bowel cancer and polyps? Lancet 1986;2:261–5.
[155] Blakeborough A, Sheridan MB, Chapman AH. Complications of barium enema examinations: a survey of UK consultant radiologists 1992 to 1994. Clin Radiol 1997;52:142–8.
[156] Rex DK, Rahmani EY, Haseman JH, Lemmel GT, Kaster S, Buckley JS. Relative sensitivity of colonoscopy and barium enema for detection of colorectal cancer in clinical practice. Gastroenterology 1997;112:17–23.
[157] Winawer SJ, Stewart ET, Zauber AG, Bond JH, Ansel H, Waye JD, et al. A comparison of colonoscopy and double-contrast barium enema for surveillance after polypectomy. National Polyp Work Group. N Engl J Med 2000;342:1766–72.
[158] Byers T, Levin B, Rothenberger D, Dodd GD, Smith RA. American Cancer Society guidelines for screening and surveillance for early detection of colorectal polyps and cancer: update 1997-American Cancer Society Detection and Treatment Advisory Group on Colorectal Cancer. CA Cancer J Clin 1997;47:154–60.
[159] Winawer S, Fletcher R, Rex D, Bond J, Burt R, Ferrucci J, et al. Colorectal cancer screening and surveillance: clinical guidelines and rationale – update based on new evidence. Gastroenterology 2003;124:544–60.
[160] Selby JV, Friedman GD, Quesenberry CP Jr, Weiss NS. A case-control study of screening sigmoidoscopy and mortality from colorectal cancer. N Engl J Med 1992;326:653–7.
[161] Bombi JA. Polyps of the colon in Barcelona, Spain: an autopsy study. Cancer 1988;66:1472–6.
[162] Lieberman DA, Weiss DG, Bond JH, Ahnen DJ, Garewal H, Chejfec G. Use of colonoscopy to screen asymptomatic adults for colorectal cancer. Veterans Affairs Cooperative Study Group. N Engl J Med 2000;343:162–8.

[163] Kee F, Wilson RH, Gilliland R, Sloan JM, Rowlands BJ, Moorehead RJ. Changing site distribution of colorectal cancer. BMJ 1992;305:158.
[164] Anderson JC, Alpern Z, Messina CR, Lane B, Hubbard P, Grimson R, et al. Predictors of proximal neoplasia in patients without distal adenomatous pathology. Am J Gastroenterol 2004;99:472–7.
[165] Lewis JD, Ng K, Hung KE, Bilker WB, Berlin JA, Brensinger C, et al. Detection of proximal adenomatous polyps with screening sigmoidoscopy: a systematic review and meta-analysis of screening colonoscopy. Arch Intern Med 2003;163:413–20.
[166] Keating J, Pater P, Lolohea S, Wickremesekera K. The epidemiology of colorectal cancer: what can we learn from the New Zealand Cancer Registry? N Z Med J 2003;116: U437.
[167] Oya M, Takahashi S, Okuyama T, Yamaguchi M, Ueda Y. Synchronous colorectal carcinoma: clinico-pathological features and prognosis. Jpn J Clin Oncol 2003;33: 38–43.
[168] Rex DK, Cutler CS, Lemmel GT, Rahmani EY, Clark DW, Helper DJ, et al. Colonoscopic miss rates of adenomas determined by back-to-back colonoscopies. Gastroenterology 1997;112:24–8.
[169] Detsky AS. Screening for colon cancer: can we afford colonoscopy? N Engl J Med 2001;345: 607–8.
[170] Kolata G. 50 and ready for a colonoscopy? Doctors say there is often a wait. New York Times. December 8, 2003. Pages A1, A23.
[171] Jentschura D, Raute M, Winter J, Henkel T, Kraus M, Manegold BC. Complications in endoscopy of the lower gastrointestinal tract: therapy and prognosis. Surg Endosc 1994;8: 672–6.
[172] Nelson DB, McQuaid KR, Bond JH, Lieberman DA, Weiss DG, Johnston TK. Procedural success and complications of large-scale screening colonoscopy. Gastrointest Endosc 2002; 55:307–14.
[173] Kavin H, Sinicrope F, Esker AH. Management of perforation of the colon at colonoscopy. Am J Gastroenterol 1992;87:161–7.
[174] Young GP, MacRae FA. Neoplastic and nonneoplastic polyps of the colon and rectum. In: Yamada T, Alpers D, Kaplowitz N, et al, editors. Textbook of gastroenterology. 4th edition. Philadelphia: Lippincott Williams & Wilkins; 2003. p. 1883–913.
[175] Axelrad AM, Fleischer DE, Geller AJ, Nguyen CC, Lewis JH, Al-Kawas FH, et al. High-resolution chromoendoscopy for the diagnosis of diminutive colon polyps: implications for colon cancer screening. Gastroenterology 1996;110:1253–8.
[176] Mitooka H, Fujimori T, Maeda S, Nagasako K. Minute flat depressed neoplastic lesions of the colon detected by contrast chromoscopy using an indigo carmine capsule. Gastrointest Endosc 1995;41:453–9.
[177] Soravia C, Berk T, Madlensky L, Mitri A, Cheng H, Gallinger S, et al. Genotype-phenotype correlations in attenuated adenomatous polyposis coli. Am J Hum Genet 1998; 62:1290–301.
[178] Ambroze WL Jr, Orangio GR, Lucas G. Surgical options for familial adenomatous polyposis. Semin Surg Oncol 1995;11:423–7.
[179] Desai DC, Neale KF, Talbot IC, Hodgson SV, Phillips RK. Juvenile polyposis. Br J Surg 1995;82:14–7.
[180] Mathus-Vliegen EM, Tytgat GN. Peutz-Jeghers syndrome: clinical presentation and new therapeutic strategy. Endoscopy 1985;17:102–4.
[181] Gallo SH, McClave SA. Blue rubber bleb nevus syndrome: gastrointestinal involvement and its endoscopic presentation. Gastrointest Endosc 1992;38:72–6.
[182] Varano VJ, Bonanno CA. Colonoscopic findings in pneumatosis cystoides intestinalis. Am J Gastroenterol 1973;59:353–60.
[183] Kim EC, Lance P. Colorectal polyps and their relationship to cancer. Gastroenterol Clin North Am 1997;26:1–17.

[184] Zerhouni EA, Rutter C, Hamilton SR, Balfe DM, Megibow AJ, Francis IR, et al. CT and MR imaging in the staging of colorectal carcinoma: report of the Radiology Diagnostic Oncology Group II. Radiology 1996;200:443–51.
[185] McAndrew MR, Saba AK. Efficacy of routine preoperative computed tomography scans in colon cancer. Am Surg 1999;65:205–8.
[186] Kinkel K, Lu Y, Both M, Warren RS, Thoeni RF. Detection of hepatic metastases from cancers of the gastrointestinal tract by using noninvasive imaging methods (US, CT, MR imaging, PET): a meta-analysis. Radiology 2002;224:748–56.
[187] Vidri A, Carpanese L, Annibale MD, Caterino M, Cosimelli M, Zeuli M, et al. Evaluation of hepatic metastases from colorectal carcinoma with MR-superparamagnetic oxide. J Exp Clin Cancer Res 2004;23:53–60.
[188] McFarland EG, Mayo-Smith WW, Saini S, Hahn PF, Goldberg MA, Lee MJ. Hepatic hemangiomas and malignant tumors: improved differentiation with heavily T2-weighted conventional spin-echo MR imaging. Radiology 1994;193:43–7.
[189] Hawighorst H, Knapstein PG, Schaeffer U, Knopp MV, Brix G, Hoffmann U, et al. Pelvic lesions in patients with treated cervical carcinoma: efficacy of pharmacokinetic analysis of dynamic MR images in distinguishing recurrent tumors from benign conditions. AJR Am J Roentgenol 1996;166:401–8.
[190] Dobos N, Rubesin SE. Radiologic imaging modalities in the diagnosis and management of colorectal cancer. Hematol Oncol Clin North Am 2002;16:875–95.
[191] Harewood GC, Wiersema MJ, Nelson H, MacCarty RL, Olson JE, Clain JE, et al. A prospective, blinded assessment of the impact of preoperative staging on the management of rectal cancer. Gastroenterology 2002;123:24–32.
[192] Boyce GA, Sivak MV Jr, Lavery IC, Fazio JW, Church JM, Milsom J, et al. Endoscopic ultrasound in the pre-operative staging of rectal carcinoma. Gastrointest Endosc 1992;38: 468–71.
[193] Herzog U, von Flue M, Tondelli P, Schuppisser JP. How accurate is endorectal ultrasound in the preoperative staging of rectal cancer? Dis Colon Rectum 1993;36:127–34.
[194] Rosch T. Endoscopic ultrasonography. Endoscopy 1994;26:148–68.
[195] Ahmad NA, Kochman ML, Ginsberg GG. Endoscopic ultrasound and endoscopic mucosal resection for rectal cancers and villous adenomas. Hematol Oncol Clin North Am 2002;16:897–906.
[196] Saitoh N, Okui K, Sarashina H, Suzuki M, Arai T, Nunomura M. Evaluation of echographic diagnosis of rectal cancer using intrarectal ultrasonic examination. Dis Colon Rectum 1986;29:234–42.
[197] Kimmey MB, Vilmann P. Endoscopic ultrasonography. In: Yamada T, Alpers D, Kaplowitz N, et al, editors. Textbook of gastroenterology. 4th edition. Philadelphia: Lippincott Williams & Wilkins; 2003. p. 3139–59.
[198] Wiersma MJ, Harewood GC. Endoscopic ultrasound for rectal cancer. Gastroenterol Clin North Am 2002;31:1093–105.
[199] Woodward T, Menke D. Diagnosis of recurrent rectal carcinoma by EUS-guided fine-needle aspiration. Gastrointest Endosc 2000;51:223–5.
[200] Rotondano G, Esposito P, Pellecchia L, Novi A, Romano G. Early detection of locally recurrent rectal cancer by endosonography. Br J Radiol 1997;70:567–71.
[201] Bozzetti F, Bertario L, Rossetti C, Gennari L, Andreola S, Baratti D, et al. Surgical treatment of locally recurrent rectal carcinoma. Dis Colon Rectum 1997;40:1421–4.
[202] Matsumoto T, Hizawa K, Esaki M, Kurahara K, Mizuno M, Hirakawa K, et al. Comparison of EUS and magnifying colonoscopy for assessment of small colorectal cancers. Gastrointest Endosc 2002;56:354–60.
[203] Tseng LJ, Jao YT, Mo LR. Preoperative staging of colorectal cancer with a balloon-sheathed miniprobe. Endoscopy 2002;34:564–8.
[204] Turini ME, BuBois RN. Primary prevention: phytoprevention and chemoprevention of colorectal cancer. Hematol Oncol Clin North Am 2002;16:811–40.

[205] Reddy BS, Maruyama H, Kellof G. Dose related inhibition of colon carcinogenesis by dietary piroxicam, a non-steroidal anti-inflammatory drug, during different stages of rat tumor development. Cancer Res 1987;47:5340–60.
[206] Beazer-Barclay Y, Levy DB, Moser AR, Dove WF, Hamilton SR, Vogelstein B, et al. Sulindac suppresses tumorigenesis in the Min mouse. Carcinogenesis 1996;17:1757–60.
[207] Gann PH, Manson JE, Glynn RJ, Buring JE, Hennekens CH. Low-dose aspirin and incidence of colorectal tumors in a randomized trial. J Natl Cancer Inst 1993;85:1220–4.
[208] Thun MJ, Namboodiri MM, Heath CW Jr. Aspirin use and reduced risk of fatal colon cancer. N Engl J Med 1991;325:1593–6.
[209] Giovannucci E, Egan KM, Hunter DJ, Stampfer MJ, Colditz GA, Willett WC, et al. Aspirin and the risk of colorectal cancer in women. N Engl J Med 1995;333:609–14.
[210] Rosenberg L, Louck C, Shapiro S. Non-steroidal anti-inflammatory drug use and reduced risk of large bowel carcinoma. Cancer 1998;82:2326–33.
[211] Waddell WR, Ganser GF, Cerise EJ, Loughry RW. Sulindac for prophylaxis of the colon. Am J Surg 1989;157:175–9.
[212] Marnett LJ. Aspirin and the potential role of prostaglandins in colon cancer. Cancer Res 1992;52:5575–89.
[213] Cappell MS, Schein JR. Diagnosis and treatment of nonsteroidal anti-inflammatory drug-associated upper gastrointestinal toxicity. Gastroenterol Clin North Am 2000;29: 97–124.
[214] Jacoby RF, Cole CE, Tutsch K, Newton MA, Kelloff G, Hawk ET, et al. Chemopreventive efficiency of combined piroxicam and difluoromethylornithine treatment of APC mutant Min mouse adenomas and selective toxicity against APC mutant embryos. Cancer Res 2000;60:1864–70.
[215] Steinbach G, Lynch PM, Phillips RKS, Wallace MH, Hawk E, Gordon GB, et al. The effect of celecoxib, a cyclooxygenase-2 inhibitor, in familial adenomatous polyposis. N Engl J Med 2001;342:1946–52.
[216] Mann NS, Mann SK, Alam I. The safety of hot biopsy forceps in the removal of small colonic polyps. Digestion 1999;60:74–6.
[217] Weston AP, Campbell DR. Diminutive colonic polyps: histopathology, spatial distribution, concomitant significant lesions, and treatment complications. Am J Gastroenterol 1995;90:24–8.
[218] Waye JD. New methods of polypectomy. Gastrointest Endosc Clin N Am 1997;7:413–22.
[219] Williams CB, Saunders BP, Talbot IC. Endoscopic management of polypoid early colon cancer. World J Surg 2000;24:1047–51.
[220] Dell'Abate P, Iosca A, Galimberti A, Piccolo P, Soliani P, Foggi E. Endoscopic treatment of colorectal benign-appearing lesions 3 cm or larger: techniques and outcome. Dis Colon Rectum 2001;44:112–8.
[221] Waye JD, Kahn O, Auerbach ME. Complications of colonoscopy and flexible sigmoidoscopy. Gastrointest Endosc Clin N Am 1996;6:343–77.
[222] Waye JD. Management of complications of colonoscopic polypectomy. Gastroenterologist 1993;1:158–64.
[223] Winawer SJ, Zauber AG, Ho MN, O'Brien MJ, Gottlieb LS, Sternberg SS, et al. Prevention of colorectal cancer by colonoscopic polypectomy. N Engl J Med 1993;329:1977–81.
[224] Soetikno RM, Gotoda T, Nakanishi Y, Soehendra N. Endoscopic mucosal resection. Gastrointest Endosc 2003;57:567–79.
[225] Ishiguro A, Uno Y, Ishiguro Y, Munakata A, Morita T. Correlation of lifting versus non-lifting and microscopic depth of invasion in early colorectal cancer. Gastrointest Endosc 1999;50:329–33.
[226] Muto T, Oya M. Recent advances in diagnosis and treatment of colorectal T1 carcinoma. Dis Colon Rectum 2003;46:S89–93.
[227] Muto T, Sawada T, Sugihara K. Treatment of carcinoma in adenomas. World J Surg 1991; 15:35–40.

[228] Cress RD, Morris CR, Wolfe BM. Cancer of the colon and rectum in California: trends in incidence by race/ethnicity, stage, and subsite. Prev Med 2000;31:447–53.
[229] Ahlquist DA, Shuber AP. Stool screening for colorectal cancer: evolution from occult blood to molecular markers. Clin Chim Acta 2002;315:157–68.
[230] Ahlquist DA, Skoletsky JE, Boynton KA, Harrington JJ, Mahoney DW, Pierceall WE, et al. Colorectal cancer screening by detection of altered human DNA in stool: feasibility of a multitarget assay panel. Gastroenterology 2000;119:1219–27.
[231] Ahlquist DA. Molecular stool screening for colorectal cancer: using DNA markers may be beneficial, but large scale evaluation is needed. BMJ 2000;321:254–5.
[232] Dong SM, Traverso G, Johnson C, Geng L, Favis R, Boynton K, et al. Detecting colorectal cancer in stool with the use of multiple genetic targets. J Natl Cancer Inst 2001;93:858–65.
[233] Atkin W, Martin JP. Stool DNA-based colorectal cancer detection: finding the needle in the haystack [editorial]. J Natl Cancer Inst 2001;93:798–9.
[234] Gocke CD, Benko FA, Kopreski MS, McGarrity TJ. P53 and APC mutations are detectable in the plasma and serum of patients with colorectal cancer (CRC) or adenomas. Ann N Y Acad Sci 2000;906:44–50.
[235] Lauschke H, Caspari R, Friedl W, Schwarz B, Mathiak M, Propping P, et al. Detection of APC and k-ras mutations in the serum of patients with colorectal cancer. Cancer Detect Prev 2001;25:55–61.
[236] Dachman A, editor. Atlas of virtual colonoscopy. New York: Springer-Verlag; 2003.
[237] Zalis ME, Hahn PF. Digital subtraction bowel cleansing in CT colonography. AJR Am J Roentgenol 2001;176:646–8.
[238] Kamar M, Portnoy O, Bar-Dayan A, Amitai M, Munz Y, Ayalon A, et al. Actual colonic perforation in virtual colonoscopy: report of a case. Dis Colon Rectum 2004;47:1242–6.
[239] Pickhardt PJ, Choi JR, Hwang I, Butler JA, Puckett ML, Hildebrandt HA, et al. Computed tomographic virtual colonoscopy to screen for colorectal neoplasia in asymptomatic adults. N Engl J Med 2003;349:2191–200.
[240] Hara AK, Johnson CD, MacCarty RL, Welch TJ. Incidental extracolonic findings on CT colonography. Radiology 2000;215:353–7.
[241] Cotton PB, Durkalski VL, Pineau BC, Palesch YY, Mauldin PD, Hoffman B, et al. Computed tomographic colonography (virtual colonoscopy): a multicenter comparison with standard colonoscopy for detection of colorectal neoplasia. JAMA 2004;29:1713–9.
[242] Ransohoff DF. Virtual colonoscopy: what it can do vs. what it will do [editorial]. JAMA 2004;291:1772–4.
[243] Fenlon HM, Nunes DP, Schroy PC III, Barish MA, Clarke PD, Ferrucci JT. A comparison of virtual and conventional colonoscopy for the detection of colorectal polyps. N Engl J Med 1999;341:1496–503.
[244] Yee J, Akerkar GA, Hung RK, Steinauer-Gebauer AM, Wall SD, McQuaid KR. Colorectal neoplasia: performance characteristics of CT colonography for detection in 300 patients. Radiology 2001;219:685–92.
[245] Royster AP, Fenlon HM, Clarke PD, Nunes DP, Ferrucci JT. CT colonoscopy of colorectal neoplasms: two-dimensional and three-dimensional virtual-reality techniques with colonoscopic correlation. AJR Am J Roentgenol 1997;169:1237–42.
[246] Lewis BS. Small intestinal bleeding. Gastroenterol Clin North Am 2000;29:67–95.
[247] Lewis B, Goldfarb N. Review article: the advent of capsule endoscopy. A not-so-futuristic approach to obscure gastrointestinal bleeding. Aliment Pharmacol Ther 2003;17:1085–96.
[248] Lewis BS, Swain P. Capsule endoscopy in the evaluation of patients with suspected small intestinal bleeding: results of a pilot study. Gastrointest Endosc 2002;56:349–53.
[249] Zwas FR, Bonheim NA, Berken CA, Gray S. Diagnostic yield of routine ileoscopy. Am J Gastroenterol 1995;90:1441–3.
[250] MacKenzie J. Push enteroscopy. Gastrointest Endosc Clin N Am 1999;9:29–36.
[251] Appleyard M, Glukhovsky A, Swain P. Wireless-capsule diagnostic endoscopy for recurrent small-bowel bleeding. N Engl J Med 2001;344:232–3.

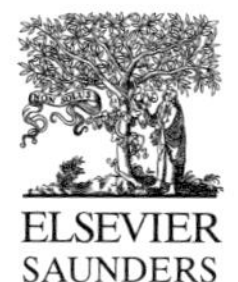

ELSEVIER
SAUNDERS

Med Clin N Am 89 (2005) 43–59

THE MEDICAL
CLINICS
OF NORTH AMERICA

# Screening of patients at average risk for colon cancer

Jack S. Mandel, PhD, MPH

*Department of Epidemiology, Rollins School of Public Health, Emory University, 1518 Clifton Road NE, Atlanta, GA 30322, USA*

Despite the availability of numerous screening tests to detect colonic adenomas or early stage colorectal cancer, screening rates are unacceptably low among all ethnic groups in the United States [1]. Only 9.8% of Hispanic-Latinos, 14.5% of American Indians and Alaskan Natives, 14.9% of African-Americans, and 18.3% of whites reported having a fecal occult blood test (FOBT) during the past year. These groups reported somewhat higher percentages (19.2%–31.3%) for undergoing any lower gastrointestinal endoscopic examination during the past 5 years. Those with no health insurance, fewer years of education, and recent immigrants were less likely to report having FOBT within the past year or lower gastrointestinal endoscopy within the past 5 years [1]. By geographic area, rates for FOBT and sigmoidoscopy were as low as 9.9% and 17.3%, respectively [2]. More attention and resources need to be spent on understanding why screening rates are so low and how they can be increased. Secondary prevention of colorectal cancer through screening can significantly reduce both the incidence and mortality of this disease.

Colorectal cancer is the third most common cancer among men and women in the United States and accounts for about 11% of all incident cancers and about 10% of all cancer mortality [3]. Throughout the world about 1 million new cases and about 500,000 deaths occur per annum [4]. The highest incidence rates occur in North America and Europe (30–50 per 100,000 population), and the lowest incidence rates occur in Africa (2–12 per 100,000), India (3–7 per 100,000), and Thailand and Vietnam (6–17 per 100,000) [5]. In the United States, about 6% of the population develops colorectal cancer during their lifetime [3]. It is estimated that in 2004, there will be about 150,000 new cases and 56,700 deaths caused by colorectal cancers in the United States [3].

*E-mail address:* jsmande@emory.edu

0025-7125/05/$ - see front matter 
doi:10.1016/j.mcna.2004.08.009

Colorectal cancer incidence in the United States increased from 1973 to 1985 from about 59 to 66 per 100,000 [6], but has recently declined to about 51 per 100,000. The trend was similar for men and women, although men had a 30% to 40% higher annual incidence. The trend was similar for blacks and whites, although blacks had a 20% higher annual incidence.

Colorectal cancer mortality has steadily decreased in the United States from about 28 per 100,000 in the late 1970s to about 20 per 100,000 in 2000, a decline of 29% [7]. The rate of decline was somewhat faster in the mid-1980s. The patterns were similar for men and women. Although the mortality declined by about 31% for white men and women, the mortality has hardly changed for black men and women. Since 1990, however, the rate in blacks has decreased from about 30 to 28 per 100,000. The mortality is higher in men than women and higher in blacks than whites.

Although 5-year survival has improved, the survival is only 63% for whites and 53% for blacks [3]. Nineteen percent of all colorectal cancers (19% for whites, 24% for blacks) have distant metastases at diagnosis. The prognosis for these cancers is poor, with only a 5% 5-year survival.

Both the incidence and the mortality from colorectal cancer can be substantially reduced by primary and secondary prevention. There are many screening tests for colorectal cancer, and any test should result in a reduction in colorectal cancer incidence and mortality. Only the guaiac FOBT has been shown to be effective in randomized controlled clinical trials. Although other screening tests have not been subjected to randomized controlled trials, the evidence is sufficient based on observational studies to encourage use of these tests. If the age-eligible population undergoes these screening tests, the burden of colorectal cancer should be substantially reduced. The scientific evidence related to secondary prevention, specifically screening of individuals at average risk for colorectal cancer, is presently reviewed.

## Screening tests

Screening is the application of a test to asymptomatic people to identify those who are likely to have (or have a precursor of) the disease [8]. A diagnostic test can then be performed on patients with a positive screening test to identify those who truly have the disease (true-positives) and those who were incorrectly identified as likely having the disease (false-positives). The ability of a screening test to identify true-positives and true-negatives (those with a negative screening test who do not have the disease) is referred to as "sensitivity" and "specificity," respectively. Ideally, a test should be 100% sensitive and 100% specific but, unfortunately, no actual cancer screening test meets these criteria. All the tests have false-positives and false-negatives (people with a negative screening test who have the disease). Applying a screening test that is highly sensitive but poorly specific yields a high number of false-positives, and subjects many people to an unnecessary diagnostic examination, incurring the examination costs and risks. Increasing specificity at the cost of sensitivity increases the number of false-negatives (ie, people with undetected cancer). Although many different studies of sensitivity and specificity have been reported, the critical measure of the effectiveness of a screening test is a reduction in colorectal cancer mortality. Merely evaluating test sensitivity is insufficient because diagnosis of incurable advanced cancers is not helpful clinically.

Several screening tests are currently available, including FOBTs (guaiac or immunochemical); flexible sigmoidoscopy; colonoscopy; and virtual colonoscopy. Other tests, such as fecal DNA tests that screen for DNA mutations and videocapsule endoscopy, are in development and might potentially be effective. The current data do not warrant use of these tests for mass screening. The role of double-contrast barium enema (DCBE) in screening is questionable given the higher sensitivity and specificity and the therapeutic potential of colonoscopy.

Three randomized controlled trials have reported consistent results for FOBT. Evidence for flexible sigmoidoscopy is largely from observational (case-control) studies, although clinical trials are in progress. There is little direct evidence for colonoscopy, but it is likely to be effective as a screening test. The main question with colonoscopy is the extent of its effectiveness. Although flexible sigmoidoscopy should be effective, the extent of its effectiveness is also unknown. The evidence for virtual colonoscopy is largely from studies comparing it with colonoscopy, the results of which are controversial. A randomized trial is needed for both colonoscopy and virtual colonoscopy to determine the extent of their effectiveness.

## Fecal occult blood tests

### *Guaiac tests*

#### *Effect on colorectal cancer mortality*

The most widely used FOBT is a guaiac-based test, Hemoccult (Beckman Coultier, Palo Alto, California). Guaiac tests detect pseudoperoxidase activity present in heme. Fecal excretion of heme is an indicator of gastrointestinal pathology. Most colorectal cancers bleed, but the bleeding is intermittent and the blood is unevenly distributed in stool. Multiple samples increase the likelihood of detecting blood from an adenoma or a cancer. A single in-office FOBT during a digital rectal examination is not very effective and not a reliable screening test.

The early development of FOBT resulted from the perceived failure of sigmoidoscopy. In 1967, Greegor [9] reported that only one malignant polyp was detected in 2500 sigmoidoscopic examinations, whereas the expected yield was one carcinoma per every 300 to 500 examinations. In a review of eight colorectal cancers, he reported that all patients but one had a positive FOBT in at least one of three stool specimens submitted at the initial visit. He noted that testing one portion of one specimen was inadequate, and testing at least two or three portions of three different stools was preferable.

In this study patients with a false-positive screening test had gastrointestinal diseases, such as diverticulitis, duodenal ulcer, and hemorrhoids, which might have caused the bleeding. Greegor [9] noted that FOBT is a test for blood in stool and not a specific test for cancer. He believed that the test, if applied frequently, should detect most of the cancers because most cancers bleed intermittently. In 1971, Greegor [10] presented a further study supporting the need for multiple guaiac tests. Because of the large number of false-positives (27 of 29 test positives), Greegor [10] added the requirement of a meat-free diet during stool collection. Most of the cancers in his series were detected at a curable stage.

Although Greegor is often credited with popularizing the use of FOBT for colon cancer screening, references to detecting small amounts of blood in stool go back over 120 years [11,12]. Greegor, however, provided the data to stimulate research to evaluate Hemoccult as a screening test for colorectal cancer. In 1975, the University of Minnesota initiated the first randomized controlled clinical trial (the Colon Cancer Control Study) to evaluate the effectiveness of Hemoccult in reducing colorectal cancer mortality. The initial study design included three groups: (1) one screened twice per year; (2) one screened once per year; and (3) a usual care (control) group. Before study implementation, however, the biannual group was changed to a biennial group to improve patient compliance with the clinical protocol. It remains unknown whether applying the test biannually, as opposed to annually, substantially improves the benefits.

The benefit of FOBT was controversial until 1993 [13]. During the 1980s colonoscopy became the diagnostic procedure of choice and many papers appeared discussing adenomas and their importance as precursors to cancer [14–20]. Some adenomas also bleed and are detectable by FOBT [21]. Interest subsequently shifted from detecting cancers at an early stage to also detecting adenomas, the precursor lesion. More attention was focused on flexible sigmoidoscopy, colonoscopy, or barium enema to detect adenomas. This added to the controversy about FOBT because it was unclear whether FOBT was effective in identifying adenomas.

Randomized trials provide the best evaluation of screening effectiveness and are far better than observational studies. In randomized trials, eligible participants are randomly assigned to a screen or a control (usual care) group to help eliminate the effects of confounding variables. In such trials, the primary measure of screening effectiveness is a reduction in mortality from colorectal cancer.

The most common observational study is the case-control study in which cases are typically deaths from colorectal cancer and controls are people who do not die from this disease. These studies tend to overestimate the benefit of screening because of selection and information bias or systematic error. Observed differences in screening histories between cases and controls must be interpreted cautiously.

In the University of Minnesota trial published in 1993, 46,551 people aged 50 to 80 were randomly assigned to one of the three groups [22]. The annual group was offered 11 screening tests and the biennial group six screening tests. The control or usual care group was not instructed to obtain or not obtain screening.

During the 13 years of follow-up colorectal cancer mortality was reduced by 33% and 6% in the annual and biennial groups, respectively. The decrease in the annual group was statistically significant, but it was not in the biennial group. The large difference between annual and biennial screening led to questions about the validity of the findings, even though the investigators stated that the biennial result was consistent with the annual result and intermediate between the cumulative colorectal cancer mortality in the annual and usual care groups. They suggested that further follow-up is necessary to determine if the biennial group significantly differed from the usual care group.

These results led in 1996 to the recommendation by the Preventive Services Task Force for annual FOBT for colorectal cancer [23]. Later that year, two randomized controlled European trials corroborated the Minnesota findings [24,25]. In a subsequently published 18-year follow-up of the Minnesota study, the biennial group had a statistically significant 21% reduction in colorectal cancer mortality [26]. Similar reductions were reported in the European trials [27,28].

The features of the three trials are summarized in Table 1. Over 250,000 people were enrolled in the three studies. The trials were conducted in Minnesota, United States; Funen, Denmark; and Nottingham, England. Although all the trials randomly assigned participants, the study designs were different. The Minnesota study solicited volunteers who were randomly assigned to one of the three study groups. This design provided very good internal validity of the results. The European trials randomly assigned age-eligible people in the community. This design results in lower compliance but permits generalization of the result to the population. All the trials used Hemoccult as the screening test (Funen used Hemoccult II); incorporated certain dietary restrictions; used colorectal cancer mortality as the primary end point; and included a biennial test group. There were some other differences, such as most of the Hemoccult tests were rehydrated before processing to enhance sensitivity in Minnesota, and for some duration of time participants with a positive test were asked to retake the test while on a restricted diet in Nottingham. The results were consistent and statistically significant. The colorectal cancer mortality reductions for the biennial screened group were 21%, 15%, and 18% for the Minnesota, Nottingham, and Funen trials, respectively. The somewhat larger reduction in the Minnesota trial could be caused by greater compliance, rehydration of the slides, longer

Table 1
Summary of the randomized controlled clinical trials of fecal occult blood testing

| Study characteristics | Minnesota, United States Trial | Nottingham, England Trial | Funen, Denmark Trial |
|---|---|---|---|
| Year started | 1975 | 1981 | 1985 |
| Number of subjects | 46,551 | 152,850 | 61,933 |
| Age in years | 50–80 | 45–74 | 45–75 |
| Screening test | Hemoccult | Hemoccult | Hemoccult II |
| Diagnostic test | Colonoscopy | Colonoscopy | Colonoscopy |
| Rehydration | Yes[a] | No | No |
| Dietary restrictions | Yes | Yes[b] | Yes |
| Screening frequency | Annual or biennial | Biennial | Biennial |
| Number of screens | Annual-11, biennial-6 | 3–6 | 5 |
| Median years follow-up | 13 | 8 | 10 |
| Compliance | | | |
| First screen (%) | 85 | 53 | 67 |
| Average for rescreen (%) | 75 | 60 | 54 |
| Test positivity (%) | 9.8 | 1.7 | 1.2 |
| Sensitivity (%) | 92 | 54 | 51 |
| Specificity (%) | 90 | 98 | 99 |
| *Initial results* | | | |
| Annual group mortality ratio (95% CI) | 0.67 (0.5–.87) | — | — |
| Biennial group mortality ratio (95% CI) | 0.94 (0.68–1.31) | 0.85 (0.74–0.98) | 0.82 (0.68–0.99) |
| *Follow-up results* | | | |
| Years of follow-up | 18 | 11 | 13 |
| Annual group mortality ratio (95% CI) | 0.67 (0.51–0.83) | — | — |
| Biennial group mortality ratio (95% CI) | 0.79 (0.62–0.97) | 0.87 (0.78–0.97) | 0.85 (0.73–1) |

[a] 82.5% of the Hemoccult slides were rehydrated.
[b] Dietary restrictions applied at retesting after a positive test.

follow-up, or chance. Biennial testing with Hemoccult significantly reduced colorectal cancer mortality. In addition, the Minnesota trial reported a larger mortality reduction in the annual (33%) compared with the biennial (21%) group.

A fourth randomized controlled clinical trial randomized 68,308 inhabitants of Goteborg, Sweden, born between 1918 and 1931 into a screen and a control group [29]. Screen group participants were screened every 16 to 24 months with rehydrated Hemoccult II. Compliance was 67% in the initial screen and 60% in the rescreen. The positivity rate was 4.4%. Although final results from this trial have not been published, preliminary results were provided in a review paper by Towler et al [30]. After 8 years of follow-up, colorectal cancer mortality was reduced by 12% (relative risk = 0.88, 95% confidence interval [CI]: 0.69–1.12). This result is consistent with the biennial results in the other three trials.

Towler et al [30] conducted a meta-analysis of the four randomized trials using the biennial screening rate reductions of 6% (rather than 21%) from Minnesota; 15% from Nottingham; 18% from Funen; and 12% from Sweden. They reported a 16% colorectal cancer mortality reduction (95% CI: 0.77–0.93) in the combined results and a 23% reduction (95% CI: 0.57–0.89) if only people actually screened were analyzed. The mortality reduction would be somewhat larger if the most recent result of a 21% reduction from the Minnesota trial was used in the meta-analysis.

The observational studies of Hemoccult have generally shown less screening occurred in cases than in controls, providing results consistent with the randomized trials [31–35]. The Winawer et al [31] study used a controlled prospective design to demonstrate a benefit of FOBT. The other studies were conventional case-control designs and showed fairly consistent results [32–35].

### *Effect on colorectal cancer incidence*

Guaiac tests, namely Hemoccult, have also been shown to reduce the incidence of colorectal cancer [36]. In the Minnesota randomized trial there were 20% (95% CI: 0.7–0.9) and 17% (95% CI: 0.73–0.94) reductions in colorectal cancer incidence in the annual and biennial groups, respectively. The most plausible explanation for this reduction was that adenomas were identified and removed and patients were placed in a surveillance protocol. The National Polyp Study showed that removing adenomas results in a significant decrease in colorectal cancer incidence [37]. The other randomized trials have not yet shown a reduction in the incidence of colorectal cancer. The reduction in these trials may be less than that in the Minnesota trial because fewer people in these trials underwent colonoscopy.

### *Conclusion*

Screening with Hemoccult, either annually or biennially, reduced the incidence and mortality from colorectal cancer. Many studies have evaluated the sensitivity and specificity of this screening test in detecting cancers and adenomas, but these studies are not comparable because they used different methods and different definitions. Sensitivity and specificity for Hemoccult testing only once is not very good. This test is not advocated as a one-time screen. Sensitivity and specificity when the test is repeatedly applied to a population is quite good (eg, in the Minnesota trial sensitivity of 80% to 90% and specificity of 90% to 98%) depending on whether the tests were rehydrated [38,39].

Hemoccult Sensa seems to have a higher positivity rate and greater sensitivity than Hemoccult. It behaves more like rehydrated Hemoccult [40]. No single-arm trials have analyzed the effectiveness of Hemoccult Sensa. Studies comparing Hemoccult with Hemoccult Sensa are discussed later.

### *Immunochemical tests*

Immunochemical tests are more specific than guaiac tests in that they detect only human hemoglobin from the lower gastrointestinal tract [40,41]. Moreover, they can be used without dietary restrictions because they do not react with nonhuman hemoglobin or with uncooked fruits and vegetables that may contain peroxidase activity [42]. No randomized controlled trials of an immunochemical test have been conducted, but many case-control studies or studies comparing an immunochemical test with Hemoccult have been conducted.

Mass screening with a 1-day immunochemical hemagglutination test (Immudia-Hem Sp or HemSelect, Fujirebio, Tokyo, Japan) was evaluated by case-control studies in Japan [43,44]. The studies provided consistent results showing the benefit of screening with odds ratios as low as 0.19, suggesting an 81% reduction in colorectal cancer mortality. Other studies reported that immunochemical tests performed better with greater compliance than Hemoccult or Hemoccult Sensa tests [41,45–49]. A relatively new immunochemical test, Insure (Enterix, Falmouth, Maine), using a brush-based sampling technique, quantitatively measures the amount of blood present in the stool sample [42]. In this test the participant swishes the brush in the toilet bowl and then wipes the brush on the test card. In a comparison with Hemoccult Sensa and FlexSure OBT, the compliance was highest for Insure, attributed to the simplified sampling technique and lack of dietary restrictions [49].

The Multisociety Task Force on Colorectal Cancer currently recommends annual screening using a guaiac-based test with dietary restrictions or an immunochemical test without dietary restrictions [50]. The American Cancer Society has a similar recommendation, but adds that the immunochemical tests are more acceptable to participants and may be better than guaiac-based tests [51]. Current data suggest that immunochemical tests perform better than guaiac tests, with a lower odds ratio (ie, greater benefit). In addition, the sensitivity and specificity of immunochemical tests are generally better than that of guaiac tests, particularly for adenomas.

## Flexible sigmoidoscopy

Screening flexible sigmoidoscopy every 5 years beginning at age 50 is recommended despite the absence of a randomized clinical trial demonstrating its effectiveness [23,50,51], based largely on several observational studies. Most colon cancers arise from adenomas; removing adenomas should reduce the cancer risk [37,52–56]. The reduction in incidence and mortality, however, is unknown. Only adenomas and early cancers within reach of the sigmoidoscope and synchronous lesions are affected by this screening. Between 50% and 75% of adenomas and cancers can be detected by flexible sigmoidoscopy [57–63].

Estimates of the benefit of flexible sigmoidoscopy have largely come from case-control studies [64–67], which must be cautiously interpreted [68]. Selby et al [64] conducted a case-control study to evaluate 20-cm rigid sigmoidoscopy in members of the Kaiser Permanente Medical Care Program of Northern California 45 years of age or older who were diagnosed with colorectal cancer between 1971 and 1987 and who died from the cancer by the end of 1988. Controls, matched for age, sex, and date of entry into the health plan were selected from the membership list of the health plan. The results showed that statistically significantly fewer cases than controls had one or more screening rigid sigmoidoscopy during the 10 years before the onset of symptoms or the diagnosis. This study suggested that screening rigid sigmoidoscopy could reduce colorectal cancer by 59% in the descending colon, but the reduction for the entire colon is likely to be much less. This study was the primary justification for the United States Preventive Services Task Force recommendation for flexible sigmoidoscopy screening [23]. Other observational studies, however, reported similar results [65–67].

The best analysis of flexible sigmoidoscopy screening will come from controlled randomized trials, such as the Prostate, Lung, Colorectal and Ovarian Cancer Screening Trial [69]. This trial is evaluating the effectiveness of two flexible sigmoidoscopy screening examinations conducted at 3- or 5-year intervals. About 150,000 men and women age 55 to 74 were enrolled in the trial. Trials in the United Kingdom and Norway are evaluating a single flexible sigmoidoscopy screening test [70,71]. Results of these trials should be available in about 5 years.

The recommended screening interval of every 5 years for flexible sigmoidoscopy [50,51] has recently been questioned because 13.9% of returning participants in the Prostate, Lung, Colorectal and Ovarian trial had a polyp or mass detected 3 years after the initial screening sigmoidoscopy [72]. About 80% (58 out of 72) of the advanced adenomas detected at the year 3 examination were in an area of the colon adequately examined at the initial sigmoidoscopy. The overall incidence of these lesions was 0.8%, a modest, but nevertheless sufficiently large effect to raise concern about follow-up examination at 5 years.

Newcombe et al [73], however, reported that the incidence of distal cancers was reduced by 70% among those reporting a single flexible sigmoidoscopy and by 76% among those who had one or more flexible sigmoidoscopy. The investigators suggested the currently recommended interval of 5 years could be increased. Mandel [74], however, warned that such a change is currently ill-advised in view of the problems with a case-control study.

About half of significant lesions may be missed by flexible sigmoidoscopy. Lieberman et al [62] performed colonoscopy on 3121 adults and found that 52% of advanced proximal lesions would have been missed if the patients had been screened with only flexible sigmoidoscopy. Imperiale et al [63] in a colonoscopy study of 1994 adults found that about half of the patients with proximal lesions had no distal polyps. Further study is needed to quantify the effectiveness of flexible sigmoidoscopy screening and the optimal screening interval.

### *Fecal occult blood test with flexible sigmoidoscopy*

No studies have evaluated the mortality reduction from the combination of FOBT with flexible sigmoidoscopy. A study reported a reduction in colorectal cancer mortality ($P = .053$) with rigid sigmoidoscopy and FOBT compared with rigid sigmoidoscopy alone [31]. Two randomized controlled trials reported that with the combined test four to five times more large polyps and cancers were detected than with FOBT alone [75,76]. In another trial, however, more polyps and cancers were not diagnosed in patients who had both FOBT and sigmoidoscopy compared with patients who had only sigmoidoscopy [77]. Although the current data are inadequate, the current recommendation of flexible sigmoidoscopy every 5 years and FOBT annually seems reasonable based on data regarding performance of the individual tests. FOBT should be performed first because colonoscopy, rather than flexible sigmoidoscopy, is recommended if the FOBT is positive.

## Colonoscopy

Colonoscopy has been proposed for either one-time or periodic screening [78–82]. Despite the absence of any randomized controlled clinical trials, colonoscopy screening is likely effective in reducing the incidence and mortality of colorectal cancer. This is supported by the fecal occult blood screening trials, which used colonoscopy as the diagnostic test, and from two cohort studies, the National Polyp Study and the Italian Multicenter Study, which showed reductions in colorectal cancer incidence among patients who had adenomatous polyps detected and removed during colonoscopy [37,83]. Inadomi and Sonnenberg [84] using a mathematical model showed that the estimated extension of life through colonoscopy screening is two times longer than that with flexible sigmoidoscopy and three times longer than that with FOBT. The model depends on assumptions regarding screening performance and must be interpreted cautiously.

The interval for screening colonoscopy for average-risk individuals is undetermined. The American Cancer Society and the American Gastroenterology Association recommend 10-year intervals, although data in support of specific screening intervals are lacking [50,51].

Colonoscopy is the diagnostic test of choice for colorectal cancer. It was initially implemented to follow-up a positive screening test or for symptomatic or high-risk individuals. Its use to screen for colorectal cancer must be evaluated carefully because of procedure risks and costs. More than 90% of average-risk people undergoing screening colonoscopy incur the procedure costs and risks without benefit (negative examination). The risks come mainly from sedation, hemorrhage, and perforation. Lieberman et al

[62] and Nelson et al [85] found that 0.3% (10 out of 3121) patients had major complications, including bleeding, myocardial infarction, and stroke. Three patients died within 1 month of colonoscopy. Imperiale et al [63] found that 1 (0.05%) of the 1994 people undergoing screening colonoscopy had a perforation that did not require surgery, and 3 (0.15%) had bleeding that required treatment. Dafnis et al [86] reported that 0.4% of 6066 colonoscopies resulted in a complication, mostly bleeding and perforation. No deaths were attributed to the colonoscopy. The overall complication rate is between 1 and 3 per 1000 colonoscopies based on studies that abstracted data on complication from medical records [22,87–93].

## Double-contrast barium enema

There are no randomized trials of DCBE but there are several observational studies. Scheitel et al [94] in a case-control study reported a 33% reduction in colorectal cancer mortality, but this estimate was imprecise. Rex et al [95] found the sensitivity of DCBE for cancer was 85% compared with 95% for colonoscopy. Winawer et al [96] reported that the sensitivity of DCBE (using colonoscopy as the standard) was 32% for polyps less than 0.5 cm, 53% for polyps 0.6 to 1 cm, and 48% for polyps greater than 1 cm. DCBE was positive in 83 of 470 patients (specificity = 85%) who had no polyps detected by colonoscopy. Fletcher [97] suggested that given the relatively poor performance of DCBE, it should be used only when colonoscopy is unavailable or contraindicated. DCBE has relatively low risks of about 1 per 10,000 examinations for major complications, including about 1 perforation in 25,000 examinations and 1 death in 55,000 examinations [98,99]. Although less effective than colonoscopy, DCBE screening every 5 years is a recommended alternative screening test [50,51].

## CT colonography (virtual colonoscopy)

In CT colonography two- or three-dimensional images of the colon are created by combining multiple helical CT scans by computerized analysis [42]. Patients must undergo a colonic preparation, although methods of performing the procedure without preparation are under investigation [100]. Patients with an identified lesion are referred for colonoscopy. Earlier studies found that CT colonography did not perform well, particularly for small lesions [101], but a recent study showed it can perform well under optimal circumstances [102]. This study, using three-dimensional imaging, reported sensitivities of 93.8% for polyps at least 10 mm in diameter, 93.9% for polyps at least 8 mm, and 88.7% for polyps at least 6 mm. These sensitivities were somewhat higher than those for colonoscopy for the two groups with larger polyps. The specificities were 96%, 92.2%, and 79.6% for the three groups, respectively. This study showed that CT colonography was an accurate method for detecting adenomatous polyps [103]. A study published a few months later suggested, however, that CT colonography was not ready for widespread use because the sensitivity for lesions at least 6 mm in diameter was 39% and for lesions at least 10 mm was 55% [104]. The specificity was 91% and 96%, respectively, for these sized lesions. Conventional colonoscopy performed much better with sensitivities of 99% and 100%, respectively. These two studies show CT colonography is a potentially useful screening tool under optimal circumstances, but is not very useful under current general practice conditions. After the technical issues are resolved, CT colonography should become a useful alternative screening test.

## Other tests: molecular screening

There are many DNA mutations associated with colorectal cancer. Stool can be examined for specific molecular markers to identify people at risk of developing the disease or having early stage disease [105–109]. These promising tests are in development and are not yet at a stage to be applied routinely to asymptomatic average-risk people. They are appealing in that they do not require special preparation and are noninvasive.

## Cost effectiveness

Pignone et al [110] reported the costs of screening ranged from $10,000 to $25,000 per life-year saved, depending on the type of screening test. Annual FOBT was the least expensive and colonoscopy every 10 years or DCBE every 5 years were the most expensive. Variability in cost estimates depends on assumptions regarding test effectiveness, test adverse effects, cancer biology, and patient compliance. Nevertheless, the costs of colorectal cancer screening compares favorably with those for mammography for breast cancer screening.

## Summary

Fortunately, many screening tests can profoundly impact on colorectal cancer. The great challenge is to implement more widely the available technology. An increase in implementation will result in a decline in colorectal cancer incidence and mortality.

## References

[1] Ward E, Jemal A, Cokkinides V, Singh GK, Cardinez C, Ghafoor A, et al. Cancer disparities by race/ethnicity and socioeconomic status. CA Cancer J Clin 2004;54:78–93.

[2] Nelson DE, Bolen J, Marcus S, Wells HE, Meissner H. Cancer screening estimates for US metropolitan areas. Am J Prev Med 2003;24:301–9.

[3] Jemel A, Ram CT, Murray T, Ghafoor A, Samuels A, Ward E, et al. Cancer statistics, 2004. CA Cancer J Clin 2004;54:8–29.
[4] Boyle P, Leon ME. Epidemiology of colorectal cancer. Br Med Bull 2002;64:1–25.
[5] Parkin DM, Whelan SL, Ferlay J, Teppo L, Thomas DB, editors. Cancer incidence in five continents, vol. 8. Lyon, France: International Agency for Research on Cancer; 2002.
[6] Surveillance. Epidemiology and end results. Available at: http://seer.cancer.gov/.
[7] National Center for Health Statistics. Division of Vital Statistics, Centers for Disease Control. Available at: www.cdc.gov.
[8] Morrison AS. Screening in chronic diseases. New York: Oxford University Press; 1992.
[9] Greegor DH. Diagnosis of large-bowel cancer in the asymptomatic patient. JAMA 1967; 201:123–5.
[10] Greegor DH. Occult blood testing for detection of asymptomatic colon cancer. Cancer 1971;28:131–4.
[11] Needham CD, Simpson RG. The benzidine test for occult blood in faeces. Q J Med 1952;21: 123–33.
[12] Irons GV, Kirsner JB. Routine chemical tests of the stool for occult blood: an evaluation. Am J Med Sci 1965;249:247–60.
[13] Simon JB. Occult blood screening for colorectal cancer: a critical review. Gastroenterology 1985;88:820–37.
[14] Jass JR. Do all colorectal cancers arise in preexisting adenomas. World J Surg 1989;13:45–51.
[15] Tierney RP, Balantyne GH, Modlin IM. The adenoma to carcinoma sequence. Surg Gynecol Obstet 1990;171:81–94.
[16] Eide TJ. Natural history of adenomas. World J Surg 1990;15:3–6.
[17] Itzkowitz SH. The adenomatous polyp. Semin Gastrointest Dis 1992;3:3–12.
[18] Bedenne L, Faivre J, Boutron MC, Picard F, Cauvin JM, Hillon P. Adenoma-carcinoma sequence or de novo carcinogenesis? A study of adenomatous remnants in a population-based series of large bowel cancers. Cancer 1992;60:883–8.
[19] Simons BD, Morrison AS, Lev R, Verhoek-Oftedahl W. Relationship of polyps to cancer of the large intestine. J Natl Cancer Inst 1992;84:962–6.
[20] O'Brien MJ, O'Keane JC, Zauber A, Gottleib LS, Winawer SJ. Precursors of colorectal carcinoma. Cancer 1992;70:1317–27.
[21] Young GP, St. John DJB. Selecting an occult blood test for use as a screening tool for large bowel cancer. In: Rozen P, Reich CD, Winower SJ, editors. Large bowel cancer: policy, prevention, research and treatment. Frontiers of gastrointestinal research, vol. 18. Basel: Krager; 1991. p. 135–6.
[22] Mandel JS, Bond JH, Church TR, Snover DC, Bradley M, Schuman LM, et al. Reducing mortality from colorectal cancer by screening for fecal occult blood. N Engl J Med 1993; 328:1365–71.
[23] United States Preventive Services Task Force. Guide to clinical preventive services. 2nd edition. Baltimore: Williams & Wilkins; 1996.
[24] Kronborg O, Fenger C, Olsen J, Jorgensen OD, Sondergaard O. Randomised study of screening for colorectal cancer with faecal-occult-blood test. Lancet 1996;348:1467–71.
[25] Hardcastle JD, Chamberlain JO, Robinson MHE, Moss SM, Amar SS, Balfour TW, et al. Randomised controlled trial of faecal-occult-blood screening for colorectal cancer. Lancet 1996;348:1472–7.
[26] Mandel JS, Church TR, Ederer F, Bond JH. Colorectal cancer mortality: effectiveness of biennial screening for fecal occult blood. J Natl Cancer Inst 1999;91:434–7.
[27] Jorgensen OD, Kronborg O, Fenger C. A randomised study of screening for colorectal cancer using faecal occult blood testing: results after 13 years and seven biennial screening rounds. Gut 2002;50:29–32.
[28] Scholefield JH, Moss S, Sufi F, Mangham CM, Hardcastle JD. Effect of faecal occult blood screening on mortality from colorectal cancer: results from a randomized controlled trial. Gut 2002;50:840–4.

[29] Kewenter J, Brevinge H, Engaras B, Haglind E, Ahren C. Results of screening, rescreening, and follow-up in a prospective randomized study for detection of colorectal cancer by fecal occult blood testing. Scand J Gastroenterol 1994;29:468–73.
[30] Towler B, Irwig L, Gasziou P, Kewenter J, Weller D, Silagy C. A systematic review of the effects of screening for colorectal cancer using the faecal occult blood test. Hemoccult. BMJ 1998;317:559–65.
[31] Winawer SJ, Flehinger BJ, Schottenfeld D, Miller DG. Screening for colorectal cancer with fecal occult blood testing and sigmoidoscopy. J Natl Cancer Inst 1993;85:1311–8.
[32] Selby JV, Friedman GD, Quesenberry CP, Weiss NS. Effects of fecal occult blood testing on mortality from colorectal cancer: a case-control study. Ann Intern Med 1993;118:1–6.
[33] Wahrendorf J, Robra BP, Wiebelt H, Oberhausen R, Weiland M, Dhom G. Effectiveness of colorectal cancer screening: results from a population-based case-control evaluation in Saarland, Germany. Eur J Cancer Prev 1993;2:221–7.
[34] Lazovich D, Weiss NS, Stevens NG, White E, McKnight B, Wagner EH. A case-control study to evaluate the efficacy of screening for fecal occult blood. J Med Screen 1995;2:84–9.
[35] Zappa M, Catiglione G, Grazzini G, Falini P, Giorgi D, Paci E, et al. Effects of faecal occult blood testing on colorectal mortality: results of a population-based case-control study in the district of Florence, Italy. Int J Cancer 1997;73:208–10.
[36] Mandel JS, Church TR, Bond JH, Ederer F, Geisser MS, Mongin SJ, et al. The effect of fecal occult-blood screening on the incidence of colorectal cancer. N Engl J Med 2000;343:1603–7.
[37] Winawer SJ, Zauber AG, Ho MN, O'Brien MJ, Gottlieb LS, Sternberg SS, et al. Prevention of colorectal cancer by colonoscopic polypectomy. N Engl J Med 1993;329:1977–81.
[38] Mandel JS, Bond JH, Bradley M, Snover DC, Church TR, Williams S, et al. Sensitivity, specificity and positive predictivity of the Hemoccult test in screening for colorectal cancers. Gastroenterology 1989;97:597–600.
[39] Church TR, Ederer F, Mandel JS. Fecal occult blood screening in the Minnesota study: sensitivity of the screening test. J Natl Cancer Inst 1997;89:1440–8.
[40] St. John DJB, Young GP, Alexeyeff MA, Deacon MC, Cuthbertson AM, Macrae FA, et al. Evaluation of new occult blood tests for detection of colorectal neoplasia. Gastroenterology 1993;104:1661–8.
[41] Ko CW, Dominitz JA, Nguyen TD. Fecal occult blood testing in a general medical clinic: comparison between guaiac-based and immunochemical-based tests. Am J Med 2003;115:111–4.
[42] Levin B, Brooks D, Smith RA, Stone A. Emerging technologies in screening for colorectal cancer: CT colonography, immunochemical fecal occult blood tests and stool screening using molecular markers. CA Cancer J Clin 2003;53:44–55.
[43] Saito H, Soma Y, Koeda J, Wada T, Kawaguchi H, Sobue T, et al. Reduction in risk of mortality from colorectal cancer by fecal occult blood screening with immunochemical hemagglutination test: a case-control study. Int J Cancer 1995;61:465–9.
[44] Saito H, Soma M, Nakajima M, Koeda J, Kawaguchi H, Kakizaki R, et al. A case-control study evaluating occult blood screening for colorectal cancer with Hemoccult test and immunochemical hemagglutination test. Oncol Rep 2000;7:815–9.
[45] Young GP, St John DJB, Winawer SJ, Rozen P. Choice of fecal occult blood tests for colorectal cancer screening: recommendations based on performance characteristics in population studies. Am J Gastroenterol 2002;97:2499–507.
[46] Allison JE, Tekawa IS, Ransom LJ, Adrian AL. A comparison of fecal-occult blood tests for colorectal cancer screening. N Engl J Med 1996;334:155–9.
[47] Zappa M, Castiglione G, Paci E, Grazzini G, Rubeca T, Turco P, et al. Measuring interval cancers in population-based screening using different assays of fecal occult blood testing: the District of Florence experience. Int J Cancer 2001;92:151–4.

[48] Cole S, Smith A, Bampton P, Sandford J, Morcom J, Young GP. Screening for colorectal cancer: direct comparison of a brush-sampling fecal immunochemical test for hemoglobin with Hemoccult. Gastroenterology 2003;124:A80.
[49] Cole SR, Young GP, Esterman A, Cadd B, Morcom J. A randomized trial of the impact of new fecal hemoglobin test technologies on population participation in screening for colorectal cancer. J Med Screen 2003;10:117–22.
[50] Winawer S, Fletcher R, Rex D, Bond J, Burt R, Ferrucci JT, et al. Colorectal cancer screening and surveillance: clinical guidelines and rationale–update based on new evidence. Gastroenterology 2003;124:544–60.
[51] Smith R, Cokkinides V, Eyre H. American Cancer Society guidelines for the early detection of cancer. CA Cancer J Clin 2003;53:27–43.
[52] Muto T, Bussey HJ, Morson BC. The evolution of cancer of the colon and rectum. Cancer 1975;36:2251–70.
[53] Stryker SJ, Wolff BG, Culp CE. Natural history of untreated colonic polyps. Gastroenterology 1987;93:1009–13.
[54] Spencer RJ, Melton LJ, Ready RL, Ilstrup DM. Treatment of small colorectal polyps: a population-based study of the risk of subsequent carcinoma. Mayo Clin Proc 1984;59: 305–10.
[55] Atkin WS, Morson BC, Cuzick J. Long-term risk of colorectal cancer after excision of rectosigmoid adenomas. N Engl J Med 1992;326:658–62.
[56] Saitoh Y, Waxman I, West AB, Popnikolov NK, Gatalica Z, Watari J, et al. Prevalence and distinctive biologic features of flat colorectal adenomas in North American populations. Gastroenterology 2001;120:1657–65.
[57] Cajucom CC, Barrios GC, Cruz L, Varin C, Herrera L. Prevalence of colorectal polyps in Filipinos: an autopsy study. Dis Colon Rectum 1992;35:676–80.
[58] Eide TJ. The age-, sex- and site-specific occurrence of adenomas and carcinomas of the large intestine within a defined population. Scand J Gastroenterol 1986;21:1083–8.
[59] Rickert RR, Auerbach O, Garfinkel L, Hammond EC, Frasca JM. Adenomatous lesions of the large bowel: an autopsy survey. Cancer 1979;43:1847–57.
[60] Sato E, Ouchi A, Sasano N, Ishidate T. Polyps and diverticulosis of the large bowel in autopsy population of Akita prefecture compared with Miyagi: high risk for colorectal cancer in Japan. Cancer 1976;37:1316–21.
[61] Bombi JA. Polyps of the colon in Barcelona, Spain: an autopsy study. Cancer 1988;66: 1472–6.
[62] Lieberman DA, Weiss DG, Bond JH, Ahnen DJ, Garewal H, Chejfec G. Use of colonoscopy to screen asymptomatic adults for colorectal cancer. Veterans Affairs Cooperative Study Group. N Engl J Med 2000;343:162–8.
[63] Imperiale TF, Wagner DR, Lin CY, Larkin GN, Rogge JD, Ransohoff DF. Risk of advanced proximal neoplasms in asymptomatic adults according to the distal colorectal findings. N Engl J Med 2000;343:169–74.
[64] Selby JV, Friedman GD, Quesenberry CP Jr, Weiss NS. A case-control study of screening sigmoidoscopy and mortality from colorectal cancer. N Engl J Med 1992;326:653–7.
[65] Newcombe PA, Norfleet RG, Storer BE, Surawicz T, Marcus PM. Screening sigmoidoscopy and colorectal cancer mortality. J Natl Cancer Inst 1992;84:1572–5.
[66] Muller AD, Sonnenberg A. Protection by endoscopy against death from colorectal cancer: a case-control study among veterans. Arch Intern Med 1995;155:1741–8.
[67] Kavanaugh AM, Giaovannucci EL, Fuchs CS, Colditz GA. Screening endoscopy and risk of colorectal cancer in United States men. Cancer Causes Control 1998;9:455–62.
[68] Church TR. A novel form of ascertainment bias in case-control studies of cancer screening. J Clin Epidemiol 1999;52:837–47.
[69] Prorok PC, Andriole GL, Bresalier RS, Buys SS, Chia D, Crawford ED, et al. Design of the Prostate, Lung, Colorectal and Ovarian (PLCO) Cancer Screening Trial. Control Clin Trials 2000;21:273S–309S.

[70] Atkin WS, Crook CF, Cuzick J, Edwards R, Northover JMA, Wardle J. Single flexible sigmoidoscopy screening to prevent colorectal cancer: baseline findings of a UK multicentre randomized trial. Lancet 2002;359:1291–300.
[71] Bretthauer M, Skovlund E, Grotmol T, Thiis-Evensen E, Gondal G, Huppertz-Hauss G, et al. Inter-endoscopist variation in polyp and neoplasia pick-up rates in flexible sigmoidoscopy screening for colorectal cancer. Scand J Gastroenterol 2003;38: 1268–74.
[72] Schoen RE, Pinsky PF, Weissfeld JL, Church T, Prorok P, Gohagan JK. Results of repeat sigmoidoscopy 3 years after a negative examination. JAMA 2003;290:41–8.
[73] Newcombe PA, Storer BE, Morimoto LM, Templeton A, Potter JD. Long-term efficacy of sigmoidoscopy in the reduction of colorectal cancer incidence. J Natl Cancer Inst 2003;95: 622–5.
[74] Mandel JS. Sigmoidoscopy screening probably works, but how well is still unknown. J Natl Cancer Inst 1993;95:571–3.
[75] Berry DP, Clarke P, Hardcastle JD, Vellacott KD. Randomized trial of the addition of flexible sigmoidoscopy to fecal occult blood testing for colorectal neoplasia population screening. Br J Surg 1997;84:1274–6.
[76] Rasmussen M, Kronborg O, Fenger C, Jorgensen OD. Possible advantages and drawbacks of adding flexible sigmoidoscopy to Hemoccult-II in screening for colorectal cancer. Scand J Gastroenterol 1999;34:73–8.
[77] Verne JE, Aubrey R, Love SB, Talbot IC, Northover JM. Population based randomized study of uptake and yield of screening by flexible sigmoidoscopy compared with screening by faecal occult blood testing. BMJ 1998;317:182–5.
[78] Lieberman DA, Weiss DG, and the VACSP Study Group. One-time screening for colorectal cancer with combined fecal occult-blood testing and examination of the distal colon. N Engl J Med 2001;345:555–60.
[79] Lieberman DA, Smith FW. Screening for colon malignancy with colonoscopy. Am J Gastroenterol 1991;86:946–51.
[80] Rex DK, Cummings OW, Helper DJ, Nowak TV, McGill JM, Chiao GZ, et al. 5-year incidence of adenomas after negative colonoscopy in asymptomatic average-risk persons. Gastroenterology 1996;111:1178–81.
[81] Lieberman DA. Endoscopic colon screening: is less more? Gastroenterology 1996;111: 1385–7.
[82] Rogge JD, Elmore MF, Mahoney SJ, Brown ED, Troiano FP, Wagner DR, et al. Low-cost office-based screening colonoscopy. Am J Gastroenterol 1994;89:1775–80.
[83] Citarda F, Tomaselli G, Capocaccia R, Barcherini S, Crespi M. Efficacy in standard clinical practice of colonoscopic polypectomy in reducing colorectal cancer incidence. Gut 2001;48: 812–5.
[84] Inadomi JM, Sonnenberg A. The impact of colorectal cancer screening on life expectancy. Gastrointest Endosc 2000;51:517–23.
[85] Nelson DB, McQuaid KR, Bond JH, Lieberman DA, Weiss DG, Johnston TK. Procedural success and complications of large-scale screening colonoscopy. Gastrointest Endosc 2002; 55:307–14.
[86] Dafnis G, Ekbom A, Pahlman L, Blomqvist P. Complications of diagnostic and therapeutic colonoscopy within a defined population in Sweden. Gastrointest Endosc 2001;54:302–9.
[87] Anderson ML, Pasha TM, Leighton JA. Endoscopic perforation of the colon: lessons from a 10-year study. Am J Gastroenterol 2000;95:3418–22.
[88] Eckardt VF, Kanzler G, Schmitt T, Eckardt AJ, Bernhard G. Complications and adverse effects of colonoscopy with selective sedation. Gastrointest Endosc 1999;49:560–5.
[89] Wexner SD, Forde KA, Sellers G, Geron N, Lopes A, Weiss EG, et al. How well can surgeons perform colonoscopy? Surg Endosc 1998;12:1410–4.
[90] Ure T, Dehghan K, Vernava AM, Longo WE, Andrus CA, Daniel GL. Colonoscopy in the elderly: low risk, high yield. Surg Endosc 1995;9:505–8.

[91] Zubarik R, Fleischer DE, Mastropietro C, Lopez J, Carroll J, Benjamin S, et al. Prospective analysis of complications 30 days after outpatient colonoscopy. Gastrointest Endosc 1999; 50:322–8.

[92] Lo AY, Beaton HL. Selective management of colonoscopic perforations. J Am Coll Surg 1994;179:333–7.

[93] Webb WA, McDaniel L, Jones L. Experience with 1000 colonoscopic polypectomies. Ann Surg 1985;201:626–32.

[94] Scheitel SM, Ahlquist DA, Wollan PC, Hagen PT, Silverstein M. Colorectal cancer screening: a community case-control study of proctosigmoidoscopy, barium enema radiography and fecal occult blood test efficacy. Mayo Clin Proc 1999;74:1207–13.

[95] Rex DK, Rahmani EY, Haseman JH, Lemmel GT, Kaster S, Buckley JS. Relative sensitivity of colonoscopy and barium enema for detection of colorectal cancer in clinical practice. Gastroenterology 1997;112:17–23.

[96] Winawer SJ, Stewart ET, Zauber AG, Bond JH, Ansel H, Waye JD, et al. A comparison of colonoscopy and double-contrast barium enema for surveillance after polypectomy. National Polyp Work Group. N Engl J Med 2000;342:1766–72.

[97] Fletcher RH. The end of barium enema? N Engl J Med 2000;342:1823–5.

[98] Kewenter J, Brevinge H. Endoscopic and surgical complications of work-up in screening for colorectal cancer. Dis Colon Rectum 1996;39:676–80.

[99] Blakeborough A, Sheridan MB, Chapman AH. Complications of barium enema examinations: a survey of UK Consultant Radiologists 1992 to 1994. Clin Radiol 1997; 52:142–8.

[100] Zalis ME, Hahn PF. Digital subtraction bowel cleansing in CT colonography. AJR Am J Roentgenol 2001;176:646–8.

[101] Rex DK, Vining MD, Kopecky K. An initial experience with screening for colon polyps using spiral CT with and without CT colography (virtual colonoscopy). Gastrointest Endosc 1999;50:309–13.

[102] Prickhardt PJ, Choi JR, Hwang I, Butler JA, Puckett ML, Hildebrandt HA, et al. Computed tomographic virtual colonoscopy to screen for colorectal neoplasia in asymptomatic adults. N Engl J Med 2003;349:2191–200.

[103] Morrin MM, LaMont T. Screening virtual colonoscopy: ready for prime time? N Engl J Med 2003;349:2261–4.

[104] Cotton PB, Durkalski VL, Pineau BC, Palesch YY, Mauldin PD, Hoffman B, et al. Computed tomographic colonography (virtual colonoscopy): a multicenter comparison with standard colonoscopy for detection of colorectal neoplasia. JAMA 2004;291:1713–8.

[105] Fearon ER, Vogelstein BA. A genetic model for colorectal tumorigenesis. Cell 1990;61: 759–67.

[106] Traverso G, Shuber A, Levin B, Johnson C, Olsson L, Schoetz DJ Jr, et al. Detection of APC mutations in fecal DNA from patients with colorectal tumors. N Engl J Med 2002; 346:311–20.

[107] Ahlquist DA, Skoletsky JE, Boynton KA, Harrington JJ, Mahoney DW, Pierceall WE, et al. Colorectal cancer screening by detection of altered human DNA in stool: feasibility of a multitarget assay panel. Gastroenterology 2000;119:1219–27.

[108] Traverso G, Shuber A, Olsson L, Levin B, Johnson C, Hamilton SR, et al. Detection of proximal colorectal cancers through analysis of faecal DNA. Lancet 2002;359:403–4.

[109] Dong SM, Traverso G, Johnson C, Geng L, Favis R, Boynton K, et al. Detecting colorectal cancer in stool with the use of multiple genetic targets. J Natl Cancer Inst 2001;93: 858–65.

[110] Pignone M, Somnath S, Hoerger T, Mandelblatt J. Cost-effectiveness analyses of colorectal cancer screening: a systematic review for the US Preventive Services Task Force. Ann Intern Med 2002;137:96–104.

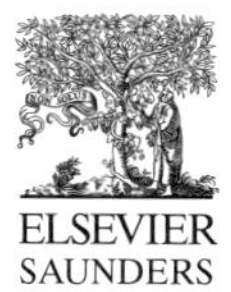
ELSEVIER
SAUNDERS

Med Clin N Am 89 (2005) 61–84

THE MEDICAL CLINICS OF NORTH AMERICA

# Surveillance of patients at high risk for colorectal cancer

Sapna Syngal, MD, MPH[a,b,c],
Prathap Bandipalliam, MD[c], C. Richard Boland, MD[d,*]

[a]*Division of Gastroenterology, Brigham and Women's Hospital, Boston, MA, USA*
[b]*Population Sciences Division, Dana-Farber Cancer Institute, Boston, MA, USA*
[c]*Harvard Medical School, Boston, MA, USA*
[d]*Division of Gastroenterology, Baylor University Medical Center, H-250, 3500 Gaston Avenue, Dallas, TX 75246, USA*

Colorectal cancer (CRC) is a common disease, and its incidence increases dramatically with advancing age. There will be an estimated 140,000 new cases of CRC in 2004, and 57,000 deaths attributable to this disease, making it a major public health concern [1]. CRC mortality may be greatly reduced by clinically feasible screening programs (Table 1). The reduction in mortality may be as great as 80% when colonoscopy and colonoscopic polypectomy programs are implemented, because this technique not only screens for cancer, but prevents cancer from developing by ablating premalignant (adenomatous) lesions [2].

Two programs can reduce morbidity and mortality from CRC: screening programs for healthy, asymptomatic individuals greater than 50 years of age, and surveillance programs for groups at increased risk of developing CRC, including a personal history of CRC or colorectal adenomas, a family history of CRC or gastrointestinal cancer syndromes, and inflammatory bowel disease.

The benefits of surveillance of high-risk groups are evident. Cancer mortality can be dramatically reduced by eradication of precursor lesions and by detection of cancer at an early and highly curable stage. Few rigorous studies of CRC surveillance in high-risk groups, however, have been performed. The main uncertainty and challenge is to determine the appropriate intervals between surveillance by randomized clinical trials.

* Corresponding author.
*E-mail address:* Rickbo@baylorhealth.edu (C.R. Boland).

0025-7125/05/$ - see front matter 
doi:10.1016/j.mcna.2004.08.013

Table 1
Summary of surveillance guidelines for individuals at moderate to high-risk for colorectal cancer

| Screening guidelines | HNPCC | FAP | IBD | Personal or family history of colon polyps or CRC |
|---|---|---|---|---|
| American Gastroenterological Association | Colonoscopy every 1–2 y beginning at 20–25 y of age or 10 y earlier than the youngest case in the family, whichever is first[a] | Annual sigmoidoscopy beginning at 10–12 y (in AFAP, colonoscopy should be used beginning in the late teens or early 20s)[a] | Ulcerative colitis: No direct evidence in the literature; however, accepted practice is to perform surveillance colonoscopy every 1–2 y following 8 y of disease in patients with pancolitis or after 15 y in those with left-sided colitis. Biopsy should be taken every 10 cm in all four quadrants and of strictures and mass lesions other than pseudopolyps[a] | *Personal history*<br>1. Individuals with a history of polyps should have a follow-up colonoscopy in ~3 y. The subsequent surveillance interval depends on the number and type of polyps found. Patients with large (>1 cm) adenomas or those with a villous pathology should have more frequent colonoscopic surveillance.<br>2. Patients with a history of CRC should have a preoperative colonoscopy to rule out synchronous tumors elsewhere in the colon. If this is not feasible they should have a colonoscopy within 1 y of colonic resection, and if normal, subsequent examinations may be performed once every 3–6 y.[a]<br>*Family history*<br>1. One first-degree relative with CRC or adenoma (<60 y) or two or more first-degree relatives with CRC: colonoscopy every 5 y beginning at age 40, or 10 y earlier than the youngest age of the diagnosis of colon cancer in the family, whichever is earlier. |

| | | | | |
|---|---|---|---|---|
| | | | | 2. One first-degree relative with CRC or adenoma (>60 y) or two second-degree relatives with CRC: same as average risk but beginning at age 40.<br>3. One second-degree or any third degree relative with CRC: same as average-risk individuals.[a] |
| American College of Gastroenterology | Colonoscopy beginning at age 20–25 y, and once every 2 y until age 40, and then annually[b] | Sigmoidoscopy screening every 1–2 y beginning at 10–12 y of age. Older unscreened relatives of a person newly diagnosed with FAP should have full colonoscopy for the first screening examination in view of the more fully developed polyposis. Screening should continue until age 40, and then be replaced with standard risk screening. AFAP - colonoscopy[b] | Crohn's disease: Despite increasing evidence of the carcinogenic potential of long-standing Crohn's disease, surveillance guidelines for CRC have yet to be defined.[c]<br>Ulcerative colitis: After 8–10 y of colitis, annual colonoscopy (avoiding periods of clinical relapse) with multiple biopsies at 10cm intervals to detect dysplasia.[d] | *Personal history*<br>Following a complete clearing colonoscopy after an initial polypectomy, follow-up colonoscopy should be performed after 3 y in patients at high risk for developing metachronous advanced adenomas (includes those who at baseline examination have multiple [>2] adenomas, a large [≥1 cm] adenoma, an adenoma with villous histology or high-grade dysplasia, or have a family history of colorectal cancer) and at 5 years for most patients at low risk for developing advanced adenomas (includes those who at baseline colonoscopy have only one or two small tubular adenomas [<1 cm] and no family history of colorectal cancer). Selected patients (elderly patients with substantial comorbidity) at low risk for metachronous advanced adenomas may not require |

(*continued on next page*)

Table 1 (*continued*)

| Screening guidelines | HNPCC | FAP | IBD | Personal or family history of colon polyps or CRC |
|---|---|---|---|---|
| | | | | follow-up surveillance colonoscopy. After one negative follow-up surveillance colonoscopy, subsequent surveillance intervals may be increased to 5 y.[e] *Family history* Individuals with a first-degree relative with adenoma (particularly if the adenoma was diagnosed before age 60, or in the case of siblings, when a parent also had colorectal cancer) should have colonoscopy at 5 y younger than the age of initial adenoma diagnosis, or at age 40 (whichever is first), and then every 3–5 y, depending on colonoscopic findings.[e] |

| | | | | |
|---|---|---|---|---|
| American Society for Gastrointestinal Endoscopy | Colonoscopic surveillance every 2 y beginning at age 25, or 5 y younger than the earliest diagnosis of CRC, whichever is earlier. Annual screening should be performed after age 40.[f] | Flexible sigmoidoscopy annually beginning at age 10 to 12 y. If no polyps are found, then annual sigmoidoscopy should be offered until age 40 and then every 3–5 y thereafter.[f] | For individuals with longstanding ulcerative colitis or Crohn's colitis (pancolitis for 8 or more y or left sided colitis for 15 or more y) colonoscopic surveillance every 1–3 y, with systematic biopsies (two to four random biopsies at 10 cm intervals throughout the entire colon and rectum). In addition, areas of mucosal irregularity and all polypoid lesions of unclear etiology should be biopsied to detect dysplasia associated lesion or mass. There are no prospective trial outcomes data, however supporting this practice; also, there is no role for colonoscopic surveillance in patients with noncolonic Crohn's disease.[f,g] | *Personal history:*<br>*CRC:* Individuals should have a preoperative colonoscopy. If this is not possible, a complete postoperative colonoscopy. Should be performed within a year of the resection. If either of these examinations is normal, then a subsequent colonoscopy may be performed after 3–6 y.<br>*Adenomas:* Individuals should have a follow-up colonoscopy after 3 y following clearance of the colon for polyps; subsequent colonoscopic surveillance depends on the number and type of polyps seen on the initial follow-up colonoscopy and the screening intervals should be individualized. Individuals with high-risk lesions (polyps >1 cm or with villous architecture) should have more frequent surveillance than individuals with small, tubular adenomas.[f]<br>*Family history*<br>Individuals with a first-degree relative diagnosed with sporadic CRC or an adenoma before age 60 or with multiple first-degree relatives diagnosed with CRC or adenomas: colonoscopy every 3–5 y beginning at an age 10 y younger than the age of the youngest affected relative.[f] |

(continued on next page)

Table 1 (*continued*)

| Screening guidelines | HNPCC | FAP | IBD | Personal or family history of colon polyps or CRC |
|---|---|---|---|---|
| SSAT, AGA, ASLD, ASGE, AHPBA consensus panel | | | Individuals with universal colitis: colonoscopy every 1–2 y starting from the 8th year of disease and annually after the 15th year of disease. Flexible sigmoidoscopy should be performed (to 60 cm with biopsy) in the alternate year when colonoscopy is done every other year. It is recommended that three-four biopsies be taken each 10 cm resulting in a total of at least 25–30 biopsies.[i] | |
| American Cancer Society | Begin colonoscopic screening at age 21, and then every 1–2 y until age 40, then annually[h] | Begin screening at puberty[h] | Colonoscopy, with biopsies to detect dysplasia, recommended every 1–2 y for patients with significant cancer risk (ie, after 8 y of onset of pancolitis or 12–15 y after onset of left-sided colitis)[h] | *Personal history*<br>1. Single small (<1 cm) adenoma: colonoscopy 3–6 y after initial polypectomy. If normal, screened as average-risk individuals.<br>2. Large (>1 cm) adenoma, villous or multiple adenomas, or adenomas with high-grade dysplasia: colonoscopy within 3 y of initial polypectomy. If normal, repeat colonoscopy in 3 y. If again normal, can be screened as average-risk individuals. |

3. Curative-intent resection of CRC: colonoscopy within 1 y of resection. If normal, repeat colonoscopy in 3 y. If normal, repeat colonoscopy every 5 y.[h]

*Family history*

CRC or adenomas in any first-degree relative before age 60 or CRC or adenomas in two or more first-degree relatives at any age (if not a hereditary syndrome): colonoscopy beginning at age 40, or 10 y earlier than the youngest case in the family, and every 5–10 y thereafter.[h]

*Abbreviations:* AFAP, attenuated familial adenomatous polyposis; AGA, American Gastroenterological Association; AHPBA, American Hepato-Pancreato-Biliary Association; ASGE, American Society for Gastrointestinal Endoscopy; ASLD, American Society for Liver Diseases; CRC, Colorectal cancer; HNPCC, hereditary nonpolyposis colon cancer; IBD, Inflammatory bowel disease; SSAT, The Society for Surgery of the Alimentary Tract.

[a] Winawer SJ, Fletcher R, Rex D, Bond JH, Burt RW, Ferrucci J, et al. Colorectal cancer screening and surveillance: clinical guidelines and rationale. Update based on new evidence. Gastroenterology 2003;124:544–60; with permission.

[b] Available at: http://www.acg.gi.org/patientinfo/ccrk/CRC2000.pdf. Accessed September 22, 2004.

[c] Hanauer SB, Sandborn W, and the Practice Parameters Committee of the American College of Gastroenterology. Management of Crohn's disease in adults. Am J Gastroenterol 2001;96:635–43; with permission.

[d] Kornbluth A, Sachar DB. ACG treatment guideline: ulcerative colitis practice guideline in adults. Am J Gastroenterol 1997;92:204–11; with permission.

[e] Bond JH. Polyp guideline: diagnosis, treatment, and surveillance for patients with colorectal polyps. Am J Gastroenterol 2000;95:3053–63; with permission.

[f] Guidelines for colorectal cancer screening and surveillance. Gastrointest Endosc 2000;51:777–82; with permission.

[g] The role of colonoscopy in the management of patients with inflammatory bowel disease. Gastrointest Endosc 1998;48:689–90; with permission.

[h] Smith RA, Cokkinides V, Eyre HJ. American Cancer Society guidelines for the early detection of cancer, 2003. CA Cancer J Clin 2003;53:27–43; with permission.

[i] SSAT, ASLD, ASGE, AHPBA Consensus Panel. Ulcerative colitis and colon carcinoma: epidemiology, surveillance, diagnosis, and treatment. J Gastrointest Surg 1998;2:305–6; with permission.

Surveillance for CRC involves two layers of testing in an asymptomatic individual who is at risk for CRC. One can elect primary surveillance colonoscopy, because this is the definitive diagnostic test. Alternatively, one can first perform a noninvasive screening test to determine whether an individual requires referral for colonoscopy.

The first-level screening tests include the fecal occult blood test (FOBT); barium enema; CT colonography (also called virtual colonoscopy); and testing for cancer-related genetic mutations in DNA shed into the feces. Each of these tests has some advantages. All have limitations and none is 100% sensitive for cancer. Unfortunately, a positive result in most of these screening tests is more likely to be a false-positive than a true-positive for CRC. Sigmoidoscopy is intermediate between a screening and diagnostic test in that it is a definitive diagnostic test for the distal colon and is a screening test for the risk of neoplasia in the proximal colon. The screening methods are discussed before reviewing their applications to specific high-risk groups.

## Screening methods

Several tests have been developed to detect colonic polyps or CRC at an early stage. Positive results require colonoscopy [3,4]. Fecal-based tests of FOBT or fecal genetic tests depend on the propensity of an early colorectal neoplasm to shed either blood or tumorous DNA into the fecal stream. Barium enema, CT colonography, sigmoidoscopy, and colonoscopy depend on detecting a mass lesion in the colon.

### *Fecal occult blood tests*

In FOBT, a sample of stool is tested for the presence of occult blood based on oxidative conversion of the colorless guaiac substrate to a blue pigment in the presence of the peroxidase activity of hemoglobin. Periodic FOBT testing can decrease the incidence of CRC by as much as 33% [5], but only when performed annually. Biannual testing reduces mortality only by 15% to 20% [6,7]. Although the test is relatively inexpensive and simple, it is relatively insensitive and has a positive predictive value as low as 2.2% [5]. Foods with peroxidase-like activity, including broccoli, cauliflower, radishes, and red meat, can produce a false-positive result and should be avoided for 3 days before testing. Conversely, prolonged storage of slides and ingestion of ascorbic acid (vitamin C) can create a false-negative result. Although technical improvements in the FOBT are being investigated, this test is unlikely ever to become highly sensitive and specific. A CRC typically sheds only about 2 mL of blood per day, which is not so much more than the normal physiologic shedding of approximately 0.7 mL of blood per day. An attempt to make the test more sensitive would perforce produce an increase in the rate of false-positives.

### *Tests for tumor DNA in stool*

Recently there have been studies investigating the possibility of detecting tumor DNA in stool, using an array of genetic markers for colon cancer, to screen for CRC [8–10]. Although early studies have yielded promising results, this approach is rapidly evolving, and further studies are necessary to define its role in screening for CRC. Early results suggest that the specificity may be high, but the sensitivity is only 50% to 70% [11]. Like the FOBT, this is a noninvasive test, and this may be the only acceptable approach for some patients.

### *Double-contrast barium enema*

Historically, radiologic examinations of the large bowel using barium contrast have been used to detect CRC. Unfortunately, these examinations are insensitive, and miss up to half of large polyps or cancers [12]. The double-contrast barium enema, in which a sticky form of barium is introduced and then followed by air to visualize the mucosa better, is a more sensitive approach to imaging. This test, however, takes more time to perform than a single-contrast study, and not all radiologists take the time to perform the test this way. Barium enema is currently reserved for instances in which colonoscopy fails for technical reasons. CT colonography has recently become the radiologic imaging procedure of choice for the colon.

### *Virtual colonoscopy*

Some studies have suggested that high-resolution CT scanning of the large bowel (also known as "CT colonography") has reasonable sensitivity for detection of large polyps. A single institutional study published in 2003 indicated that improvements in hardware (multichannel scanners), software (three-dimensional, fly-through reconstruction), preparation (tagging stool with markers that can be subtracted from the images by the software), and radiologic expertise can render these studies as sensitive as colonoscopy, missing fewer than 10% of lesions greater than or equal to 6 mm [13]. Unless all the recent technical advances are instituted, however, the test is neither more sensitive nor more specific than a barium enema, and has unacceptable performance characteristics [14]. This technology is likely to advance quickly, and CT colonography may become a major tool in CRC screening. An optimal program should link the radiologic findings with the colonoscopist, so that mass lesions identified by virtual colonoscopy may be confirmed and removed endoscopically following a single bowel preparation.

### *Sigmoidoscopy*

In sigmoidoscopy the rectum and sigmoid colon are directly visualized endoscopically and identified polyps are removed. The major drawback, however, is the inability to examine the proximal colon, which is especially important in individuals with a hereditary predisposition to CRC, because many of them have proximal colonic tumors [15]. In addition, when polyps are identified, endoscopic polypectomy should be used only if the entire colon has been prepared to prevent complications from electrocautery. Two case-control studies of sigmoidoscopy (mostly using the older rigid sigmoidoscope) demonstrated 60% to 79% reductions in cancer-related mortality in the portion of the bowel examined, and suggested that the protective effects of this screening might last as long as 10 years [16,17]. Longer, flexible sigmoidoscopies permit examination up to the splenic flexure. Most physicians prefer colonoscopy for examination of the entire colon.

### *Colonoscopy*

The dramatic impact of sigmoidoscopy prompted investigation into the feasibility of performing total colonoscopy as the initial screening examination. Colonoscopy offers an opportunity to visualize the entire colon and to remove all polyps; it remains the gold standard for CRC screening. It is the only technique in which polyps (including malignant ones) can be removed. The best evidence for reducing CRC mortality with polypectomy comes from the National Polyp Study. In this uncontrolled trial of the effect of polypectomy on CRC mortality, the investigators used historical groups as controls to estimate the natural history of unremoved colorectal adenomas, and concluded that polypectomy can reduce subsequent CRC mortality by as much as 76% to 90% [18]. This study demonstrated that repeating colonoscopy 1 year after removal of the index polyp was unnecessary, and that repeating colonoscopy after 3 years was sufficiently safe. Subsequent data have led to the recommendation that follow-up intervals are determined by the number and pathologic nature of the index polyps [2]. Several studies suggest that staining of colonic mucosa with dyes, such as indigo carmine [19,20] or methylene blue [21], during colonoscopy helps detect small, flat colorectal polyps. This technique increases the procedure time and is not routinely used.

## Identification of very high-risk groups: hereditary colorectal cancer syndromes

### *Lynch syndrome*

Lynch syndrome, or hereditary nonpolyposis colon cancer, is the most common hereditary colon cancer syndrome. It is estimated to account for approximately 3% to 5% of all CRCs. It is characterized by early onset of colon cancer, and is often associated with several different extracolonic cancers, most commonly endometrial cancer [22]. Lynch syndrome is caused by defects in the DNA mismatch repair system [23–25]. This repair system is basically the spell-checking system of DNA. It includes *MLH1*, *MSH2*, *MSH6*, *MLH3*, *MSH3*, and *PMS2* and other genes [26]. This repair system identifies and corrects base mismatches that occur during DNA replication. Defects in this repair system, which may occur as a consequence of germline mutations in the DNA mismatch repair genes, lead to the rapid accumulation of errors that occur during DNA replication. Germline mutations in the *MLH1* and *MSH2* genes account for most cases of Lynch syndrome. Defects in this repair system lead to a mutational signature in the DNA of the tumor tissue, called microsatellite instability, which is readily detected [25]. Germline mutations in the hMSH6 gene produce an attenuated form of Lynch syndrome, characterized by delayed onset of familial CRC, and a high incidence of endometrial cancer [27,28].

*Clinical features*

Lynch syndrome is clinically characterized by several early onset colon cancers in the family, many of them diagnosed before the age of 50. The cancers usually occur in the right colon, and often on histopathology have a mucinous pattern associated with tumor infiltrating lymphocytes [29]. The clinical picture also often includes several extracolonic cancers [30], such as endometrial, ovarian, urinary tract (transitional cell cancers), small intestine, brain, stomach, and hepatobiliary tract tumors and early onset adenomatous colonic polyps. These colonic polyps are usually less than 10 in number. The term "nonpolyposis" distinguishes this syndrome from the polyposis syndromes described later. The lifetime risk of developing CRC may be as high as 91% in affected individuals [31,32].

The Amsterdam criteria have traditionally been used to diagnose the Lynch syndrome [33,34]. These criteria, however, are somewhat restrictive and other criteria have been proposed, including the Modified Amsterdam and Amsterdam II criteria [35]. The Bethesda guidelines have been proposed to identify patients with CRC who should be tested for microsatellite instability to screen for Lynch syndrome [36]. The affected proband is first tested for the presence of a mutation. If a mutation is found, then that data can be used to screen at-risk blood relatives. A negative genetic test is less informative, however, because a few families with hereditary nonpolyposis colon cancer have no detectable mutation in either the *MLH1 or MSH2* genes with currently available techniques.

*Management*

Regular colonoscopic surveillance and polypectomy is the mainstay of management of individuals with the Lynch syndrome. Colonoscopy every 3 years reduces CRC mortality by 65%, but interval cancers do occur between examinations despite this surveillance [37]. Surveillance colonoscopy is recommended to begin at age 25 (or 10 years earlier than the youngest cancer in the family), and to be repeated every 1 to 2 years [38]. Annual colonoscopy is safer in terms of reducing cancer, but is more costly and increases the cumulative risk of colonoscopic complications. Colonoscopy every second year is a reasonable compromise. One must be alert to the risk of cancers of the stomach, ovaries, and urinary tract, although strict screening regimens have never been tested or validated for these cancers. Periodic examination of the stomach at the time of colonoscopy seems reasonable, but the premalignant gastric lesion is unknown, and this intervention may not necessarily reduce mortality. Periodic screening for endometrial and ovarian cancer (with endometrial biopsies and pelvic ultrasound) is also important. Prophylactic hysterectomy is an option in selected cases.

### *Management summary*

Annual history and physical examination should focus on possible cancers in numerous organ systems. Colonoscopy is recommended every 1 to 2 years, beginning at 20 to 25 years of age, or 5 to 10 years earlier than the earliest case in the family. Removal of the uterus and ovaries should be considered when childbearing is complete. Periodic esophagogastroduodenoscopy, when gastric cancer is in the family, may be indicated. Identify the germline mutation by blood testing, obtain genetic counseling for the family, and test for the proband's mutation in all first-degree relatives.

## *Familial polyposis syndromes*

### *Familial adenomatous polyposis*

Familial adenomatous polyposis (FAP) is an autosomal-dominant syndrome characterized by early onset of multiple colonic adenomatous polyps and subsequent development of colon cancer. It accounts for much less than 1% of all CRCs and is estimated to occur in 1 per 7000 to 10,000 of the general population. It is usually caused by germline mutations in the adenomatous polyposis coli (*APC*) gene [39,40]. Alternatively, an autosomal-recessive disease can be caused by inactivating mutations in the *MYH* base excision repair gene, which then permits the secondary accumulation of mutations in the *APC* gene [41–44]. In all cases, the syndromic polyps are adenomas, and their growth is triggered by inactivation of the *APC* gene, which indirectly regulates colonic epithelial growth; APC has been called the gatekeeper of the colon [45].

FAP clinically presents with hundreds to thousands of adenomatous polyps carpeting the colon, which is pathognomonic for the classic form of the syndrome. The polyps usually appear during the teenage years (median onset at age 16). Without treatment the immense number of adenomas almost invariably results in CRC, through the classic adenoma-to-carcinoma sequence, by the third or fourth decade of life. FAP is associated with small intestinal adenomas, and the periampullary region is especially prone to develop cancer, which occurs in 5% to 10% of FAP patients. The stomach frequently develops multiple polyps, but these polyps are pathologically characterized as fundic gland hyperplasia, and are associated with gastric cancer in less than 1% of cases [46]. In addition, FAP is also associated with extracolonic tumors including osteomas, and adrenal, liver, and thyroid tumors. The association of colon polyps with multiple fibromas, osteomas, dental abnormalities, and so forth was historically referred to as "Gardner's syndrome," but this is actually a variant presentation of FAP. These extracolonic abnormalities can be detected in most patients with FAP. Similarly, the combination of colonic polyps and brain tumors was previously termed "Turcot's syndrome," but this is usually a variation of FAP; a few families with brain and colon tumors have the Lynch syndrome [47].

A serious complication of FAP that occurs in 10% to 15% of patients, particularly certain kindreds, is desmoid tumors, which are dense neoplastic growths of connective tissue [48]. Many FAP families have congenital hypertrophic retinal pigment epithelium, referred to as "CHRPE lesions," which can be detected by ophthalmoscopic examination. This usually occurs only when the germline *APC* mutation is located downstream of exon 7, and is not a useful screening test for FAP, unless CHRPE lesions are known to occur in the kindred.

Because of the large number of adenomatous polyps beginning in adolescence, nearly all FAP patients eventually develop CRC. Observing hundreds to thousands of adenomatous polyps in the colon is pathognomonic. The diagnosis can be confirmed by sequencing the *APC* gene; this detects the disease-causing mutation in about 70% of cases. All disease-causing mutations create either a premature stop codon (ie, encode a truncated protein), or completely delete the gene from the genome. When a clinical scenario is most consistent with autosomal-recessive inheritance (ie, a horizontal rather than vertical family history), mutations in the MYH gene should be considered.

Genetic counseling and testing are part of the standard of care for patients with FAP. The affected proband should be tested first for the presence of a mutation. If a mutation is detected, this result can be used to screen other at-risk (first-degree) relatives. A negative result in the proband is, however, uninformative, because a mutation can sometimes be undetectable with currently available techniques. Once a pathogenic mutation is identified in a family, testing other at-risk relatives can obviate the need for ongoing colonoscopic surveillance in those who lack the mutation, or confirm the need for intensive colonoscopic surveillance, as recommended for FAP patients, in those who have the mutation. Although certain associations between the location of mutation and the phenotypic manifestations occur in FAP [49], these associations are often not consistent enough to affect clinical decision making.

Surgical removal of the colon and rectum (total proctocolectomy with ileal pouch and anal anastomosis) is the definitive treatment for FAP. Selected patients with mild forms of the disease and rectal sparing may reasonably undergo a less extensive procedure, such as a rectal-sparing colectomy, with the caveat that the rectal remnant must be regularly screened endoscopically. In addition, upper gastrointestinal surveillance every 1 to 3 years is indicated to screen for gastric or ampullary neoplasms. Because of the high prevalence of ampullary neoplasms, duodenoscopy with ampullary biopsies should be performed as part of the upper tract surveillance program. Recently, the cyclooxygenase-2 inhibitor celecoxib has been used as a chemopreventive agent for FAP, but it should be used only as an adjunct to endoscopic screening and surgery [50].

*Attenuated familial adenomatous polyposis*

Attenuated FAP is a variant form of the FAP syndrome characterized by only 10 to 100 colonic adenomas (hence the name "attenuated") [51]. The polyps occur later in life than those in classic FAP. Attenuated FAP is usually caused by mutations in the 5′ end or the 3′ end of the *APC* gene. One reason for attenuation of the phenotype is that mutations at the 5′ end of the gene can be bypassed by an internal translation initiation site in the *APC* gene [52]. It can also be associated with upper gastrointestinal or other extracolonic tumors seen in classic FAP. Indeed, the gastric polyposis may be more impressive than the colonic polyposis. Management includes surveillance colonoscopy with colonoscopic polypectomy, or surgery depending on the number of polyps and the rate of polyp formation. Colonoscopic screening of at-risk relatives is very important. The approach to genetic testing is similar to that in FAP.

An attenuated form of colonic polyposis without a vertical family history may be caused by an autosomal-recessive disorder in which both alleles of the *MYH* gene are mutated. *MYH* is a base excision repair gene, and biallelic mutations permit many G:C→T:A mutations to accumulate throughout the genome, and the *APC* gene is the clinically most relevant target of this defect. These individuals do not have germline mutations in *APC* (ie, have a negative blood test for APC mutations), and each neoplasm has a unique, acquired mutation in this gene [43,44].

*I1307K and recurrent colorectal polyps*

Essentially all *APC* mutations that cause FAP either truncate the *APC* gene or delete the entire gene through deletion of chromosome 5q. Truncating mutations at either end of the gene cause attenuated disease. Only one missense mutation has been clearly associated with an increase in polyp formation and cancer risk: I1307K. This sequence variation (T to A at nucleotide 3920) converts an isoleucine (I) to a lysine (K) at codon 1307. This mutation predisposes to colorectal neoplasia because it creates eight consecutive adenine (A) residues, which is intrinsically unstable. This mutation is prone to cause a second mutation in which one of the adenines is deleted and this second mutation creates a downstream stop codon. I1307K increases colorectal cancer risk about twofold, with a recurrent polyp phenotype, and can be managed with serial colonoscopic polypectomy. About 6% of all Ashkenazi Jews and about 28% of Ashkenazi Jews with a family history of CRC carry this polymorphism [53]. This mutation is easily detected by reference laboratories. The disease typically does not require colectomy. Because clinical recommendations for treatment and follow-up of carriers of the I1307K mutation are based on the clinical and family history rather than the genetic test result, genetic testing for this alteration is infrequently performed clinically.

*Management summary*

In classic FAP, find the germline mutation, get genetic counseling, and test all first-degree relatives. After diagnosis, the only issue is the timing of colectomy and the optimal type of surgery. In the absence of a genetic diagnosis, annual colonoscopy should begin in early adolescence and continue until age 40 in typical cases. Attenuated FAP is best managed by finding the germline mutation, because the manifestations are delayed in onset, and often subtle. Based on the number of polyps and their progression over time, patients may be managed indefinitely with annual colonoscopy and polypectomy.

## *Hamartomatous polyposis syndromes*

*Peutz-Jeghers syndrome*

Peutz-Jeghers syndrome (PJS) is a rare autosomal-dominant syndrome characterized by multiple hamartomatous polyps of the colon and small intestine described first by Peutz in 1921 and then by Jeghers in 1949 [54]. It occurs in about 1 in 120,000 births and is the second most common hamartomatous polyposis syndrome. PJS is caused by germline mutations in a serine-threonine kinase called either STK-11 or LKB-1 on chromosome 19p [55].

PJS clinically manifests with multiple hamartomatous polyps in the small and large intestine, particularly the jejunum. Most patients have characteristic mucocutaneous pigmented lesions, most obvious in and around the mouth, perioral region, and on the hands and feet. In addition to CRC, it is associated with extracolonic tumors, such as ovarian sex cord tumors; Sertoli's cell testicular tumors; breast, pancreatic, and endometrial tumors; and a rare form of cervical cancer known as "adenoma malignum." The overall risk for cancer is increased 18-fold compared with age-matched populations, with an estimated cumulative risk of cancer of 93% by age 64. Taking age into consideration, the relative risk for CRC is increased 84-fold [56–58]. The carcinogenesis pathway is sometimes referred to as the "hamartoma-adenoma-carcinoma" sequence, highlighting the progression of the hamartomatous polyp to an adenoma and to an adenocarcinoma.

The finding of multiple characteristic hamartomatous polyps with bands of arborizing smooth muscle in the lamina propria without the cystic dilatation seen in juvenile polyposis syndrome (JPS) associated with distinctive mucocutaneous pigmentation is diagnostic of PJS. Genetic testing should begin with testing the affected proband for mutations in the STK-11 gene.

Regular upper and lower gastrointestinal endoscopic surveillance with polypectomy is indicated. Small bowel enteroscopy is also essential to screen for polyps. Recent studies have advocated the use of intraoperative enteroscopy to visualize the small bowel fully in patients with PJS. Capsule endoscopy has not been studied yet in this population, but will likely play a role in their surveillance. Larger polyps may require surgical resection to prevent complications, such as obstruction, intussusception, and bleeding. Genetic testing can be used to screen blood relatives at risk, once the proband's mutation is identified.

*Management summary.* Recommendations regarding screening for CRC in PJS are not established. Upper and lower gastrointestinal endoscopy should be performed every 3 to 5 years, along with small bowel radiography or wireless capsule endoscopy. Periodic breast, pelvic, and genital examinations should be part of the surveillance program [56,59].

*Juvenile polyposis syndrome*

JPS is an autosomal-dominant syndrome characterized by multiple hamartomatous polyps of the gastrointestinal tract, first described by McColl et al in 1964 [60]. It is the most common hamartomatous polyposis syndrome. It is usually caused by germline mutations in the SMAD-4 gene on chromosome 18q21 [61,62], but can be caused by mutations in the BMPR1A gene. These patients can be confusing because of phenotypic and genetic heterogeneity [62,63].

JPS presents clinically with multiple hamartomatous polyps in the colon, small intestine, and stomach, although the rectosigmoid region is most commonly affected. It is also often associated with congenital abnormalities of the gastrointestinal tract (malrotation of the midgut), genitourinary system, and heart [59].

Affected individuals are at increased risk for developing CRC, with an estimated risk of approximately 20% at approximately age 34 and of approximately 68% at age 60 [59,64]. The syndrome generally presents with gastrointestinal bleeding, intussusception, and obstruction because of the intestinal polyps. It can present in childhood. The polyps are histopathologically characterized by cystic dilatation of epithelial-lined spaces with chronic inflammatory cells in the lamina propria. Proposed clinical diagnostic criteria include three or more juvenile colonic polyps, polyposis of the entire gastrointestinal tract, or any number of polyps in a proband with a family history of juvenile polyps [65].

Individuals with JPS need upper and lower gastrointestinal endoscopic surveillance with polypectomy. Diffuse polyposis of the colon or stomach may be an indication for colectomy or gastrectomy, respectively. If a mutation is identified in SMAD-4 or BMPR1A in the proband, genetic testing should be offered to blood relatives at risk.

*Management summary.* CRC surveillance guidelines for individuals with JPS have not been promulgated. It is, however, reasonable to begin surveillance of at-risk individuals with upper and lower endoscopy and small bowel studies in the second decade and every 3 to 5 years thereafter [59].

### *Cowden's syndrome and Bannayan-Riley-Ruvalcaba syndrome (Ruvalcaba-Myhre-Smith)*

Cowden's syndrome, a rare genetic disease first described in 1963, is characterized by hamartomas of the gastrointestinal tract and tumors of the skin (trichilemmoma), breast (including breast cancer), and thyroid [64]. Cowden's syndrome is caused by mutation of the PTEN gene on chromosome 10q [66–69], but even more than in other hamartomatoses, the phenotypic and genetic heterogeneity can render classification difficult [63,70]. Bannayan-Riley-Ruvalcaba syndrome is another rare autosomal-dominant syndrome, which is usually, but not invariably, associated with the PTEN gene [71,72]. It often presents with hamartomatous polyps of the gastrointestinal tract, characteristic skin pigmentation, macrocephaly, mental retardation, lipid storage myopathy, and Hashimoto's thyroiditis.

*Management summary.* Management of these two rare syndromes should be individualized based on the individual clinical features. CRC risk is usually not greater than that of the general population.

## Chronic colonic inflammation: inflammatory bowel disease

### *Ulcerative colitis*

Ulcerative colitis (UC) is a chronic inflammatory disease of the large intestine characterized by immune-mediated inflammation and ulceration of colorectal mucosa. The estimated incidence is 3 to 15 per 100,000 persons per year. The etiology of UC is unclear, although genetic and environmental factors are important. Colonoscopic examination reveals inflammation of the colonic mucosa, as evidenced by mucosal bleeding; mucopurulent exudate; mucosal friability; and pseudopolyps, which are the result of scarred epithelium. Distorted colonic mucosa complicates the colonoscopic detection of early colonic neoplasia.

The risk of CRC is directly related to the duration of the UC. A meta-analysis has reported the cumulative risk of CRC to be 2% at 10 years, 8% at 20 years, and 18% after 30 years of disease [73,74]. The incidence of CRC is higher in patients with pancolitis, longer disease duration, and concomitant sclerosing cholangitis. Generally, the risk increases at an annual rate of 0.5% to 2% per year after 8 to 10 years of UC.

Because of the increased risk of CRC, regular colonoscopic surveillance with systematic biopsies to detect dysplasia is performed. The commonly accepted practice, although not rigorously proved, is to perform colonoscopic surveillance every 1 to 2 years after 8 to 10 years of pancolitis or after

15 years of left-sided colitis, with systematic biopsies (four-quadrant biopsies every 10 cm) and biopsies of any suspicious masses or strictures [2]. This approach should reduce cancer mortality [75]. Administration of sulfasalazine or mesalamine for UC may protect against CRC [76].

### *Crohn's disease*

Crohn's disease is a chronic transmural inflammation of the gastrointestinal tract, which may involve any region of the alimentary tract. Individuals with this disease have a significantly increased risk of CRC [77]. As in UC, the risk for CRC increases with longer disease duration. Again, without direct evidence in the literature, periodic surveillance (every 1 to 2 years) after 8 to 10 years of Crohn's colitis is the standard of care [2].

## Groups at moderate risk for colorectal cancer

### *Personal history of adenomas or colorectal cancer*

Patients with prior adenomatous colon polyps or prior CRC are at increased risk of subsequent CRC [78]. Patients who have a history of CRC should have a complete colonoscopy before (or soon after) removal of their cancer. Once the colon has been cleared of polyps, colonoscopic surveillance should be performed at 3 years, and once there is a normal examination, every 5 years thereafter [2].

Because adenomas are neoplasms at early stages of development, patients with these lesions require chronic surveillance. Because adenomas are common in the population, surveillance intervals depend on the risk factors for CRC. The risk of CRC is especially high in individuals diagnosed with large (>1 cm) adenomas; greater than or equal to three adenomas; adenomas with villous features; and adenomas with severe dysplasia (carcinoma in situ). Patients with adenomas with these features should be managed like patients with cancer, with colonoscopy every 3 years until there are no recurrent adenomas, and then every 5 years. Patients with one or two small nonvillous adenomas can be managed safely by performing their first surveillance colonoscopy at 5 years [2].

#### *Management summary*

Whether the patient has a cancer or an advanced adenoma, surveillance colonoscopy is indicated every 3 years until the colon is clear, after which colonoscopy every 5 years is sufficient. Patients commonly have one or two small, nonadvanced adenomas, and these patients may not require intensive surveillance once their colon has been cleared of polyps.

### *Family history of adenoma or colorectal cancer*

Patients with a family history of colonic adenomas or CRC who do not meet the criteria for the previously mentioned hereditary CRC syndromes are still at increased risk for developing CRC. The risk of CRC is increased about twofold to threefold compared with the general population for individuals with one first-degree relative or two second-degree relatives with CRC, and increased threefold to fourfold for individuals with two first-degree relatives with CRC or one first-degree relative with CRC diagnosed at age less than 50 years [2]. Surveillance for such individuals is recommended commencing either at age 40 (instead of 50, which is the recommended age in the general population) or 10 years earlier than the youngest CRC in the family, and repeated every 5 years [2]. Individuals with only one second-degree (or more distant) relative with CRC do not require more intensive screening than the general population.

*Management summary*

For nonsyndromic positive family histories, screen beginning at age 40, and perform colonoscopy every 5 years.

### *Patients with ureterosigmoidostomy*

Patients who have undergone ureterosigmoidostomy, with the ureters draining into the sigmoid colon, are at increased risk for adenomas and CRC [79]. It is prudent to offer these patients lifelong colonoscopic surveillance for neoplasia at the anastomotic sites. Surveillance beginning 10 years after the surgery, and then continuing annually, is usually recommended. Suspicious lesions should be biopsied, but polypoid lesions should not be removed by colonoscopic polypectomy because this might damage the anastomosis and lead to urinary leakage. Fortunately, this operation has been replaced by other surgical approaches.

### *Acromegaly*

Individuals with acromegaly seem to be at increased risk of developing colon adenomas and CRC [80]. This is a rare disease and data concerning surveillance are unavailable. It is reasonable to offer frequent colonoscopic surveillance, but the optimal surveillance interval is not determined. Some recommend beginning surveillance at age 40. If an adenoma is found, subsequent surveillance is recommended every 3 years. If no adenoma or cancer is found, subsequent surveillance may be offered every 5 years.

### Streptococcus bovis *bacteremia*

Several reports have suggested an association between *Streptococcus bovis* bacteremia and colonic adenomas and CRC [81,82]. Because many of these patients harbor an asymptomatic CRC, it is often recommended that these patients undergo full colonoscopy to screen for CRC. If this examination is negative, subsequent surveillance is not required.

## References

[1] Jemal A, Tiwari RC, Murray T, Ghafoor A, Samuels A, Ward E, et al. Cancer statistics, 2004. CA Cancer J Clin 2004;54:8–29.

[2] Winawer S, Fletcher R, Rex D, Bond J, Burt R, Ferrucci J, et al. Colorectal cancer screening and surveillance: clinical guidelines and rationale. Update based on new evidence. Gastroenterology 2003;124:544–60.

[3] Walsh JM, Terdiman JP. Colorectal cancer screening: clinical applications. JAMA 2003;289: 1297–302.

[4] Vijan S, Hwang EW, Hofer TP, Hayward RA. Which colon cancer screening test? A comparison of costs, effectiveness, and compliance. Am J Med 2001;111:593–601.

[5] Mandel JS, Bond JH, Church TR, Snover DC, Bradley GM, Schuman LM, et al. Reducing mortality from colorectal cancer by screening for fecal occult blood. Minnesota Colon Cancer Control Study. N Engl J Med 1993;328:1365–71.

[6] Kronborg O, Fenger C, Olsen J, Jorgensen OD, Sondergaard O. Randomised study of screening for colorectal cancer with faecal-occult-blood test. Lancet 1996;348:1467–71.

[7] Hardcastle JD, Chamberlain JO, Robinson MH, Moss SM, Amar SS, Balfour TW, et al. Randomised controlled trial of faecal-occult-blood screening for colorectal cancer. Lancet 1996;348:1472–7.

[8] Traverso G, Shuber A, Levin B, Johnson C, Olsson L, Schoetz DJ Jr, et al. Detection of APC mutations in fecal DNA from patients with colorectal tumors. N Engl J Med 2002;346: 311–20.

[9] Traverso G, Shuber A, Olsson L, Levin B, Johnson C, Hamilton SR, et al. Detection of proximal colorectal cancers through analysis of faecal DNA. Lancet 2002;359:403–4.

[10] Dong SM, Traverso G, Johnson C, Geng L, Favis R, Boynton K, et al. Detecting colorectal cancer in stool with the use of multiple genetic targets. J Natl Cancer Inst 2001;93:858–65.

[11] Boland CR. Molecular basis for stool-based DNA tests for colorectal cancer: a primer for clinicians. Rev Gastroenterol Disord 2002;2(Suppl 1):S12–9.

[12] Winawer SJ, Stewart ET, Zauber AG, Bond JH, Ansel H, Waye JD, et al. A comparison of colonoscopy and double-contrast barium enema for surveillance after polypectomy. National Polyp Study Work Group. N Engl J Med 2000;342:1766–72.

[13] Pickhardt PJ, Choi JR, Hwang I, Butler JA, Puckett ML, Hildebrandt HA, et al. Computed tomographic virtual colonoscopy to screen for colorectal neoplasia in asymptomatic adults. N Engl J Med 2003;349:2191–200.

[14] Cotton PB, Durkalski VL, Pineau BC, Palesch YY, Mauldin PD, Hoffman B, et al. Computed tomographic colonography (virtual colonoscopy): a multicenter comparison with standard colonoscopy for detection of colorectal neoplasia. JAMA 2004;291:1713–9.

[15] Lynch HT, Smyrk TC, Watson P, Lanspa SJ, Lynch JF, Lynch PM, et al. Genetics, natural history, tumor spectrum, and pathology of hereditary nonpolyposis colorectal cancer: an updated review. Gastroenterology 1993;104:1535–49.

[16] Selby JV, Friedman GD, Quesenberry CP Jr, Weiss NS. A case-control study of screening sigmoidoscopy and mortality from colorectal cancer. N Engl J Med 1992;326:653–7.

[17] Newcomb PA, Norfleet RG, Storer BE, Surawicz TS, Marcus PM. Screening sigmoidoscopy and colorectal cancer mortality. J Natl Cancer Inst 1992;84:1572–5.

[18] Winawer SJ, Zauber AG, Ho MN, O'Brien MJ, Gottlieb LS, Sternberg SS, et al. Prevention of colorectal cancer by colonoscopic polypectomy. The National Polyp Study Workgroup. N Engl J Med 1993;329:1977–81.

[19] Lee JH, Kim JW, Cho YK, Sohn CI, Jeon WK, Kim BI, et al. Detection of colorectal adenomas by routine chromoendoscopy with indigocarmine. Am J Gastroenterol 2003;98: 1284–8.

[20] Eisen GM, Kim CY, Fleischer DE, Kozarek RA, Carr-Locke DL, Li TC, et al. High-resolution chromoendoscopy for classifying colonic polyps: a multicenter study. Gastrointest Endosc 2002;55:687–94.

[21] Kiesslich R, Fritsch J, Holtmann M, Koehler HH, Stolte M, Kanzler S, et al. Methylene blue-aided chromoendoscopy for the detection of intraepithelial neoplasia and colon cancer in ulcerative colitis. Gastroenterology 2003;124:880–8.

[22] Marra G, Boland CR. Hereditary nonpolyposis colorectal cancer: the syndrome, the genes, and historical perspectives. J Natl Cancer Inst 1995;87:1114–25.

[23] Lynch HT, Lynch J. Lynch syndrome: genetics, natural history, genetic counseling, and prevention. J Clin Oncol 2000;18:19S–31S.

[24] Boland CR, Thibodeau SN, Hamilton SR, Sidransky D, Eshleman JR, Burt RW, et al. A National Cancer Institute Workshop on Microsatellite Instability for cancer detection and familial predisposition: development of international criteria for the determination of microsatellite instability in colorectal cancer. Cancer Res 1998;58:5248–57.

[25] Umar A, Boland CR, Terdiman JP, Syngal S, De La CA, Ruschoff J, et al. Revised Bethesda Guidelines for hereditary nonpolyposis colorectal cancer (Lynch syndrome) and microsatellite instability. J Natl Cancer Inst 2004;96:261–8.

[26] Fishel R, Kolodner RD. Identification of mismatch repair genes and their role in the development of cancer. Curr Opin Genet Dev 1995;5:382–95.

[27] Kolodner RD, Tytell JD, Schmeits JL, Kane MF, Gupta RD, Weger J, et al. Germ-line msh6 mutations in colorectal cancer families. Cancer Res 1999;59:5068–74.

[28] Wagner A, Hendriks Y, Meijers-Heijboer EJ, de Leeuw WJ, Morreau H, Hofstra R, et al. Atypical HNPCC owing to MSH6 germline mutations: analysis of a large Dutch pedigree. J Med Genet 2001;38:318–22.

[29] Smyrk TC, Watson P, Kaul K, Lynch HT. Tumor-infiltrating lymphocytes are a marker for microsatellite instability in colorectal carcinoma. Cancer 2001;91:2417–22.

[30] Watson P, Lynch HT. Extracolonic cancer in hereditary nonpolyposis colorectal cancer. Cancer 1993;71:677–85.

[31] Aarnio M, Sankila R, Pukkala E, Salovaara R, Aaltonen LA, De La CA, et al. Cancer risk in mutation carriers of DNA-mismatch-repair genes. Int J Cancer 1999;81:214–8.

[32] Dunlop MG, Farrington SM, Carothers AD, Wyllie AH, Sharp L, Burn J, et al. Cancer risk associated with germline DNA mismatch repair gene mutations. Hum Mol Genet 1997;6:105–10.

[33] Vasen HF, Mecklin JP, Khan PM, Lynch HT. The International Collaborative Group on Hereditary Non-Polyposis Colorectal Cancer (ICG-HNPCC). Dis Colon Rectum 1991;34:424–5.

[34] Vasen HF, Mecklin JP, Watson P, Utsunomiya J, Bertario L, Lynch P, et al. Surveillance in hereditary nonpolyposis colorectal cancer: an international cooperative study of 165 families. The International Collaborative Group on HNPCC. Dis Colon Rectum 1993;36:1–4.

[35] Vasen HF, Watson P, Mecklin JP, Lynch HT. New clinical criteria for hereditary nonpolyposis colorectal cancer (HNPCC, Lynch syndrome) proposed by the International Collaborative group on HNPCC. Gastroenterology 1999;116:1453–6.

[36] Rodriguez-Bigas MA, Boland CR, Hamilton SR, Henson DE, Jass JR, Khan PM, et al. A National Cancer Institute Workshop on Hereditary Nonpolyposis Colorectal Cancer Syndrome: meeting highlights and Bethesda guidelines. J Natl Cancer Inst 1997;89:1758–62.

[37] Jarvinen HJ, Aarnio M, Mustonen H, Aktan-Collan K, Aaltonen LA, Peltomaki P, et al. Controlled 15-year trial on screening for colorectal cancer in families with hereditary nonpolyposis colorectal cancer. Gastroenterology 2000;118:829–34.

[38] Vasen HF, van Ballegooijen M, Buskens E, Kleibeuker JK, Taal BG, Griffioen G, et al. A cost-effectiveness analysis of colorectal screening of hereditary nonpolyposis colorectal carcinoma gene carriers. Cancer 1998;82:1632–7.

[39] Groden J, Thliveris A, Samowitz W, Carlson M, Gelbert L, Albertsen H, et al. Identification and characterization of the familial adenomatous polyposis coli gene. Cell 1991;66:589–600.

[40] Kinzler KW, Nilbert MC, Su LK, Vogelstein B, Bryan TM, Levy DB, et al. Identification of FAP locus genes from chromosome 5q21. Science 1991;253:661–5.
[41] Al Tassan N, Chmiel NH, Maynard J, Fleming N, Livingston AL, Williams GT, et al. Inherited variants of MYH associated with somatic G:C→T:A mutations in colorectal tumors. Nat Genet 2002;30:227–32.
[42] Lipton L, Halford SE, Johnson V, Novelli MR, Jones A, Cummings C, et al. Carcinogenesis in MYH-associated polyposis follows a distinct genetic pathway. Cancer Res 2003;63: 7595–9.
[43] Sampson JR, Dolwani S, Jones S, Eccles D, Ellis A, Evans DG, et al. Autosomal recessive colorectal adenomatous polyposis due to inherited mutations of MYH. Lancet 2003;362: 39–41.
[44] Sieber OM, Lipton L, Crabtree M, Heinimann K, Fidalgo P, Phillips RK, et al. Multiple colorectal adenomas, classic adenomatous polyposis, and germ-line mutations in MYH. N Engl J Med 2003;348:791–9.
[45] Kinzler KW, Vogelstein B. Lessons from hereditary colorectal cancer. Cell 1996;87:159–70.
[46] Burt RW. Gastric fundic gland polyps. Gastroenterology 2003;125:1462–9.
[47] Hamilton SR, Liu B, Parsons RE, Papadopoulos N, Jen J, Powell SM, et al. The molecular basis of Turcot's syndrome. N Engl J Med 1995;332:839–47.
[48] Knudsen AL, Bulow S. Desmoid tumour in familial adenomatous polyposis: a review of literature. Fam Cancer 2001;1:111–9.
[49] Giardiello FM, Petersen GM, Piantadosi S, Gruber SB, Traboulsi EI, Offerhaus GJ, et al. APC gene mutations and extraintestinal phenotype of familial adenomatous polyposis. Gut 1997;40:521–5.
[50] Steinbach G, Lynch PM, Phillips RK, Wallace MH, Hawk E, Gordon GB, et al. The effect of celecoxib, a cyclooxygenase-2 inhibitor, in familial adenomatous polyposis. N Engl J Med 2000;342:1946–52.
[51] Knudsen AL, Bisgaard ML, Bulow S. Attenuated familial adenomatous polyposis (AFAP): a review of the literature. Fam Cancer 2003;2:43–55.
[52] Heppner GK, Trzepacz C, Tuohy TM, Groden J. Attenuated APC alleles produce functional protein from internal translation initiation. Proc Natl Acad Sci U S A 2002;99: 8161–6.
[53] Laken SJ, Petersen GM, Gruber SB, Oddoux C, Ostrer H, Giardiello FM, et al. Familial colorectal cancer in Ashkenazim due to a hypermutable tract in APC. Nat Genet 1997;17: 79–83.
[54] Keller JJ, Offerhaus GJ, Giardiello FM, Menko FH. Jan Peutz, Harold Jeghers and a remarkable combination of polyposis and pigmentation of the skin and mucous membranes. Fam Cancer 2001;1:181–5.
[55] Gruber SB, Entius MM, Petersen GM, Laken SJ, Longo PA, Boyer R, et al. Pathogenesis of adenocarcinoma in Peutz-Jeghers syndrome. Cancer Res 1998;58:5267–70.
[56] Boardman LA, Thibodeau SN, Schaid DJ, Lindor NM, McDonnell SK, Burgart LJ, et al. Increased risk for cancer in patients with the Peutz-Jeghers syndrome. Ann Intern Med 1998; 128:896–9.
[57] Giardiello FM, Welsh SB, Hamilton SR, Offerhaus GJ, Gittelsohn AM, Booker SV, et al. Increased risk of cancer in the Peutz-Jeghers syndrome. N Engl J Med 1987;316:1511–4.
[58] Giardiello FM, Brensinger JD, Tersmette AC, Goodman SN, Petersen GM, Booker SV, et al. Very high risk of cancer in familial Peutz-Jeghers syndrome. Gastroenterology 2000; 119:1447–53.
[59] Dunlop MG. Guidance on gastrointestinal surveillance for hereditary non-polyposis colorectal cancer, familial adenomatous polyposis, juvenile polyposis, and Peutz-Jeghers syndrome. Gut 2002;51(Suppl 5):V21–7.
[60] McColl I, Busxey HJ, Veale AM, Morson BC. Juvenile polyposis coli. Proc R Soc Med 1964; 57:896–7.

[61] Howe JR, Roth S, Ringold JC, Summers RW, Jarvinen HJ, Sistonen P, et al. Mutations in the SMAD4/DPC4 gene in juvenile polyposis. Science 1998;280:1086–8.

[62] Sayed MG, Ahmed AF, Ringold JR, Anderson ME, Bair JL, Mitros FA, et al. Germline SMAD4 or BMPR1A mutations and phenotype of juvenile polyposis. Ann Surg Oncol 2002; 9:901–6.

[63] Zhou XP, Woodford-Richens K, Lehtonen R, Kurose K, Aldred M, Hampel H, et al. Germline mutations in BMPR1A/ALK3 cause a subset of cases of juvenile polyposis syndrome and of Cowden and Bannayan-Riley-Ruvalcaba syndromes. Am J Hum Genet 2001;69:704–11.

[64] Wirtzfeld DA, Petrelli NJ, Rodriguez-Bigas MA. Hamartomatous polyposis syndromes: molecular genetics, neoplastic risk, and surveillance recommendations. Ann Surg Oncol 2001;8:319–27.

[65] Giardiello FM, Hamilton SR, Kern SE, Offerhaus GJ, Green PA, Celano P, et al. Colorectal neoplasia in juvenile polyposis or juvenile polyps. Arch Dis Child 1991;66:971–5.

[66] Nelen MR, Padberg GW, Peeters EA, Lin AY, van den HB, Frants RR, et al. Localization of the gene for Cowden disease to chromosome 10q22–23. Nat Genet 1996;13:114–6.

[67] Arch EM, Goodman BK, Van Wesep RA, Liaw D, Clarke K, Parsons R, et al. Deletion of PTEN in a patient with Bannayan-Riley-Ruvalcaba syndrome suggests allelism with Cowden disease. Am J Med Genet 1997;71:489–93.

[68] Zori RT, Marsh DJ, Graham GE, Marliss EB, Eng C. Germline PTEN mutation in a family with Cowden syndrome and Bannayan-Riley-Ruvalcaba syndrome. Am J Med Genet 1998; 80:399–402.

[69] Nelen MR, van Staveren WC, Peeters EA, Hassel MB, Gorlin RJ, Hamm H, et al. Germline mutations in the PTEN/MMAC1 gene in patients with Cowden disease. Hum Mol Genet 1997;6:1383–7.

[70] Nelen MR, Kremer H, Konings IB, Schoute F, van Essen AJ, Koch R, et al. Novel PTEN mutations in patients with Cowden disease: absence of clear genotype-phenotype correlations. Eur J Hum Genet 1999;7:267–73.

[71] Longy M, Coulon V, Duboue B, David A, Larregue M, Eng C, et al. Mutations of PTEN in patients with Bannayan-Riley-Ruvalcaba phenotype. J Med Genet 1998;35:886–9.

[72] Carethers JM, Furnari FB, Zigman AF, Lavine JE, Jones MC, Graham GE, et al. Absence of PTEN/MMAC1 germ-line mutations in sporadic Bannayan-Riley-Ruvalcaba syndrome. Cancer Res 1998;58:2724–6.

[73] Gyde SN, Prior P, Allan RN, Stevens A, Jewell DP, Truelove SC, et al. Colorectal cancer in ulcerative colitis: a cohort study of primary referrals from three centres. Gut 1988;29: 206–17.

[74] Eaden JA, Mayberry JF. Colorectal cancer complicating ulcerative colitis: a review. Am J Gastroenterol 2000;95:2710–9.

[75] Choi PM, Nugent FW, Schoetz DJ Jr, Silverman ML, Haggitt RC. Colonoscopic surveillance reduces mortality from colorectal cancer in ulcerative colitis. Gastroenterology 1993;105:418–24.

[76] Bernstein CN, Eaden J, Steinhart AH, Munkholm P, Gordon PH. Cancer prevention in inflammatory bowel disease and the chemoprophylactic potential of 5-aminosalicylic acid. Inflamm Bowel Dis 2002;8:356–61.

[77] Ribeiro MB, Greenstein AJ, Sachar DB, Barth J, Balasubramanian S, Harpaz N, et al. Colorectal adenocarcinoma in Crohn's disease. Ann Surg 1996;223:186–93.

[78] Johns LE, Houlston RS. A systematic review and meta-analysis of familial colorectal cancer risk. Am J Gastroenterol 2001;96:2992–3003.

[79] Azimuddin K, Khubchandani IT, Stasik JJ, Rosen L, Riether RD. Neoplasia after ureterosigmoidostomy. Dis Colon Rectum 1999;42:1632–8.

[80] Jenkins PJ, Fairclough PD. Colorectal neoplasia in acromegaly. Clin Endocrinol (Oxf) 2001; 55:727–9.

[81] Burns CA, McCaughey R, Lauter CB. The association of *Streptococcus bovis* fecal carriage and colon neoplasia: possible relationship with polyps and their premalignant potential. Am J Gastroenterol 1985;80:42–6.
[82] Beeching NJ, Christmas TI, Ellis-Pegler RB, Nicholson GI. *Streptococcus bovis* bacteraemia requires rigorous exclusion of colonic neoplasia and endocarditis. Q J Med 1985;56:439–50.

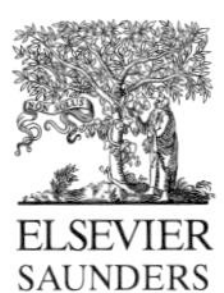


Med Clin N Am 89 (2005) 85–110

THE MEDICAL CLINICS OF NORTH AMERICA

# Prevention and therapy of colorectal cancer

Ernest T. Hawk, MD, MPH*, Asad Umar, PhD, DVM, Ellen Richmond, RN, MS, Jaye L. Viner, MD, MPH

*Gastrointestinal and Other Cancers Research Group, Division of Cancer Prevention, National Cancer Institute, EPN, Suite 2141, 6130 Executive Boulevard, Bethesda, MD 20892–7317, USA*

Colorectal cancer (CRC) accounts for about 10% of cancer mortality in the United States, causing 57,000 deaths in 2004 alone [1]. Approximately 146,000 new cases of CRC are diagnosed each year: 106,000 in the colon and the remainder in the rectum. Mortality has been declining steadily since the 1980s, most likely because of early CRC detection and intervention against early stage disease, including adenomas. Although growing knowledge of disease pathogenesis and the emergence of various screening tools and early medical and surgical interventions have made CRC one of the most preventable of all cancers, it remains the second leading cause of cancer mortality in the United States. This article focuses on established and promising classes of agents developed for CRC prevention and treatment.

## Carcinogenesis: the premise of prevention and therapy

The colorectum is the premier model for studying the molecular pathogenesis of cancer. Accessibility of the colorectum to serial assessment has led to seminal insights into the genesis of neoplasia. This largely accounts for the rapid pace of advances in CRC screening, surveillance, imaging, diagnosis (eg, testing for germline genetic mutations), treatment, and prevention. CRC is a late, nonobligate stage in a prolonged process of stepwise, cumulative changes of genetic-molecular structure and function (eg, K-*ras* oncogenes, *APC, MSH-2*, or *p53* tumor suppressor genes). These

Prepared in the authors' capacities as employees of the US federal government.

* Corresponding author.
*E-mail address:* eh51p@nih.gov (E.T. Hawk).

0025-7125/05/$ - see front matter. Published by Elsevier Inc.
doi:10.1016/j.mcna.2004.08.003

changes are expressed within and across cellular generations and manifest in cells as hyperproliferation and atypia; in local tissue as adenomatous polyps and dysplasia; and in the colorectum as a proliferating, undifferentiated mass unresponsive to apoptotic signals. Genetic mutations or epigenetic derangements of key molecular functions disrupt genomic fidelity, signal transduction, cell division, apoptosis, angiogenesis, and compartmental boundaries (eg, tissue invasion and metastasis) [2]. Neoplastic transformation from normal to hyperproliferative to dysplastic tissue has been demonstrated in abnormal colorectal crypts (ie, aberrant crypt foci) within K-*ras* mutations [3]. Progression from aberrant crypt foci to adenoma and to carcinoma has been associated with aberrant SMAD 2/4, DCC, and p53 [4].

Sporadic CRC, the most common form of the disease, results from the interplay between genetic susceptibilities and environmental insults. The major risk factor for sporadic CRC, as for most malignancies, is advanced age, starting in the fifth decade [5]. Other risk factors include a personal or family history of sporadic CRC or colorectal adenomas, diets low in fruits and vegetables or high in fat, sedentary lifestyle, and inflammatory bowel disease. By contrast, heritable factors are associated with familial disease and are relatively less common, comprising approximately 35% of CRCs [6]. Familial adenomatous polyposis (FAP) and hereditary nonpolyposis colorectal cancer account for nearly half of all heritable CRC. The etiologies, clinical manifestations, and recommendations for CRC screening and chemoprevention differ for sporadic and heritable disease.

## Cancer chemoprevention

Cancer chemoprevention is defined as the use of chemical, biologic, or nutritional compounds to prevent, inhibit, or reverse carcinogenesis before the development of invasive disease [7]. Most CRC chemoprevention trials have yielded null results; the investigational agents neither significantly increased nor decreased the risk of colorectal neoplasia during the observation period. Recent studies, however, have shown preventive efficacy with a variety of agents, suggesting advances with regard to agent and cohort prioritization and trial design. Chemoprevention trials now typically recruit patients at greater than average risk for CRC, although some trials evaluate average-risk cohorts. The steep learning curve from these trials provides direction for future inquiries in selected cohorts, for example, using combination regimens to improve the therapeutic index. Key agents in CRC prevention and treatment are reviewed.

### *Agents with null effects*

The first colorectal neoplasia chemoprevention trial evaluated vitamin C versus placebo in patients with FAP [8]. This study showed no reduction in adenoma burden, but stimulated further research. Subsequent trials demonstrated no significant impact against recurrent or incident adenomas by the following dietary interventions for 2 to 4 years: (1) reduced fat plus increased fiber, fruits, and vegetables [9]; (2) reduced fat in combination with wheat bran or beta-carotene supplements [10]; (3) supplements of wheat bran fiber and vitamins C and E [11]; and (4) supplements of calcium, beta-carotene, vitamin C, vitamin E, and selenium [12]. Most trials evaluating individual dietary supplements also yielded null results. Fiber supplementation with daily wheat bran [11,13] or ispaghula husk [14] failed to reduce adenoma recurrence in high- to moderate-risk patients. In two studies, additional fiber intake may have even increased recurrent adenomas in subsets of the study population [9,14]. Trials evaluating beta-carotene alone [10,15–17], beta-carotene combined with alpha-tocopherol [16,17], or a combination of vitamins C and E [11,15] reported null results regarding recurrent adenomas. Finally, a placebo-controlled trial showed a nonsignificant reduction in incident CRC [17], but a perplexingly significant increase in incident adenomas with alpha-tocopherol supplementation [16].

Null results have also been demonstrated with several pharmacologic agents. For example, a 5-year trial of aspirin, 325 mg every other day, versus placebo showed no reduction in advanced adenomas or CRC incidence [18]. Another study showed a negligible 4% reduction among participants randomized to receive aspirin, 325 mg/d, but a statistically significant and unexpectedly greater reduction of 19% in patients randomized to receive aspirin, 81 mg/day [19]. Similarly, a trial of ursodiol, 8 to 10 mg/kg/d, reported nonsignificant 7% and 14% reductions in incident adenomas and advanced adenomas, respectively [20].

### *Agents with protective effects*

Four classes of compounds have demonstrated efficacy in reducing recurrent colorectal adenomas or cancer in randomized, controlled trials: (1) selenium, (2) calcium carbonate, (3) hormone-replacement therapy, and (4) nonsteroidal anti-inflammatory drugs (NSAIDs) (Table 1). Although risk reductions associated with these compounds have been relatively modest, one NSAID has been approved as an adjunct to standard care for FAP patients [21].

#### *Selenium*

Selenium has been associated with preventive effects in several observational studies [22], but not in others [23–26]. One trial testing the chemopreventive efficacy of selenium supplementation versus placebo in 1312 persons with a history of skin cancer showed a statistically significant 58% reduction in CRC incidence, a secondary endpoint, among subjects randomized to selenium supplementation [27]. Further evaluation of selenium's potential as a CRC chemopreventive has been planned as a substudy within

Table 1
Randomized, double-blinded, and controlled colorectal neoplasia prevention trials demonstrating a preventive effect

| Reference | Intervention | Cohort[a] | Primary results |
|---|---|---|---|
| Baron et al, 1999 [31] | Calcium, 3 gm/d, versus placebo × 4 y | 930 patients with prior adenomas | Patients with adenomas, 19% reduction in incidence*; adenoma number, 24% reduction* |
| Bonithon-Kopp et al, 2000 [33]; Faivre et al, 1997 [136] | Calcium, 2 gm/d, versus 3.8 gm/d ispaghula husk versus placebo for 3 y | 655 patients with prior adenomas; 35–75 years old | Adenoma incidence, 34% reduction (NS) with calcium; 67% increase* with fiber |
| Clark et al, 1996 [27] | Selenium, 200 mmol/d, versus placebo for 6.4 y | 1312 patients with prior skin cancers | CRC incidence, 58% reduction* |
| Rossouw et al, 2002 [39] | Conjugated equine estrogen, 0.625 mg/d, plus medroxyprogesterone acetate, 2.5 mg/d, versus placebo for 5.2 y | 16,608 healthy women, 50–79 years old | CRC incidence, 37% reduction* |
| Baron et al, 2003 [19] | Aspirin, 81 mg versus 325 mg/d versus placebo for 3 y | 1211 patients with prior adenomas | Aspirin, 81 mg/d<br>Adenoma incidence, 19% reduction*<br>Advanced adenoma incidence, 41% reduction*<br>Aspirin, 325 mg/d<br>Adenoma incidence, 4% reduction (NS)<br>Advanced adenoma incidence, 17% reduction (NS) |
| Benamouzig et al, 2003 [58][b] | Aspirin, 160–300 mg/d, versus placebo for 4 y | 291 patients with prior adenomas | Persons with adenomas, 27% reduction ($P = .08$); adenoma > 1 cm in diameter, 83% reduction* |
| Sandler et al, 2003 [57] | Lysine acetylsalicylate, 325 mg/d, versus placebo for 3 y | 635 patients with prior resected early stage CRC | Adenoma incidence, 35% reduction*<br>Prolonged time to first adenoma* |

*Abbreviation:* NS, not statistically significant.

[a] Number randomized.

[b] Interim result at 1 year; intended duration of intervention is 4 years.

* Statistically significant ($P < .05$).

the 32,000-man Selenium and Vitamin E Cancer Prevention Trial and another trial evaluating effects against recurrent adenomas in patients at moderate risk for CRC.

*Calcium carbonate*

Calcium binds bile and fatty acids into insoluble soaps, thereby preventing mutagenic contact with colonic epithelium. Calcium may also inhibit epithelial proliferation by modulating protein kinase C activity, stabilizing membranes, or modifying K-*ras* [28–30].

Two randomized, placebo-controlled, phase III trials have reported that calcium reduces adenoma recurrence. Baron et al [31,32] showed a statistically significant 19% reduction in the recurrence rate of adenomas, and a 44% reduction in the recurrence rate of advanced adenomas, in some cases within 1 year after initiating treatment [31]. A second multicenter, randomized, placebo-controlled trial reported a nonsignificant 34% reduction in recurrent adenomas [33]. Both these studies showed that calcium supplements achieve statistically significant reductions against recurrent adenomas in patients at moderate risk for CRC. The US Women's Health Initiative is now evaluating CRC incidence in 45,000 postmenopausal women randomized to calcium and vitamin D versus placebo for an average of 9 years [34].

*Hormone-replacement therapy*

Estrogens may reduce colorectal carcinogenesis by direct or indirect reductions in secondary bile acid production and by inhibition of insulin-like growth factor I, which may stimulate epithelial proliferation [35]. Although a meta-analysis of 18 epidemiologic studies suggested that hormone-replacement therapy (composed of estrogens in combination with progestins) might reduce the risk of CRC by nearly 20% [36], these protective effects seem to wane after drug cessation [36,37].

The Women's Health Initiative reported a significant 37% reduction in CRC incidence among hormone-replacement therapy users, but this substudy was closed prematurely after the hormone-replacement therapy group was found to have higher rates of breast cancer and other adverse outcomes than the placebo group. Although the risks clearly outweighed the benefits of hormone-replacement therapy in this cohort, this demonstration of chemopreventive efficacy prompts exploration of the underlying mechanisms to improve the regimen's therapeutic index and to determine its potential use in populations at risk for CRC [38–41].

*Nonsteroidal anti-inflammatory drugs*

Numerous studies demonstrate the efficacy of NSAIDs against colorectal neoplasia, including aberrant crypt foci, adenomas, and cancer. Although incompletely understood, the chemopreventive activity of NSAIDs relates to the inhibition of one or both of the cyclooxygenase enzymes, COX-1 and COX-2. COX-2 is a target of interest because it is commonly overexpressed in human neoplasms and cancers [42]. Recent investigations correlate COX-2 overexpression with reduced survival of patients with colorectal [43] and other cancers [44–47]. Inhibition of one or both COX enzymes, by aspirin or other NSAIDs, reduces cellular proliferation, induces apoptosis, promotes immunologic surveillance, and reduces neoangiogenesis [48]. NSAIDs may also exert anticancer effects through COX-independent mechanisms, such as peroxisome proliferator-activated receptor stimulation [49] or by blocking Akt phosphorylation [50]. COX-independent effects have been demonstrated by testing COX-2 selective inhibitors in COX-2 null hematopoietic and epithelial cancer cell lines [51], albeit at concentrations far exceeding clinically feasible doses (up to 1–5 mmol/L) [5].

More than 35 epidemiologic studies over the last two decades consistently associate routine NSAID use with a 40% to 50% reduction of colorectal adenomas, cancer, and cancer-related mortality, regardless of patient age, gender, family history, nationality, health care setting, or study design [42]. More than 15 case series have reported reductions in the adenoma burden of FAP patients who were administered sulindac or other NSAIDs for as little as a few months [52], and one case series demonstrated that these effects were sustained for about 5 years [53]. In the Nurses' Health Study, in which aspirin use in 27,077 female nurses since 1980 has been analyzed, women who took two or more standard aspirin tablets weekly were 25% less likely to develop adenomas as compared with those who took it less often; and those who took the highest dose had the lowest risk of adenoma development [54].

Two trials of prephenotypic FAP patients, one administered sulindac and the other administered aspirin, showed null results with regard to adenoma prevention [55,56]. Three recent, randomized, placebo-controlled trials of aspirin have reported significant preventive effects against colorectal adenomas [19,57,58]. Two of these trials demonstrated a significant reduction in patients taking aspirin, 300 to 325 mg/day [57,58], whereas the third trial showed an unexpectedly small 4% reduction among participants receiving 325 mg/day, as compared with a significant 19% reduction among participants receiving only 81 mg/day [19]. Data from an ongoing trial, the United Kingdom only Colorectal Adenoma Prevention Trial are expected to be analyzed within the next few years [59,60].

### *COX-2 inhibitors*

COX-2 selective inhibitors are NSAID derivatives that were developed to improve the safety profile of NSAIDs, particularly by reducing the risk of gastrointestinal bleeding. Celecoxib was approved as an adjunct to standard care for FAP based on the results of a 6-month randomized, placebo-controlled trial of 83 patients. This study showed a 28% reduction in colorectal adenomas [21], and improvement in the duodenal adenoma burden [61] among patients with FAP receiving 400 mg twice a day.

Ancillary substudies have shown reduced proliferation and increased apoptosis in adenomas excised from patients randomized to celecoxib [62]. In addition, proteomic assessments have identified a protein pattern arising from exposure to celecoxib and another that may predict for agent responsiveness [63]. An Israeli case series of FAP patients showed significant reductions in the development of new adenomas among those taking the COX-2 selective inhibitor rofecoxib [64], which suggests that chemopreventive efficacy against colorectal carcinogenesis may be class rather than agent specific. Ongoing trials are assessing NSAID efficacy and durability of response, as single agents or in combination with other agents, in other cohorts at risk for CRC.

## Staging

Proper treatment and accurate prognosis of patients with CRC depends on accurate clinical staging. Preoperative surgical staging typically includes a thoracoabdominopelvic CT scan, complete blood count, urinalysis, and assessments of liver and renal function. In the case of a patient with apparently localized disease and good medical status without serious comorbidity, a serum carcinoembryonic antigen level is obtained and the patient undergoes surgical resection both for treatment and pathologic staging. Currently, such tests as fluorodeoxyglucose positron emission tomography scanning are recommended only in special circumstances (eg, to exclude metastatic disease that would rule out curative surgical resection).

The widely used TNM (tumor, node, metastases) cancer staging system classifies the extent of disease in order to assess patient prognosis. TNM staging provides objective and precise assessment of the extent of CRC, with regard to neoplastic invasion through the colonic wall, dissemination to regional nodes, and metastases to distant organs, thereby guiding treatment. Involvement of regional nodes is particularly important and requires adequate surgical sampling. In a recent study suggesting that at least eight nodes are required for accurate classification, more than half of the patients were undersampled [65]. Other groups have suggested that at least 14 [66,67] or 17 to 20 [68] nodes must be examined for accurate TNM staging. A recent Intergroup study (INT-0089) of 3411 evaluable patients with resected colon cancer supports sampling larger numbers of nodes. In this study median survival was inversely correlated with nodal involvement, and was directly correlated with the number of nodes that were evaluated, regardless of metastatic involvement [69]. The latter finding may be a surrogate for the adequacy of surgical resection or for improved intraoperative and pathologic staging. Nevertheless, these data confirm that accurate surgical and pathologic nodal evaluation plays a critical role in assessing the complete resectability and curability of CRC.

Based on surgical staging, CRC is categorized into four TNM stages (Table 2). Although the staging is relatively straightforward, distinctions

Table 2
Colorectal cancer staging system, therapy, and 5-year survival data

| Stage | Primary tumor (T) | Lymph node involvement (N) | Metastasis (M) | Therapy | 5-year survival (%) |
|---|---|---|---|---|---|
| I | Tumor invades submucosa or muscularis | None | None | Surgery ± aspirin | 96 |
| II | Tumor invades muscularis or perirectal tissue | None | None | Surgery ± clinical trial (adjuvant chemotherapy controversial) | 87 |
| III | Any | Any | None | Surgery + adjuvant chemotherapy[a] | 55 |
| IV | Any | Any | Any | Surgery or chemotherapy for palliation | 5 |

[a] Radiation therapy may be indicated for rectal primaries and considered for colonic primaries complicated by local perforation, obstruction, or involved surgical margins.

*Data from* American Cancer Society. How is colorectal cancer staged? Available at: http://coloncancer.about.com/gi/dynamic/offsite.htm?zi=1/XJ&sdn=coloncancer&zu=http%3A%2F%2Fwww.cancer.org%2Fdocroot%2FCRI%2Fcontent%2FCRI_2_4_3X_How_is_colon_and_rectum_cancer_staged.asp%3Frnav%3Dcri. Accessed August 2004.

within stages can be important. For example, within stage II of locally invasive CRC without apparent metastases, the subset with intestinal obstruction, perforation, or inadequate surgical margins has poor clinical outcomes that may warrant more aggressive management. Factors other than pathologic stage (including age, gender, histologic grade, venous-lymphatic-perineural invasion, DNA-ploidy, and S-phase fraction) may also have prognostic significance, although correlations with disease recurrence and survival are inconsistent across studies.

## Therapy

### *Surgical resection*

The mainstay of curative therapy for CRC, regardless of stage, is surgical resection of affected bowel with clear margins, along with the adjacent mesentery and at least 12 regional nodes. The specific procedure depends on the anatomic location of the cancer, but surgical treatment typically involves hemicolectomy. For rectal tumors, total mesorectal excision with a distal surgical margin of at least 2 cm is recommended. Recent data suggest that clinical outcome is a function of cancer-free margins and surgical experience [70]. For example, local recurrence rates declined to less than 5% when surgical margins were greater than 1 cm; and recurrences were significantly higher, by as much as 170%, when surgery was performed by less experienced surgeons. Tumors within 6 to 15 cm of the anal verge are usually treated by low anterior resection with end-to-end anastomosis. For tumors that are bulky, located within 6 cm of the anal verge, or involve the anal sphincter, surgeons typically recommend wide surgical resection with abdominoperineal resection and permanent colostomy. In certain settings, such as an uninvolved anal sphincter, low rectal tumors may be amenable to sphincter-sparing resection with coloanal anastomosis.

Laparoscopic resection in CRC is extremely promising [71]. The potential advantages of this relatively noninvasive approach include reduced postoperative ileus and pain, and shorter recovery time. Nevertheless, some clinicians have voiced concerns regarding inadequate resection, understaging, prolonged operative time, high operative cost, and metastatic trocar implants. A recent randomized, controlled trial of laparoscopic versus open resections provided support for laparoscopic resection by demonstrating shorter hospital stays and briefer use of narcotics and oral analgesics with comparable rates of intraoperative complications, 30-day postoperative mortality, short-term complications, and reoperation and readmission [72].

### *Radiation therapy*

Local recurrence following surgical resection is determined by tumor stage and tumor location (rectum more than colon). These two features dictate the need for adjuvant, neoadjuvant, or palliative radiotherapy. Colon cancer has a propensity to recur in distant sites, whereas rectal cancer has a propensity to recur locally in up to 50% of patients with stage II or III disease, resulting in significant management challenges, such as bowel obstruction. Postoperative radiation, with or without chemotherapy, significantly reduces local recurrence rates and has become the standard of care in this setting. A common regimen incorporates infusional 5-fluorouracil (5-FU) as a radiosensitizer to boost the efficacy of pelvic radiation, typically administered as 45 to 55 Gy over 5 weeks.

Chemoradiation has been shown to downstage distal cancers, thereby improving the likelihood of clear surgical margins and sphincter preservation, and to palliate unresectable tumors. Radiation therapy provides pain relief in 80% of patients, 20% of whom report total pain control, and may control hemorrhage in more than 70% of patients. Despite these favorable effects, improvement in overall survival has not been consistently demonstrated [73–78].

Retrospective data suggest that chemoradiation may be less acutely toxic when applied preoperatively rather than postoperatively [79]. Side effects are localized to the radiation field and are dose- and schedule-dependent. The most frequent serious toxicities occur in up to one third of patients and include diarrhea, perianal skin reactions, and cystitis. Less frequent side effects include myelosuppression, tenesmus, hemorrhage, and dysuria [80]. These toxicities usually resolve within 4 to 12 weeks.

Although less common, delayed toxicities that manifest 6 to 18 months after treatment are much more serious. Small intestinal injury results in enteritis, adhesions, and small bowel obstruction. Other side effects include large bowel dysfunction, such as diarrhea, tenesmus, and bloody or mucus discharge that occur in up to 20% of patients [81]. Other complications include abscesses, fistulas, strictures, urinary urgency, sarcomas, and sexual dysfunction [82].

*Systemic chemotherapy*

*5-Fluorouracil*

5-FU has been the mainstay of systemic chemotherapy for CRC for more than 30 years. Its efficacy derives from several mechanisms, the most important of which is the drug's ability to combine with methylenetetrahydrofolate to create a relatively stable ternary complex with thymidylate synthase, which inhibits the conversion of deoxyuridylate to thymidylate and interferes with DNA synthesis. 5-FU also directly incorporates into RNA and DNA, compromising RNA processing and translation as well as DNA synthesis and function [83]. Response rates to 5-FU monotherapy range from 10% to 15%. Coadministration of 5-FU with modulators, such as folinic acid (ie, leucovorin calcium [LV]), stabilizes the ternary complex with thymidylate synthase, prolongs 5-FU activity, boosts response rates to 20% to 25%, and marginally increases 1-year survival [84].

The short half-life and S-phase–dependent mechanism of action of 5-FU have prompted efforts to improve efficacy by prolonging drug exposure through various infusional and oral formulations. A recent meta-analysis of six randomized trials comparing bolus with continuous intravenous infusion revealed statistically significant but modest improvements in response rates and survival with continuous infusion regimens [85]. 5-FU–related toxicity seems to depend on the schedule. As compared with bolus regimens, continuous infusion 5-FU is associated with relatively fewer cytopenias but more hand-foot syndrome. These regimens have similar rates of nausea, diarrhea, and mucositis.

Adjuvant approaches using oral fluoropyrimidines potentially offer comparable or superior efficacy and greater ease of administration than intravenous delivery regimens. Capecitabine, an oral prodrug that combines 5-FU with a dihydropyrimidine dehydrogenase inhibitor, has equivalent survival efficacy and an improved toxicity profile as compared with bolus 5-FU–LV in randomized trials [86,87]. Capecitabine was approved in 2001 as first-line therapy for metastatic CRC.

*Irinotecan*

Irinotecan (Camptosar) is an alkaloid derivative that targets topoisomerase I following its conversion to the active metabolite, SN-38. SN-38 stabilizes the DNA-topoisomerase complex, resulting in replication arrest and apoptosis. Toxicities of irinotecan include an acute cholinergic syndrome characterized by salivation, lacrimation, diaphoresis, bradycardia, abdominal cramping, and delayed-onset diarrhea.

Single-agent irinotecan has been shown to improve survival when used as second-line therapy for 5-FU refractory CRC. In addition, a large, randomized, phase III trial of first-line therapy demonstrated improved progression-free and overall survival using irinotecan combined with 5-FU–LV (IFL) as compared with 5-FU–LV alone [88]. This IFL regimen, however, has been associated with death from sudden thromboembolic events and severe gastrointestinal toxicity.

*Oxaliplatin*

Oxaliplatin (Eloxatin), a third-generation platinum compound that forms DNA adducts with bulky 1,2-diaminocyclohexane rings [89], seems to retard DNA repair and induce DNA injury. The toxicity profile of oxaliplatin includes two dose-limiting neurologic syndromes: a transient, cold-induced, sensory neuropathy characterized by dysesthesias and paresthesias occurring during or soon after infusion; and a delayed, dose-dependent neuropathy, occurring in 10% to 15% of patients following a cumulative dose of 750 to 850 mg/m$^2$. Persistent toxicity partially reverses in 75% of patients within 5 months of exposure.

Single-agent oxaliplatin is active in approximately 20% of chemonaïve patients, but is active in only 10% of patients previously treated with 5-FU. Recent randomized, controlled trials have reported improved response rates and longer times to progression with combined oxaliplatin and 5-FU–LV as compared to 5-FU–LV alone (see below).

*Bevacizumab*

Vascular endothelial growth factor is commonly overexpressed in CRC and plays a crucial role in regulating angiogenesis, which is required for tumor growth beyond 1 to 2 mm$^3$. Bevacizumab (Avastin) is a murine antihuman monoclonal antibody against vascular endothelial growth factor that inhibits angiogenesis. This agent may also exert antitumor effects by reducing tumor perfusion, vascular volume, and interstitial pressure; improving delivery of chemotherapeutics; and by sensitizing tumor cells to cytotoxics [90,91]. A regimen combining bevacizumab with bolus IFL was shown to achieve statistically and clinically significant improvements in overall survival, progression-free survival, and response rates among patients with metastatic CRC as compared with an IFL-placebo regimen [92]. The Food and Drug Administration recently approved intravenous bevacizumab, 5 mg/kg, administered every 14 days in combination with intravenous 5-FU–based chemotherapy as first-line therapy for patients with metastatic CRC based on data from two randomized trials. The pivotal trial randomized 813 patients with metastatic CRC to IFL plus bevacizumab versus IFL. Median overall survival was 20.3 versus 15.6 months ($P < .001$) for the IFL plus bevacizumab versus IFL groups. The bevacizumab-treated patients also had a prolonged median progression-free survival (10.6 versus 6.2 months, $P < .001$); improved overall response rate (44.8% versus 34.8%, $P = .004$); and prolonged duration of response (10.4 versus 7.1 months, $P = .001$). A companion trial randomized an additional 104 patients to 5-FU–LV versus 5-FU–LV with bevacizumab, 5 mg/kg every 2 weeks, versus 5-FU–LV with bevacizumab, 10 mg/kg every 2 weeks. Overall survival and response rates were not significantly improved with bevacizumab, but progression-free survival improved from 5.2 months to 9 months at the 5 mg/kg dose level. The reason for the lack of efficacy at the higher dose is unknown.

Bevacizumab is generally well-tolerated. The risk of grade 3 hypertension was fourfold greater with bevacizumab (11% versus 2.3%) in the pivotal trial, but it was generally controlled with standard oral antihypertensives. The most common severe side effects among 1032 patients receiving bevacizumab were gastrointestinal perforation, impaired wound healing, hemorrhage, hypertension, proteinuria, and congestive heart failure. Additional studies of this agent as adjuvant therapy in combination with other agents (eg, oxaliplatin) are ongoing.

*Cetuximab*

Another good target for CRC therapy and possibly prevention is epidermal growth factor receptor, which is thought to play a critical role in intracellular signaling required for tumor growth and progression [93]. Cetuximab (Erbitux) is one of several small molecules and antibodies that have been developed to target epidermal growth factor receptor. Cetuximab is a recombinant, human-mouse chimeric monoclonal antibody that binds specifically and competitively to the extracellular domain of human epidermal growth factor receptor on normal and tumor cells, thereby blocking normal epidermal growth factor receptor ligands [94]. It blocks phosphorylation and activation of receptor-associated kinases, thereby inhibiting cell proliferation, stimulating apoptosis, and decreasing matrix metalloproteinase and vascular endothelial growth factor production.

In a trial of 329 patients with metastatic CRC refractory to irinotecan-based treatment, patients were randomized to receive cetuximab with irinotecan versus cetuximab alone [95]. Objective response rates were greater (22.9% versus 10.8%, $P = .007$) with the combination regimen, and the median time to progression was prolonged (4.1 months versus 1.5 months, $P < .001$). The most serious adverse reactions associated with cetuximab included infusion reactions, dermatologic toxicity, interstitial lung disease, fever, sepsis, kidney failure, pulmonary embolus, dehydration, and diarrhea. These data, among others, led the Food and Drug Administration to grant accelerated approval for cetuximab in combination with irinotecan for patients with epidermal growth factor receptor-expressing metastatic CRC that is refractory to irinotecan-based chemotherapy, and for cetuximab alone in patients with epidermal growth factor receptor-expressing CRC who are unable to tolerate irinotecan-based chemotherapy. Ongoing trials are evaluating the long-term impact of cetuximab on disease progression and survival.

## Multimodal management of colorectal cancer by stage

Multimodal therapy for CRC includes surgery, chemotherapy, or radiation therapy to improve clinical outcomes and palliation, achieve local control, and reduce toxicity, depending on the stage of disease and the clinical setting. An overview of standard therapies for CRC follows according to stage of disease.

### *Stage I*

Approximately 15% of patients present with stage I CRC and have an excellent prognosis. Following complete open surgical resection, 5-year survival exceeds 95%. Although adjuvant therapy has not been shown to reduce the risk of cancer recurrence in this population, a recent randomized, placebo-controlled trial of aspirin, 325 mg/d, in 635 early stage CRC patients suggests that an adjuvant/preventive strategy may complement endoscopic surveillance [57]. At a median follow-up of 12.8 months, this study showed a 35% reduction (from 27% to 17%, $P = .004$) in recurrent adenomas and a 36% increase in the time to detection of the first adenoma ($P = .022$) among those treated with aspirin. Toxicities were comparable between the two groups. These data support a role for chemoprevention in early stage cancer and suggest a promising path for future investigations.

### *Stage II*

Approximately 20% to 30% of patients present with stage II CRC. Following complete surgical resection, 5-year survival is approximately 75% to 85%. The benefit of adjuvant therapy for stage II cancer is controversial, even for patients with unfavorable tumor anatomy, including adherence to adjacent structures, perforation, and obstruction; with unfavorable biology, including aneuploidy, high proliferative fraction, microsatellite instability, and deletion of chromosome 18q; or with unfavorable clinical parameters, such as emergent presentation. Adjuvant chemotherapy was first shown to improve survival in patients with stage II or III disease in 1990, when Moertel et al [96] reported a 33% reduction in mortality among stage III patients treated with 1 year of 5-FU and levamisole. Subsequent randomized trials established 6 months of 5-FU and LV as the standard adjuvant regimen (see stage III, below). Nevertheless, no single trial has demonstrated that 5-FU–based chemotherapy improves survival in stage II patients, even among high-risk subsets. This may be caused by the relatively low-risk of disease recurrence; the limited efficacy of chemotherapy in this setting; or the paucity of stage II patients enrolled in most adjuvant trials.

A recent pooled analysis of five trials testing 5-FU–based therapy versus observation reported a nonsignificant 2% improvement in survival from 80% to 82% at 5 years [97]. NSABP recently compiled data from four adjuvant trials and reported a 30% reduction in mortality among stage II patients [98]. Another independent analysis of pooled data from seven studies involving 3341 patients with stage II or III CRC suggests similar benefits from chemotherapy across all subgroups [99]. Finally, a systematic review of 37 trials and 11 meta-analyses reported a 13% reduction in mortality among stage II CRC patients treated with adjuvant therapy [100]. In clinical practice, patients with stage II cancer are often considered for adjuvant chemotherapy, but the final decision is individualized based on their risk factors, comorbidities, and the toxicity of the proposed regimen. The standard 5-FU–based adjuvant regimen has a 0.5% to 1% treatment-related mortality [101] and new agents or different methods of administration may improve treatment options for patients with stage II CRC and decrease treatment toxicity.

Patients with stage II rectal cancer are at relatively high risk of local relapse, and the benefits of adjuvant chemotherapy and radiation are more established. Adjuvant radiation, given at 45 to 55 Gy either preoperatively or postoperatively, reduces locoregional failure rates [102–104], but the risk of chronic bowel dysfunction mandates scrupulous technique. 5-FU–based chemotherapy combined with radiation increases the disease-free interval, improves disease-free survival, and improves the overall survival for patients with stage II rectal cancer [105,106]. Recent work has established that 5-FU is more effective in this setting when administered by continuous infusion than by intravenous bolus as evidenced by a 10% improved survival [107].

### *Stage III*

Approximately 30% to 40% of patients present with stage III CRC. They have a 55% 5-year survival following surgical resection and adjuvant chemotherapy. Adjuvant chemotherapy or radiation therapy is administered to decrease the risk of local recurrence, eradicate micrometastases, and improve disease-free and overall survival. Intergroup 0035 demonstrated that adjuvant chemotherapy reduces the risk of cancer recurrence and death by approximately 30%, leading to the recommendation for 12 months of adjuvant 5-FU–based chemotherapy for patients with stage III disease [96,108]. A subsequent phase III trial involving 3759 patients with stage II or III disease showed no significant survival differences when 6 months of 5-FU–LV was delivered by either the Mayo or Roswell Park regimens, both of which were superior to 12 months of 5-FU with levamisole [109]. Because of these data, 6 months of 5-FU–LV administered within 3 to 8 weeks of surgery became the standard adjuvant therapy. Investigators have recently evaluated two new agents, irinotecan and oxaliplatin, in the adjuvant setting.

The MOSAIC trial randomized 2246 patients with stage II or III colon cancer to infusional 5-FU with LV or to the same regimen with oxaliplatin (FOLFOX) bimonthly for 12 cycles [110–112]. The FOLFOX-treated patients had significantly improved 3-year disease-free survival (78.2% versus 72.9%), but no survival advantage has been identified to date. Patients receiving FOLFOX had a significantly increased risk of cytopenias; gastrointestinal side effects of nausea, diarrhea, and vomiting; allergic reactions; and sensory neuropathy, most of which were transient. About 12% of patients experienced grade 3 paresthesia during treatment with oxaliplatin, but dropped to 1.1% within 1 year of follow-up.

Currently, 5-FU–LV administered over 6 months is standard adjuvant therapy for stage III patients. Many clinicians, however, now treat patients with adjuvant FOLFOX, based on preliminary evidence of improved disease-free survival and tolerable toxicity from the MOSAIC trial, and expectations of improved survival with longer-term follow-up. Importantly, a recent pooled analysis of trial data indicates that the benefit of adjuvant treatment in patients over 70 years of age is comparable to that observed in younger patients [113].

Patients with stage III rectal cancer are at an increased risk of locoregional recurrence, and often receive radiation therapy, typically with concurrent infusional 5-FU, a known radiation sensitizer [114]. In certain cases, neoadjuvant radiation therapy, with or without chemotherapy, may also be administered to preserve sphincter function [115,116].

### *Stage IV*

Approximately 20% to 25% of patients present with stage IV CRC, which has an average 5-year survival of less than 5%. Treatment of these patients depends on the extent and the location of disease. Although surgical options are very limited, they provide the only potential for cure. The most common site of tumor recurrence is the liver, with up to 50% of patients developing hepatic metastases during the course of their disease. Patients with disease limited to a small number of liver (or lung) metastases, adequate liver (or lung) reserve, and good performance status may benefit from resection of the CRC primary and metastatic foci with curative intent [117]. It is unclear whether adjuvant chemotherapy confers additional benefit. One study of adjuvant chemotherapy following resection of hepatic metastases reported reductions in hepatic recurrence, but no impact on survival [118].

Unresectable hepatic metastases may be treated with radiofrequency or cryosurgical ablation to achieve long-term local control [119,120]. These patients may also benefit from chemotherapy intended to prolong and improve the quality of life by controlling local disease and reducing the burden of systemic disease. Hepatic intra-arterial chemotherapy with floxuridine achieves higher response rates, but is associated with liver function abnormalities and, in some cases, fatal biliary sclerosis. Overall, studies have failed to demonstrate a survival advantage of local therapy over systemic therapy, and this intervention is recommended only within the scope of a clinical trial [103].

Systemic chemotherapy with 5-FU–based regimens provides palliation for patients with locally advanced, metastatic, or recurrent cancer. Two randomized trials of 5-FU–based therapies documented increased partial responses and prolonged time-to-progression among treated patients as compared with those receiving supportive care [121,122]. Other trials have also documented improved survival and quality of life among patients with advanced disease who received 5-FU–based regimens [123,124].

More recently, patients treated with various three-drug combinations, such as IFL, have had improved survival rates, but with greater, although still manageable, toxicity [125,126]. A recent trial of IFL versus 5-FU–LV in patients with advanced CRC demonstrated significantly longer progression-free survival (7.9 versus 4.3 months, $P = .004$); a higher response rate (39% versus 21%, $P < .001$); and prolonged overall median survival (14.8 months versus 12.6 months, $P = .04$) [88]. The irinotecan-containing AIO regimen has demonstrated similar efficacy and is considered a standard first-line regimen in the United States [127].

Recent approval of oxaliplatin for the treatment of metastatic CRC was based on data from several trials suggesting improved progression-free survival, response rates, and overall survival [128–130]. The most recently reported comparative trial documented a median time to progression of 8.7 months, a response rate of 45%, and median survival of 19.5 months with FOLFOX, as well as lower rates of gastrointestinal side effects, febrile neutropenia, and dehydration. This regimen was found to be superior to IFL and IROX (irinotecan and oxaliplatin) in terms of both efficacy and toxicity. Based on these data, FOLFOX was recommended as a new first-line standard of care for patients with advanced CRC [130]. European investigators have reported data from a single-arm trial of XELOX with excellent response rates and median survival (55% and 19.5 months, respectively), and low rates of myelosuppression (grade 3 or 4 neutropenia in 7% of treated patients), suggesting that intravenous oxaliplatin combined with oral capecitabine may be effective and convenient for certain patients [131]. Confirmation in a large definitive phase III trial is needed before adopting this regimen as a standard first-line approach for the management of advanced CRC.

The choice of first-line CRC therapeutic regimens for patients with locally advanced, unresectable, or metastatic cancer is complex because few trials have compared the different regimens. Treatment decisions often depend on multiple factors (physician experience, patient preference, comorbidities, cost, reimbursement, and convenience) rather than efficacy alone. Currently, the menu of available treatment options includes AIO; FOLFOX4; FOLFOX6; FOLFIRI; IFL (or Saltz regimen); IFL plus bevacizumab; NCCTG 5-FU–LV regimen (low-dose LV); and NSABP 5-FU–LV regimen (high-dose LV) (Table 3). Many practitioners use FOLFOX as a first choice for patients with a good medical status, but recent data showing the superiority of IFL plus bevacizumab suggest another good, albeit expensive, option [132].

The choice of second-line treatment depends on the patient's initial therapy. For example, patients previously treated with irinotecan-based regimens should receive FOLFOX; and those treated with FOLFOX should receive irinotecan-based regimens. The recent approval of cetuximab provides another acceptable option. Indeed, in the pivotal trial roughly 23% of irinotecan-refractory patients had an objective response to the combination of irinotecan plus cetuximab [95]. An ongoing study is exploring whether bevacizumab is also effective in this setting [132].

Table 3
Drug combinations for colorectal cancer chemotherapy

| Regimen | Agents and schedule |
| --- | --- |
| AIO | Irinotecan as a 2-h infusion on day 1; leucovorin as a 2-h infusion on day 1; followed by 5-FU IV bolus by ambulatory pump over 24 h weekly × 4 every 52 wk |
| FOLFOX4 | Oxaliplatin as a 2-h infusion on day 1; leucovorin as a 2-h infusion on days 1 and 2; followed by a loading dose of 5-FU IV bolus, then 5-FU by ambulatory pump over 22 h on days 1 and 2, every 2 wk |
| FOLFOX6 | Oxaliplatin as a 2-h infusion on day 1; leucovorin as a 2-h infusion on day 1; followed by a loading dose of 5-FU IV bolus on day 1, then 5-FU by ambulatory pump over 46 h every 2 wk |
| FOLFIRI | Irinotecan as a 2-h infusion on day 1; leucovorin as a 2-h infusion on day 1; followed by a loading dose of 5-FU IV bolus on day 1, then 5-FU by ambulatory pump over 46 h every 2 wk |
| IFL (or Saltz) | Irinotecan, 5-FU IV bolus, and leucovorin IV bolus weekly for 4 out of 6 wk |
| IFL plus bevacizumab | Irinotecan, 5-FU, and leucovorin IV once weekly for 4 out of 6 wk, with bevacizumab IV every 2 wk |
| NCCTG 5-FU–LV (low-dose LV) | Bolus 5-FU plus leucovorin daily for 5 d, every 28 d |
| NSABP 5-FU–LV (high-dose LV) | Bolus 5-FU plus leucovorin weekly for 6 consecutive wk, every 8 wk |

*Abbreviations:* IV, intravenous; NCCTG, North Central Cancer Treatment Group; NSABP, National Surgical Adjuvant Breast and Bowel Project.

## Future directions in colorectal cancer prevention and therapy

Rapid progress in CRC treatment during the last 5 years has led to novel treatments and public health quandaries. Multiple regimens have gained scientific and regulatory acceptance, but the relative merits of these regimens are difficult to discern because of a paucity of comparative trials. Moreover, therapy tailored according to CRC risk and responsiveness based on a biologic characterization of disease is in its infancy. Finally, the impact of emerging CRC therapies on medical expenditures has yet to be tallied. For example, adding bevacizumab to standard combination chemotherapy for the 30,000 to 40,000 new patients diagnosed with advanced CRC annually is expected to cost $1.5 billion [132]. Prolongation of survival, even when cure is unattainable as in most cases of metastatic CRC, is a worthy goal, but ultimately the cost must be borne by a healthcare system that is already overburdened.

Despite advances in therapy, the allure of cancer screening and prevention is undeniable; and these have emerged as dominant strategies for combating CRC. These twin strategies are logical and effective, and a growing body of data demonstrates meaningful reductions in CRC incidence and mortality with readily available approaches [133]. Four randomized, controlled trials including several hundred thousand individuals have shown 15% to 30% reductions in CRC mortality with annual fecal occult blood testing [134,135], and even better tools are under development. Newer screening tests, such as CT colonography and molecularly-based stool tests, are likely to improve test sensitivity and specificity, as well as efficacy and safety. In addition, these new technologies are providing insights into molecular carcinogenesis, which can then be transformed into targets for cancer chemoprevention.

Clinical testing remains the rate-limiting step in the translation of new technologies into tools for clinical practice. The participation of practicing physicians and their patients in this process has been meager to date. This issue, perhaps more than any other, limits the pace and progress of clinical research. Creative ideas have been promoted to address this persistent challenge (eg, new research infrastructures, incentives for health care professionals and patients, and education and marketing strategies), none of which can match the power of this simple message: CRC should be preventable or highly treatable when prevention fails. The reason we fall short of this goal has more to do with lack of commitment than any lack of insight. Participation in clinical trials, as patients and practitioners, may provide some of our best opportunities to shape public health now and for the future.

## References

[1] Jemal A, Tiwari RC, Murray T, Ghafoor A, Samuels A, Ward E, et al. Cancer statistics, 2004. CA Cancer J Clin 2004;54:8–29.

[2] Hanahan D, Weinberg RA. The hallmarks of cancer. Cell 2000;100:57–70.
[3] Takayama T, Ohi M, Hayashi T, Miyanishi K, Nobuoka A, Nakajima T, et al. Analysis of K-ras, APC, and beta-catenin in aberrant crypt foci in sporadic adenoma, cancer, and familial adenomatous polyposis. Gastroenterology 2001;121:599–611.
[4] Ilyas M, Straub J, Tomlinson IP, Bodmer WF. Genetic pathways in colorectal and other cancers. Eur J Cancer 1999;35:1986–2002.
[5] Hawk ET, Limburg PJ, Viner JL. Epidemiology and prevention of colorectal cancer. Surg Clin North Am 2002;82:905–41.
[6] Lichtenstein P, Holm NV, Verkasalo PK, Iliadou A, Kaprio J, Koskenvuo M, et al. Environmental and heritable factors in the causation of cancer: analyses of cohorts of twins from Sweden, Denmark, and Finland. N Engl J Med 2000;343:78–85.
[7] Sporn MB. Approaches to prevention of epithelial cancer during the preneoplastic period. Cancer Res 1976;36(7 pt 2):2699–702.
[8] Bussey HJ, DeCosse JJ, Deschner EE, Eyers AA, Lesser ML, Morson BC, et al. A randomized trial of ascorbic acid in polyposis coli. Cancer 1982;50:1434–9.
[9] Schatzkin A, Lanza E, Corle D, Lance P, Iber F, Caan B, et al. Lack of effect of a low-fat, high-fiber diet on the recurrence of colorectal adenomas. Polyp Prevention Trial Study Group. N Engl J Med 2000;342:1149–55.
[10] MacLennan R, Macrae F, Bain C, Battistutta D, Chapuis P, Gratten H, et al. Randomized trial of intake of fat, fiber, and beta carotene to prevent colorectal adenomas. The Australian Polyp Prevention Project. J Natl Cancer Inst 1995;87:1760–6.
[11] DeCosse JJ, Miller HH, Lesser ML. Effect of wheat fiber and vitamins C and E on rectal polyps in patients with familial adenomatous polyposis. J Natl Cancer Inst 1989;81:1290–7.
[12] Hofstad B, Almendingen K, Vatn M, Andersen SN, Owen RW, Larsen S, et al. Growth and recurrence of colorectal polyps: a double-blind 3-year intervention with calcium and antioxidants. Digestion 1998;59:148–56.
[13] Alberts DS, Martinez ME, Roe DJ, Guillen-Rodriguez JM, Marshall JR, van Leeuwen JB, et al. Lack of effect of a high-fiber cereal supplement on the recurrence of colorectal adenomas. Phoenix Colon Cancer Prevention Pysicians' Network. N Engl J Med 2000;342:1156–62.
[14] Faivre J, Bonithon-Kopp C. Effect of fibre and calcium supplementation on adenoma recurrence and growth. IARC Sci Publ 2002;156:457–61.
[15] Greenberg ER, Baron JA, Tosteson TD, Freeman DH Jr, Beck GJ, Bond JH, et al. A clinical trial of antioxidant vitamins to prevent colorectal adenoma. Polyp Prevention Study Group. N Engl J Med 1994;331:141–7.
[16] Malila N, Virtamo J, Virtanen M, Albanes D, Tangrea JA, Huttunen JK. The effect of alpha-tocopherol and beta-carotene supplementation on colorectal adenomas in middle-aged male smokers. Cancer Epidemiol Biomarkers Prev 1999;8:489–93.
[17] Albanes D, Malila N, Taylor PR, Huttunen JK, Virtamo J, Edwards BK, et al. Effects of supplemental alpha-tocopherol and beta-carotene on colorectal cancer: results from a controlled trial (Finland). Cancer Causes Control 2000;11:197–205.
[18] Gann PH, Manson JE, Glynn RJ, Buring JE, Hennekens CH. Low-dose aspirin and incidence of colorectal tumors in a randomized trial. J Natl Cancer Inst 1993;85:1220–4.
[19] Baron JA, Cole BF, Sandler RS, Haile RW, Ahnen D, Bresalier R, et al. A randomized trial of aspirin to prevent colorectal adenomas. N Engl J Med 2003;348:891–9.
[20] Alberts DS, Martinez ME, Roe D, Einspahr JG, Guillen J, Clouser M, et al. Proving the bile acid hypothesis for colon carcinogenesis: mature results from a phase III chemoprevention trial of ursodeoxycholic acid versus placebo to prevent colorectal adenoma recurrence. ASCO Proceedings 2003;363.
[21] Steinbach G, Lynch PM, Phillips RK, Wallace MH, Hawk E, Gordon GB, et al. The effect of celecoxib, a cyclooxygenase-2 inhibitor, in familial adenomatous polyposis. N Engl J Med 2000;342:1946–52.
[22] Shamberger RJ, Tytko SA, Willis CE. Antioxidants and cancer. Part VI. Selenium and age-adjusted human cancer mortality. Arch Environ Health 1976;31:231–5.

[23] Knekt P, Aromaa A, Maatela J, Alfthan G, Aaran RK, Teppo L, et al. Serum vitamin E, serum selenium and the risk of gastrointestinal cancer. Int J Cancer 1988; 42:846–50.
[24] Knekt P, Aromaa A, Maatela J, Alfthan G, Aaran RK, Hakama M, et al. Serum selenium and subsequent risk of cancer among Finnish men and women. J Natl Cancer Inst 1990;82: 864–8.
[25] Clark LC, Hixson LJ, Combs GF Jr, Reid ME, Turnbull BW, Sampliner RE. Plasma selenium concentration predicts the prevalence of colorectal adenomatous polyps. Cancer Epidemiol Biomarkers Prev 1993;2:41–6.
[26] Nelson RL, Davis FG, Sutter E, Kikendall JW, Sobin LH, Milner JA, et al. Serum selenium and colonic neoplastic risk. Dis Colon Rectum 1995;38:1306–10.
[27] Clark LC, Combs GF Jr, Turnbull BW, Slate EH, Chalker DK, Chow J, et al. Effects of selenium supplementation for cancer prevention in patients with carcinoma of the skin: a randomized controlled trial. Nutritional Prevention of Cancer Study Group. JAMA 1996; 276:1957–63 [published erratum appears in JAMA 1997;277:1520].
[28] Giovannucci E, Goldin B. The role of fat, fatty acids, and total energy intake in the etiology of human colon cancer. Am J Clin Nutr 1997;66(Suppl 6):1564S–71S.
[29] Narisawa T, Magadia NE, Weisburger JH, Wynder EL. Promoting effect of bile acids on colon carcinogenesis after intrarectal instillation of N-methyl-N'-nitro-N-nitrosoguanidine in rats. J Natl Cancer Inst 1974;53:1093–7.
[30] Bautista D, Obrador A, Moreno V, Cabeza E, Canet R, Benito E, et al. Ki-*ras* mutation modifies the protective effect of dietary monounsaturated fat and calcium on sporadic colorectal cancer. Cancer Epidemiol Biomarkers Prev 1997;6:57–61.
[31] Baron JA, Beach M, Mandel JS, van Stolk RU, Haile RW, Sandler RS, et al. Calcium supplements for the prevention of colorectal adenomas. Calcium Polyp Prevention Study Group. N Engl J Med 1999;340:101–7.
[32] Baron JA, Cole BF, Mott LA. Group FtPPS: aspirin chemoprevention of colorectal adenomas. Proc AACR 2002;43:669.
[33] Bonithon-Kopp C, Kronborg O, Giacosa A, Rath U, Faivre J. Calcium and fibre supplementation in prevention of colorectal adenoma recurrence: a randomised intervention trial. European Cancer Prevention Organization Study Group. Lancet 2000;356: 1300–6.
[34] Design of the Women's Health Initiative clinical trial and observational study. The Women's Health Initiative Study Group. Control Clin Trials 1998;19:61–109.
[35] Borgelt L, Umland E. Benefits and challenges of hormone replacement therapy. J Am Pharm Assoc (Wash) 2000;40(5 Suppl 1):S30–1.
[36] Grodstein F, Martinez ME, Platz EA, Giovannucci E, Colditz GA, Kautzky M, et al. Postmenopausal hormone use and risk for colorectal cancer and adenoma. Ann Intern Med 1998;128:705–12.
[37] Calle EE, Miracle-McMahill HL, Thun MJ, Heath CWJ. Estrogen replacement therapy and risk of fatal colon cancer in a prospective cohort of postmenopausal women. J Natl Cancer Inst 1995;87:517–23.
[38] Guo JY, Li X, Browning JD Jr, Rottinghaus GE, Lubahn DB, Constantinou A, et al. Dietary soy isoflavones and estrone protect ovariectomized ERalphaKO and wild-type mice from carcinogen-induced colon cancer. J Nutr 2004;134:179–82.
[39] Rossouw JE, Anderson GL, Prentice RL, LaCroix AZ, Kooperberg C, Stefanick ML, et al. Risks and benefits of estrogen plus progestin in healthy postmenopausal women: principal results From the Women's Health Initiative randomized controlled trial. JAMA 2002;288: 321–33.
[40] MacLennan SC, MacLennan AH, Ryan P. Colorectal cancer and oestrogen replacement therapy: a meta-analysis of epidemiological studies. Med J Aust 1995;162:491–3.
[41] Nanda K, Bastian LA, Hasselblad V, Simel DL. Hormone replacement therapy and the risk of colorectal cancer: a meta-analysis. Obstet Gynecol 1999;93(5 Pt 2):880–8.

[42] Hawk ET, Viner JL, Umar A, Anderson WF, Sigman CC, Guyton KZ. Cancer and the cyclooxygenase enzyme: implications for the treatment and prevention. Am J Cancer 2003; 2:27–55.

[43] Sheehan KM, Sheahan K, O'Donoghue DP, MacSweeney F, Conroy RM, Fitzgerald DJ, et al. The relationship between cyclooxygenase-2 expression and colorectal cancer. JAMA 1999;282:1254–7.

[44] Ristimaki A, Sivula A, Lundin J, Lundin M, Salminen T, Haglund C, et al. Prognostic significance of elevated cyclooxygenase-2 expression in breast cancer. Cancer Res 2002;62: 632–5.

[45] Gaffney DK, Holden J, Davis M, Zempolich K, Murphy KJ, Dodson M. Elevated cyclooxygenase-2 expression correlates with diminished survival in carcinoma of the cervix treated with radiotherapy. Int J Radiat Oncol Biol Phys 2001;49:1213–7.

[46] Buskens CJ, Van Rees BP, Sivula A, Reitsma JB, Haglund C, Bosma PJ, et al. Prognostic significance of elevated cyclooxygenase 2 expression in patients with adenocarcinoma of the esophagus. Gastroenterology 2002;122:1800–7.

[47] Khuri FR, Wu H, Lee JJ, Kemp BL, Lotan R, Lippman SM, et al. Cyclooxygenase-2 overexpression is a marker of poor prognosis in stage I non-small cell lung cancer. Clin Cancer Res 2001;7:861–7.

[48] Marnett LJ, DuBois RN. COX-2: a target for colon cancer prevention. Annu Rev Pharmacol Toxicol 2002;42:55–80.

[49] Lehmann JM, Lenhard JM, Oliver BB, Ringold GM, Kliewer SA. Peroxisome proliferator-activated receptors alpha and gamma are activated by indomethacin and other non-steroidal anti-inflammatory drugs. J Biol Chem 1997;272:3406–10.

[50] Hsu AL, Ching TT, Wang DS, Song X, Rangnekar VM, Chen CS. The cyclooxygenase-2 inhibitor celecoxib induces apoptosis by blocking Akt activation in human prostate cancer cells independently of Bcl-2. J Biol Chem 2000;275:11397–403.

[51] Waskewich C, Blumenthal RD, Li H, Stein R, Goldenberg DM, Burton J. Celecoxib exhibits the greatest potency amongst cyclooxygenase (COX) inhibitors for growth inhibition of COX-2-negative hematopoietic and epithelial cell lines. Cancer Res 2002;62: 2029–33.

[52] Hawk E, Lubet R, Limburg P. Chemoprevention in hereditary colorectal cancer syndromes. Cancer 1999;86:2551–63.

[53] Cruz-Correa M, Hylind LM, Romans KE, Booker SV, Giardiello FM. Long-term treatment with sulindac in familial adenomatous polyposis: a prospective cohort study. Gastroenterology 2002;122:641–5.

[54] Chan AT, Giovannucci EL, Schernhammer ES, Colditz GA, Hunter DJ, Willett WC, et al. A prospective study of aspirin use and the risk for colorectal adenoma. Ann Intern Med 2004;140:157–66.

[55] Giardiello FM, Yang VW, Hylind LM, Krush AJ, Petersen GM, Trimbath JD, et al. Primary chemoprevention of familial adenomatous polyposis with sulindac. N Engl J Med 2002;346:1054–9.

[56] Burn J, Chapman PD, Bishop DT, Dixon R, Turner F, Coaker J, et al. Results of the CAPP1 Study: aspirin and resistant starch are beneficial in familial adenomatous polyposis. Familial Cancer 2003;2(Suppl 1):42.

[57] Sandler RS, Halabi S, Baron JA, Budinger S, Paskett E, Keresztes R, et al. A randomized trial of aspirin to prevent colorectal adenomas in patients with previous colorectal cancer. N Engl J Med 2003;348:883–90.

[58] Benamouzig R, Deyra J, Martin A, Girard B, Jullian E, Piednoir B, et al. Daily soluble aspirin and prevention of colorectal adenoma recurrence: one-year results of the APACC trial. Gastroenterology 2003;125:328–36.

[59] Muir K, Logan R, Armitage N. The United Kingdom colorectal adenoma prevention trial (ukCAP): trial description and recruited patient characteristics. In: Frontiers in cancer prevention research. Boston: 2002.

[60] Rexrode KM, Lee IM, Cook NR, Hennekens CH, Buring JE. Baseline characteristics of participants in the Women's Health Study. J Womens Health Gend Based Med 2000;9: 19–27.
[61] Phillips RK, Wallace MH, Lynch PM, Hawk E, Gordon GB, Saunders BP, et al. A randomised, double blind, placebo controlled study of celecoxib, a selective cyclooxygenase 2 inhibitor, on duodenal polyposis in familial adenomatous polyposis. Gut 2002;50:857–60.
[62] Sinicrope FA, Half EO, Morris JS, Lynch PM, Morrow JD, Levin B, et al. Cell proliferation and apoptotic indices predict adenoma regression in a placebo-controlled trial of celecoxib in familial adenomatous polyposis (FAP) patients. Cancer Epidemiol Biomarkers Prev 2004;13.
[63] Xiao Z, Luke BT, Izmirlian G, Umar A, Lynch PM, Phillips RK, et al. Serum proteomic profiles suggest celecoxib-modulated targets and response predictors. Cancer Res 2004;64: 2904–9.
[64] Hallak A, Alon-Baron L, Shamir R, Moshkowitz M, Bulvik B, Brazowski E, et al. Rofecoxib reduces polyp recurrence in familial polyposis. Dig Dis Sci 2003;48:1998–2002.
[65] Maurel J, Launoy G, Grosclaude P, Gignoux M, Arveux P, Mathieu-Daude H, et al. Lymph node harvest reporting in patients with carcinoma of the large bowel: a French population-based study. Cancer 1998;82:1482–6.
[66] Wong JH, Severino R, Honnebier MB, Tom P, Namiki TS. Number of nodes examined and staging accuracy in colorectal carcinoma. J Clin Oncol 1999;17:2896–900.
[67] Wong JH. Improved methods to stage cancer: the evolving role of sentinel node staging in solid malignancies. Hawaii Med J 2002;61:260.
[68] Goldstein NS, Sanford W, Coffey M, Layfield LJ. Lymph node recovery from colorectal resection specimens removed for adenocarcinoma: trends over time and a recommendation for a minimum number of lymph nodes to be recovered. Am J Clin Pathol 1996;106:209–16.
[69] Le Voyer TE, Sigurdson ER, Hanlon AL, Mayer RJ, Macdonald JS, Catalano PJ, et al. Colon cancer survival is associated with increasing number of lymph nodes analyzed: a secondary survey of intergroup trial INT-0089. J Clin Oncol 2003;21:2912–9.
[70] Hodgson DC, Fuchs CS, Ayanian JZ. Impact of patient and provider characteristics on the treatment and outcomes of colorectal cancer. J Natl Cancer Inst 2001;93:501–15.
[71] Hahnloser D, Nelson H. Laparoscopic colectomy for colon cancer. Minerva Chir 2003;58: 431–8.
[72] A comparison of laparoscopically assisted and open colectomy for colon cancer. N Engl J Med 2004;350:2050–9.
[73] Gunderson LL, Sosin H. Areas of failure found at reoperation (second or symptomatic look) following "curative surgery" for adenocarcinoma of the rectum: clinicopathologic correlation and implications for adjuvant therapy. Cancer 1974;34:1278–92.
[74] Rich T, Gunderson LL, Lew R, Galdibini JJ, Cohen AM, Donaldson G. Patterns of recurrence of rectal cancer after potentially curative surgery. Cancer 1983;52:1317–29.
[75] Mendenhall WM, Million RR, Pfaff WW. Patterns of recurrence in adenocarcinoma of the rectum and rectosigmoid treated with surgery alone: implications in treatment planning with adjuvant radiation therapy. Int J Radiat Oncol Biol Phys 1983;9:977–85.
[76] Prolongation of the disease-free interval in surgically treated rectal carcinoma. Gastrointestinal Tumor Study Group. N Engl J Med 1985;312:1465–72.
[77] Wolmark N, Wieand HS, Hyams DM, Colangelo L, Dimitrov NV, Romond EH, et al. Randomized trial of postoperative adjuvant chemotherapy with or without radiotherapy for carcinoma of the rectum: National Surgical Adjuvant Breast and Bowel Project Protocol R-02. J Natl Cancer Inst 2000;92:388–96.
[78] Improved survival with preoperative radiotherapy in resectable rectal cancer. Swedish Rectal Cancer Trial. N Engl J Med 1997;336:980–7.
[79] Minsky BD, Cohen AM, Kemeny N, Enker WE, Kelsen DP, Reichman B, et al. Combined modality therapy of rectal cancer: decreased acute toxicity with the preoperative approach. J Clin Oncol 1992;10:1218–24.

[80] Bosset JF, Calais G, Daban A, Berger C, Radosevic-Jelic L, Maingon P, et al. Preoperative chemoradiotherapy versus preoperative radiotherapy in rectal cancer patients: assessment of acute toxicity and treatment compliance. Report of the 22921 randomised trial conducted by the EORTC Radiotherapy Group. Eur J Cancer 2004;40: 219–24.
[81] Vigliotti A, Rich TA, Romsdahl MM, Withers HR, Oswald MJ. Postoperative adjuvant radiotherapy for adenocarcinoma of the rectum and rectosigmoid. Int J Radiat Oncol Biol Phys 1987;13:999–1006.
[82] Johnston MJ, Robertson GM, Frizelle FA. Management of late complications of pelvic radiation in the rectum and anus: a review. Dis Colon Rectum 2003;46:247–59.
[83] Pinedo HM, Peters GF. Fluorouracil: biochemistry and pharmacology. J Clin Oncol 1988; 6:1653–64.
[84] Buroker TR, Oconnell MJ, Wieand HS, Krook JE, Gerstner JB, Mailliard JA, et al. Randomized comparison of 2 schedules of fluorouracil and leucovorin in the treatment of advanced colorectal-cancer. J Clin Oncol 1994;12:14–20.
[85] Efficacy of intravenous continuous infusion of fluorouracil compared with bolus administration in advanced colorectal cancer. Meta-Analysis Group in Cancer. J Clin Oncol 1998;16:301–8.
[86] Hoff PM, Ansari R, Batist G, Cox J, Kocha W, Kuperminc M, et al. Comparison of oral capecitabine versus intravenous fluorouracil plus leucovorin as first-line treatment in 605 patients with metastatic colorectal cancer: results of a randomized phase III study. J Clin Oncol 2001;19:2282–92.
[87] Van Cutsem E, Twelves C, Cassidy J, Allman D, Bajetta E, Boyer M, et al. Oral capecitabine compared with intravenous fluorouracil plus leucovorin in patients with metastatic colorectal cancer: results of a large phase III study. J Clin Oncol 2001;19: 4097–106.
[88] Saltz LB, Cox JV, Blanke C, Rosen LS, Fehrenbacher L, Moore MJ, et al. Irinotecan plus fluorouracil and leucovorin for metastatic colorectal cancer. Irinotecan Study Group. N Engl J Med 2000;343:905–14.
[89] Tashiro T, Kawada Y, Sakurai Y, Kidani Y. Antitumor-activity of a new platinum complex, oxalato (trans-L- 1,2-diaminocyclohexane)platinum(Ii): new experimental data. Biomed Pharmacother 1989;43:251–60.
[90] Willett CG, Boucher Y, di Tomaso E, Duda DG, Munn LL, Tong RT, et al. Direct evidence that the VEGF-specific antibody bevacizumab has antivascular effects in human rectal cancer. Nat Med 2004;10:145–7.
[91] Jain RK. Normalizing tumor vasculature with anti-angiogenic therapy: a new paradigm for combination therapy. Nat Med 2001;7:987–9.
[92] Hurwitz H, Fehrenbacher L, Novotny W, Cartwright T, Hainsworth J, Heim W, et al. Bevacizumab plus irinotecan, fluorouracil, and leucovorin for metastatic colorectal cancer. N Engl J Med 2004;350:2335–42.
[93] Mendelsohn J. Targeting the epidermal growth factor receptor for cancer therapy. J Clin Oncol 2002;20(Suppl 18):1S–13S.
[94] Baselga J. The EGFR as a target for anticancer therapy: focus on cetuximab. Eur J Cancer 2001;37(Suppl 4):S16–22.
[95] Cunningham D, Humblet Y, Siena S, Khayat D, Bleiberg H, Santoro A, et al. Cetuximab monotherapy and cetuximab plus irinotecan in irinotecan-refractory metastatic colorectal cancer. N Engl J Med 2004;351:337–45.
[96] Moertel CG, Fleming TR, Macdonald JS, Haller DG, Laurie JA, Goodman PJ, et al. Levamisole and fluorouracil for adjuvant therapy of resected colon carcinoma. N Engl J Med 1990;322:352–8.
[97] Efficacy of adjuvant fluorouracil and folinic acid in B2 colon cancer. International Multicentre Pooled Analysis of B2 Colon Cancer Trials (IMPACT B2) Investigators. J Clin Oncol 1999;17:1356–63.

[98] Mamounas E, Wieand S, Wolmark N, Bear HD, Atkins JN, Song K, et al. Comparative efficacy of adjuvant chemotherapy in patients with Dukes' B versus Dukes' c colon cancer: results from four national surgical adjuvant breast and bowel project adjuvant studies (C-01, C-02, C-03, and C-04). J Clin Oncol 1999;17:1349–55.
[99] Gill S, Loprinzi CL, Sargent DJ, Thome SD, Alberts SR, Haller DG, et al. Pooled analysis of fluorouracil-based adjuvant therapy for stage II and III colon cancer: who benefits and by how much? J Clin Oncol 2004.
[100] Figueredo A, Charette ML, Maroun J, Brouwers MC, Zuraw L. Adjuvant therapy for stage II colon cancer: a systematic review from the Cancer Care Ontario Program in Evidence-Based Care's Gastrointestinal Cancer Disease Site Group. J Clin Oncol 2004.
[101] Moertel CG, Fleming TR, Macdonald JS, Haller DG, Laurie JA, Tangen CM, et al. Intergroup study of fluorouracil plus levamisole as adjuvant therapy for stage II/Dukes' B2 colon cancer. J Clin Oncol 1995;13:2936–43.
[102] Local recurrence rate in a randomised multicentre trial of preoperative radiotherapy compared with operation alone in resectable rectal carcinoma. Swedish Rectal Cancer Trial. Eur J Surg 1996;162:397–402.
[103] Reappraisal of hepatic arterial infusion in the treatment of nonresectable liver metastases from colorectal cancer. Meta-Analysis Group in Cancer. J Natl Cancer Inst 1996;88: 252–8.
[104] Randomised trial of surgery alone versus surgery followed by radiotherapy for mobile cancer of the rectum. Medical Research Council Rectal Cancer Working Party. Lancet 1996;348:1610–4.
[105] Thomas PR, Lindblad AS. Adjuvant postoperative radiotherapy and chemotherapy in rectal carcinoma: a review of the Gastrointestinal Tumor Study Group experience. Radiother Oncol 1988;13:245–52.
[106] Krook JE, Moertel CG, Gunderson LL, Wieand HS, Collins RT, Beart RW, et al. Effective surgical adjuvant therapy for high-risk rectal carcinoma. N Engl J Med 1991;324:709–15.
[107] O'Connell MJ, Martenson JA, Wieand HS, Krook JE, Macdonald JS, Haller DG, et al. Improving adjuvant therapy for rectal cancer by combining protracted-infusion fluorouracil with radiation therapy after curative surgery. N Engl J Med 1994;331:502–7.
[108] NIH consensus conference. Adjuvant therapy for patients with colon and rectal cancer. JAMA 1990;264:1444–50.
[109] Haller DG, Catalano PJ, Macdonald JS, Mayer RJ. Fluorouracil (FU), leucovorin (LV) and levamisole (LEV) adjuvant therapy for colon cancer: five year final report of INT-0089. Presented at the Annual Meeting of American Society of Clinical Oncology, 1998.
[110] Maindrault-Goebel F, Tournigand C, Andre T, Carola E, Mabro M, Artru P, et al. Oxaliplatin reintroduction in patients previously treated with leucovorin, fluorouracil and oxaliplatin for metastatic colorectal cancer. Ann Oncol 2004;15:1210–4.
[111] Andre T, Louvet C, Raymond E, Tournigand C, de Gramont A. Bimonthly high-dose leucovorin, 5-fluorouracil infusion and oxaliplatin (FOLFOX3) for metastatic colorectal cancer resistant to the same leucovorin and 5-fluorouracil regimen. Ann Oncol 1998;9: 1251–3.
[112] O'Connell MJ. Current status of adjuvant therapy for colorectal cancer. Oncology (Huntingt) 2004;18:751–5 [discussion: 5–8].
[113] Sargent DJ, Goldberg RM, Jacobson SD, Macdonald JS, Labianca R, Haller DG, et al. A pooled analysis of adjuvant chemotherapy for resected colon cancer in elderly patients. N Engl J Med 2001;345:1091–7.
[114] Oconnell M, Martenson JA, Wieand HS, Krook JE, Macdonald JS, Haller DG, et al. Improving adjuvant therapy for rectal-cancer by combining protracted-infusion fluorouracil with radiation-therapy after curative surgery. N Engl J Med 1994;331:502–7.
[115] Mohiuddin M, Regine WF, Marks GJ, Marks JW. High-dose preoperative radiation and the challenge of sphincter-preservation surgery for cancer of the distal 2 cm of the rectum. Int J Radiat Oncol Biol Phys 1998;40:569–74.

[116] Valentini V, Coco C, Cellini N, Picciocchi A, Genovesi D, Mantini G, et al. Preoperative chemoradiation for extraperitoneal T3 rectal cancer: acute toxicity, tumor response, and sphincter preservation. Int J Radiat Oncol Biol Phys 1998;40:1067–75.

[117] Harmon KE, Ryan JA Jr, Biehl TR, Lee FT. Benefits and safety of hepatic resection for colorectal metastases. Am J Surg 1999;177:402–4.

[118] Kemeny MM, Adak S, Gray B, Macdonald JS, Smith T, Lipsitz S, et al. Combined-modality treatment for resectable metastatic colorectal carcinoma to the liver: surgical resection of hepatic metastases in combination with continuous infusion of chemotherapy–an intergroup study. J Clin Oncol 2002;20:1499–505.

[119] Oshowo A, Gillams A, Harrison E, Lees WR, Taylor I. Comparison of resection and radiofrequency ablation for treatment of solitary colorectal liver metastases. Br J Surg 2003;90:1240–3.

[120] Sotsky TK, Ravikumar TS. Cryotherapy in the treatment of liver metastases from colorectal cancer. Semin Oncol 2002;29:183–91.

[121] Petrelli N, Herrera L, Rustum Y, Burke P, Creaven P, Stulc J, et al. A prospective randomized trial of 5-fluorouracil versus 5-fluorouracil and high-dose leucovorin versus 5-fluorouracil and methotrexate in previously untreated patients with advanced colorectal carcinoma. J Clin Oncol 1987;5:1559–65.

[122] Petrelli N, Douglass HO Jr, Herrera L, Russell D, Stablein DM, Bruckner HW, et al. The modulation of fluorouracil with leucovorin in metastatic colorectal carcinoma: a prospective randomized phase III trial. Gastrointestinal Tumor Study Group. J Clin Oncol 1989;7:1419–26.

[123] Scheithauer W, Rosen H, Kornek GV, Sebesta C, Depisch D. Randomised comparison of combination chemotherapy plus supportive care with supportive care alone in patients with metastatic colorectal cancer. BMJ 1993;306:752–5.

[124] Expectancy or primary chemotherapy in patients with advanced asymptomatic colorectal cancer: a randomized trial. Nordic Gastrointestinal Tumor Adjuvant Therapy Group. J Clin Oncol 1992;10:904–11.

[125] Rothenberg ML, Eckardt JR, Kuhn JG, Burris HA III, Nelson J, Hilsenbeck SG, et al. Phase II trial of irinotecan in patients with progressive or rapidly recurrent colorectal cancer. J Clin Oncol 1996;14:1128–35.

[126] Rougier P, Van Cutsem E, Bajetta E, Niederle N, Possinger K, Labianca R, et al. Randomised trial of irinotecan versus fluorouracil by continuous infusion after fluorouracil failure in patients with metastatic colorectal cancer. Lancet 1998;352:1407–12.

[127] Douillard JY, Cunningham D, Roth AD, Navarro M, James RD, Karasek P, et al. Irinotecan combined with fluorouracil compared with fluorouracil alone as first-line treatment for metastatic colorectal cancer: a multicentre randomised trial. Lancet 2000;355: 1041–7.

[128] de Gramont A, Bosset JF, Milan C, Rougier P, Bouche O, Etienne PL, et al. Randomized trial comparing monthly low-dose leucovorin and fluorouracil bolus with bimonthly high-dose leucovorin and fluorouracil bolus plus continuous infusion for advanced colorectal cancer: a French intergroup study. J Clin Oncol 1997;15:808–15.

[129] Giacchetti S, Perpoint B, Zidani R, Le Bail N, Faggiuolo R, Focan C, et al. Phase III multicenter randomized trial of oxaliplatin added to chronomodulated fluorouracil-leucovorin as first-line treatment of metastatic colorectal cancer. J Clin Oncol 2000;18: 136–47.

[130] Goldberg RM, Sargent DJ, Morton RF, Fuchs CS, Ramanathan RK, Williamson SK, et al. A randomized controlled trial of fluorouracil plus leucovorin, irinotecan, and oxaliplatin combinations in patients with previously untreated metastatic colorectal cancer. J Clin Oncol 2004;22:23–30.

[131] Cassidy J, Tabernero J, Twelves C, Brunet R, Butts C, Conroy T, et al. XELOX (capecitabine plus oxaliplatin): active first-line therapy for patients with metastatic colorectal cancer. J Clin Oncol 2004;22:2084–91.

[132] Mayer RJ. Two steps forward in the treatment of colorectal cancer. N Engl J Med 2004;350: 2406–8.
[133] Viner JL, Umar A, Hawk ET. Chemoprevention of colorectal cancer: problems, progress, and prospects. Gastroenterol Clin North Am 2002;31:971–99.
[134] Towler B, Irwig L, Glasziou P, Kewenter J, Weller D, Silagy C. A systematic review of the effects of screening for colorectal cancer using the faecal occult blood test, hemoccult. BMJ 1998;317:559–65.
[135] Faivre J, Dancourt V, Lejeune C, Tazi MA, Lamour J, Gerard D, et al. Reduction in colorectal cancer mortality by fecal occult blood screening in a French controlled study. Gastroenterology 2004;126:1674–80.
[136] Faivre J, Couillault C, Kronborg O, Rath U, Giacosa A, De Oliveira H, et al. Chemoprevention of metachronous adenomas of the large bowel: design and interim results of a randomized trial of calcium and fibre. ECP Colon Group. Eur J Cancer Prev 1997;6:132–8.

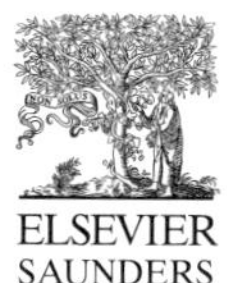


THE MEDICAL CLINICS OF NORTH AMERICA

Med Clin N Am 89 (2005) 111–138

# The emerging role of virtual colonoscopy

Zvi Lefkovitz, MD[a,*], Robert Shapiro, MD[a], Stephen Koch, MD[a], Mitchell S. Cappell, MD, PhD, FACG[b]

[a]*Department of Radiology, Mount Sinai School of Medicine, Mount Sinai Medical Center, 1190 Fifth Avenue, New York, NY 10029, USA*

[b]*Division of Gastroenterology, Department of Medicine, Albert Einstein Medical Center, 5501 Old York Road, Philadelphia, PA 19141-3098, USA*

Colon cancer is largely preventable by appropriate screening, surveillance, and treatment of precancerous adenomatous polyps [1]. Yet, colon cancer still causes substantial morbidity and mortality in America. Nearly 60,000 Americans die annually from colon cancer and many more undergo colon cancer surgery or chemotherapy [2]. This human tragedy and public health challenge has persisted because less than one fourth of the eligible population in the United States undergoes any method of colon cancer screening [3].

The decision by Medicare in 2001 and subsequently by other insurance carriers to reimburse for screening colonoscopy for the average-risk population has removed financial barriers for colon cancer screening [4]; however, other barriers to screening colonoscopy persist. Colonoscopy has undesirable features for a screening test of required sedation, test invasiveness, potential procedure complications, and high total cost. Moreover, the current demand for colonoscopy for colon cancer screening far exceeds the available supply of colonoscopists [5]. Virtual colonoscopy has desirable features for a screening test of no required sedation, minimal test invasiveness, and rare test complications. Moreover, with rapid technologic advances, virtual colonoscopy should become more readily available, cheaper, and more accurate. Virtual colonoscopy may become a viable alternative to conventional colonoscopy not only for patients with incomplete or failed conventional colonoscopy, but also for screening the general population for colon cancer.

* Corresponding author.
*E-mail address:* zvi.lefkovitz@msnyuhealth.org (Z. Lefkovitz).

0025-7125/05/$ - see front matter 
doi:10.1016/j.mcna.2004.08.004

A review of the current status of virtual colonoscopy is germane and topical. First, clinicians need to be knowledgeable about this rapidly evolving and clinically relevant technology to understand the test benefits and limitations and to refer patients for this test appropriately. Second, a critical review of the exponentially expanding literature on this subject is important. Recent studies of this test report widely divergent results because of differences in CT technology, adjunctive techniques, CT colonographic interpretation, and study design. This article describes the imaging methods, adjunctive techniques, and radiologic interpretation of CT colonography, and comprehensively and critically reviews the clinical data to help the clinician evaluate the current and potential applications of this technology.

## Principles of screening

Colon cancer is a suitable disease for screening because it is highly fatal when advanced but easily treatable and curable when detected early or in a precursor phase, and it is very common in the United States. A screening test should be relatively inexpensive, widely available, noninvasive, simple, well tolerated, and safe. A screening test should be highly sensitive, with sensitivity defined as the percent of patients with the condition diagnosed by the screening test, in order not to miss patients who have the condition (false-negatives). A screening test need not be quite as specific, with specificity defined as the percent of patients without the condition correctly diagnosed as being disease-free. A poorly specific screening test, however, subjects many people (false-negatives) to an unnecessary second (diagnostic) test, increasing the total costs and risks of screening the population.

The benefits of a screening test depend not only on test sensitivity and specificity, but on the prevalence of the disease in the study population. The positive predictive value is defined as the percentage of patients with a positive screening test that actually has the disease. The positive predictive value decreases as the disease prevalence decreases in a study population; this indicates reduced clinical reliability of a positive screening test in a study population with low disease prevalence.

Patients with a positive screening test are subjected to a definitive diagnostic (reference) test. The diagnostic test must be highly reliable, with very high sensitivity and specificity, because clinical decisions are based on this test. The diagnostic test may, however, be more expensive, invasive, and complicated than the screening test because it is applied to a subset of the general population prescreened and at high risk for the disease.

## History of colon cancer screening and CT colonography

The rationale for screening to detect colon cancer at an early and highly curable stage dates back about a century. Cuthbert Dukes in the 1920s and

1930s developed a pathologic staging system for colorectal cancer, showed that the prognosis was highly correlated with the pathologic cancer stage, and concluded that cancers detected earlier have a better prognosis [6,7]. The rationale for screening to detect and eradicate premalignant adenomatous polyps to prevent colon cancer is relatively recent. By the mid 1970s several investigators, including Morson [8] and Enterline [9], established that colon cancer nearly always develops from benign adenomatous polyps. This universally accepted adenoma-to-carcinoma sequence provides the pathophysiologic basis for screening tests to detect and eradicate polyps and to reduce colon cancer mortality. Wolff and Shinya [10,11] first applied electrocautery to a wire snare for colonoscopic polypectomy in 1969. Gilbertsen [12] in 1974 provided clinical evidence that endoscopic polypectomy reduces the incidence of colon cancer by eradication of precursor adenomas.

The historically most important screening test for colon cancer in the general population was fecal occult blood testing. This test was first recommended in 1914 by Boas [13], the first gastroenterologist in history. The pathophysiologic basis of this test is that colon cancer tends to cause intermittent occult gastrointestinal bleeding [14]. Greegor [15] underlined the importance of guaiac testing for colon cancer in 1967, when he noted in a review of eight patients with colon cancer that all but one had fecal occult blood. Greegor [16] reported in 1972 that 85% of colon cancers initially detected by guaiac testing were confined to the colonic wall and occurred in asymptomatic patients. These studies suggested that fecal occult blood might be useful to detect colon cancer at an early and highly curable stage. Mass screening of the general population for fecal occult blood was implemented based on the simplicity, convenience, low cost, and safety of the test. Several studies demonstrate significant benefits from fecal occult blood testing. For example, in 1993 Mandel et al [17] demonstrated in a large, prospective, randomized, controlled study that annual screening by fecal occult blood testing results in reduced mortality from colon cancer.

Fecal occult blood testing, however, has severe drawbacks as a screening test. First, it is only moderately highly sensitive. The sensitivity is increased somewhat by testing three stool specimens on three different occasions for occult blood and by rehydrating the specimens before testing [18]. Even under ideal circumstances in research protocols, however, the sensitivity for colon cancer is only about 85% and the sensitivity for clinically significant adenomatous polyps is much lower [14,19]. Insufficient sensitivity results in patients with the disease being undiagnosed (false-negatives) and not receiving potentially life-saving treatment. Second, the test is poorly specific. The specificity is moderately increased by such measures as instructing the patient to avoid eating red meat, broccoli, or cauliflower before the test, and to avoid taking aspirin before the test. Even under ideal circumstances in research protocols, however, the specificity is only about 30% [20].

Because of these deficiencies, other screening tests have been proposed and implemented. Flexible sigmoidoscopy is simpler, safer, and less invasive than colonoscopy. It often does not require sedation and analgesia. Sigmoidoscopy every 3 to 5 years in combination with fecal occult blood testing every year has been recommended for screening of patients more than 50 years old. In 1992, Selby et al [21] reported that sigmoidoscopy reduces the risk of fatal rectosigmoid cancer. Yet, sigmoidoscopy has an unsatisfactory sensitivity for colonic polyp or cancer detection of only 50% to 75% [22–25]. Only about half the colon is visualized at sigmoidoscopy and colonic polyps or cancers beyond the reach of the sigmoidoscope often go undetected [22].

Although approved as an option for colon cancer screening by Medicare, double-contrast barium enema is poorly sensitive for detection of moderate-sized polyps. For example, Winawer et al [26] reported a sensitivity of double-contrast barium enema of 32% for polyps less than 0.6 cm, 53% for polyps 0.6 to 1 cm, and 48% for polyps greater than 1 cm.

The previously mentioned problems with these screening tests led to investigation of colonoscopy for colon cancer screening in patients more than 50 years old. Colonoscopy is a superb diagnostic test for colon cancer and colonic polyps. It is a highly reliable test, with a relatively high sensitivity and specificity. Nonetheless, up to 27% of adenomas less than 6 mm in diameter and about 6% of adenomas greater than 10 mm in diameter are missed on colonoscopy [27]. At colonoscopy polyps are removed and masses biopsied for a pathologic diagnosis. Moreover, colonoscopy with colonoscopic polypectomy is usually therapeutic and diagnostic for colonic polyps. Definitive therapy at diagnosis during one procedure is a highly desirable feature of colonoscopy. Both the National Polyp Study in 1993 [1] and the Italian Multicenter Study in 2000 [28] demonstrated reductions in colorectal cancer incidence among patients who had adenomatous polyps detected and eradicated during colonoscopy.

Colonoscopy, however, has some flaws as a screening test for colon cancer for populations at low risk of significant disease (Table 1). Colonoscopy is expensive, particularly when performed in a hospital or ambulatory surgery center. It requires a team including a technician, nurse, and highly trained colonoscopist. The test is not readily available, with long waiting times because of a shortage of highly trained colonoscopists. Colonoscopic equipment is expensive to buy and maintain. Colonoscopy is not readily accepted by patients, a factor that affects patient compliance. The test requires patient preparation for 24 hours before the procedure. The test is uncomfortable and sometimes painful. Sedation and analgesia are generally required. Because of the sedation and analgesia, the patient requires postprocedure monitoring and accompaniment by a chaperone after discharge. Because of the postprocedure recovery time, the patient typically loses a day of gainful employment for the test. Colonoscopy has small but significant risks, particularly colonic perforation and gastrointestinal bleeding, which occur in about 3 per 1000 colonoscopies [29,30].

Table 1
Comparison of colonoscopy and CT colonography as a screening test for colonic polyps and colon cancer

| Feature | Ideal screening test | Colonoscopy | CT colonography |
|---|---|---|---|
| Low cost | ++++ | + | +++ (potentially) |
| Simple test | ++++ | + | +++ |
| Minimal loss of gainful employment | ++++ | + (1 d) | +++ |
| Ready test availability | ++++ | ++ (long weight) | ++++ (potentially) |
| No patient preparation | ++++ | ++ | ++[a] |
| Minimal procedure invasiveness | ++++ | + | +++ |
| Patient acceptance | ++++ | ++ | +++ |
| Minimal procedure pain | ++++ | ++ | ++ |
| No need for sedation and analgesia | ++++ | + | ++++ |
| No monitoring of patient after test | ++++ | + | ++++ |
| Minimal procedure risks | ++++ | ++ | +++ |
| Patient compliance | ++++ | ++ | ++ |
| Sensitivity for large polyps | ++++ | ++++ | ++++ (?) |
| Sensitivity for small polyps | ++++ | +++ | ++ (?) |
| Sensitivity for cancers | ++++ | ++++ | ++++ |
| Rapidly available test result | ++++ | ++++ | +++ |

Scale ranges from + (poor) to ++++ (excellent). (?) denotes sensitivity of test is controversial.
[a] Potentially ++++ if laxative or cathartic administration becomes unnecessary with digital stool subtraction.

Yet, colonoscopy is currently recommended by the American Gastroenterological Association [31], the American Cancer Society [32], the American College of Gastroenterology [33], and the American Society for Gastrointestinal Endoscopy [34] as the primary screening test for colonic polyps and cancer in patients more than 50 years old, a population at low risk for colonic disease. Although details vary slightly among the individual organizations, all the organizations recommend colonoscopy for screening of patients at average risk of colon cancer beginning at age 50, and colonoscopy to be repeated 10 years later if the initial colonoscopy reveals no colonic adenomas or cancers [35,36]. Patients with colonic adenomas detected during screening colonoscopy are entered into a surveillance colonoscopy program with repeat colonoscopy in approximately 3 to 5 years, depending on the number, size, and type of adenomatous polyps [35,37]. The flaws as a screening test are most evident when colonoscopy is applied to such a population with low disease prevalence. For example, if the population of patients more than 50 years old without risk factors for colon cancer has a one in five risk of having colonic polyps [38], four out of five patients subjected to the risks, costs, and discomfort of colonoscopy receive no test benefit.

The profusion of available colon cancer screening tests, the alternative recommended screening regimens, the controversy in the literature, and the intense search for better screening tests all testify to the inadequacy of the current screening tests and regimens. What is needed is a better screening test than colonoscopy, to restrict colonoscopy to its most appropriate role as a superb diagnostic (reference) test for patients with a positive screening test. Vining introduced virtual colonoscopy in 1994 [39] to fill this clinical void by developing a radiologic test that preserves much of the desirable features of colonoscopy of high test reliability while eliminating it's undesirable features of test invasiveness, procedural risks, and need for analgesia and sedation (see Table 1). The first virtual colonoscopy took 50 seconds for data acquisition, and 8 hours for computer processing [39]. Revolutionary advances in CT technology and computer processing have reduced the CT scan time to about 30 seconds, using multidetector (multislice) CT scanners, and the computer processing time to about 10 minutes. Virtual colonoscopy has become technically and economically feasible.

Early studies [40–42] reported that two-dimensional CT colonography, with relatively thick CT sections and without stool tagging agents, was poorly sensitive at detecting polyps. Virtual colonoscopy has rapidly evolved because of advances in CT, especially multidetector technology and three-dimensional computer software for flythrough imaging. A recent large, multicenter, prospective study by Pickhardt et al [43] demonstrated that CT virtual colonoscopy is an accurate screening method to detect colonic polyps in an asymptomatic average-risk adult population. The results of virtual colonoscopy compared favorably with the results of conventional colonoscopy. A more recent study using less sophisticated technology, however, reported CT colonography was poorly sensitive in the detection of colonic polyps [44]. The accuracy of CT colonography should improve further with more sophisticated software, increasingly advanced multislice CT technology, and more training and experience by radiologists.

## Technique

CT colonography depends on (1) an adequately cleansed and distended colon, (2) a rapid thin-section CT examination to obtain colonic volumetric data, and (3) computerized processing of the data into two-dimensional images in the axial, sagittal, and coronal planes or three-dimensional virtual colonoscopy images.

### *Colonic preparation*

Thorough bowel cleansing is essential. Residual stool can be mistaken for a polyp or mass [45]. Standard bowel preparations, if properly performed, provide adequate bowel cleansing. Bowel cleansing includes limiting oral intake to clear liquids or a low-residue diet beginning 24 hours before the test, and ingesting a laxative or cathartic to promote colonic evacuation [46]. The patient should be advised of the importance of taking the entire colonic preparation as directed. Magnesium citrate and bisacodyl tablets or suppositories (Lo So Preparation, E-Z-EM, Westbury, New York) provide colonic cleansing with little residual fluid, an advantage for image interpretation. Polyethylene glycol electrolyte solution (Go-Lytely, Braintree Laboratories, Braintree, Massachusetts) provides better evacuation of stool, but leaves more fluid within the colon. This wet preparation may interfere with image interpretation. Orally administered sodium phosphate or phosphosoda (24-hour Fleet 1 preparation, Fleet Pharmaceuticals, Lynchburg, Virginia) is also used for bowel cleansing. It typically leaves the colon relatively dry [46]. This cathartic can cause electrolyte imbalances and should be avoided in patients with renal failure, pre-existing electrolyte abnormalities, congestive heart failure, ascites, or ileus [46,47]. Patients administered sodium phosphate should drink adequate amounts of water to prevent dehydration. The patient evacuates any residual fluid immediately before the examination.

### *Patient examination*

The examination is performed by a well-trained, licensed CT technologist under the supervision of a radiologist. The patient is placed in a decubitus position on the CT scanning table. A small plastic or flexible rubber catheter is inserted into the rectum. Air is gently pumped into the colon using a small hand-held bulb pump or, occasionally, an automatic insufflator. Colonic distention with room air provides a low-density background to identify more easily medium-density colonic polyps and masses. Approximately 2 L of air are required for adequate colonic distention, but the precise amount varies with each patient [46]. The initial insufflation is 40 pumps, but may be less if limited by patient intolerance. Patient-controlled air insufflation may optimize colonic distention with minimal patient discomfort [43]. The patient is turned to the supine position to film a scout CT image that resembles a conventional radiograph to determine whether the colon was adequately distended (Fig. 1). More air is added if necessary. After adequate colonic distention, CT images are obtained in the supine position. The patient is then turned to the prone position, several additional puffs of air are administered, and CT images are obtained in this position. Images in both prone and supine positions are obtained from the level of the diaphragm to the level of the perineum during a breathhold (of 30 seconds) [48]. The rectal tube is then withdrawn. This completes the patient scanning and patient involvement in the examination.

### *Optional adjunctive techniques*

Carbon dioxide is an alternative to room air for colonic distention. It is absorbed about 35-fold faster than room air from the colonic lumen [46],

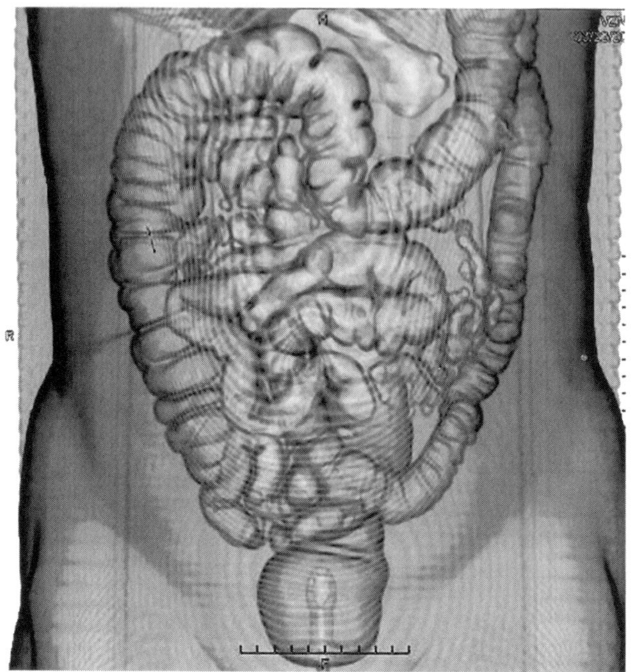

Fig. 1. CT scout image demonstrates an evenly and adequately distended colon.

and is rapidly eliminated by the lungs [46,49]. Faster colonic deflation after the examination using carbon dioxide improves procedure tolerance. Deflation during the examination, however, can affect CT resolution; this deflation is prevented by constant colonic insufflation of carbon dioxide at a preset pressure during the procedure.

Glucagon administration has been proposed to decrease patient discomfort and promote colonic distention. Glucagon, a single-chain polypeptide hormone, increases serum glucose levels and relaxes gastrointestinal smooth muscle [46]. The colon is the least sensitive part of the gastrointestinal tract to glucagon [50]. One study reported no significant improvement in colonic distention with intravenous glucagon administration before CT colonography [51]. Other muscle relaxants used to promote colonic distention include hyoscine butylbromide or butylscopolamine.

Oral contrast agents can be used to tag and identify retained feces. In a sophisticated application of this technique, barium is administered to coat and tag particulate stool and iodinated contrast is administered to diffuse into and opacify retained colonic fluid. For example, 500 mL of 2.1% barium contrast material (Scan C, Lafayette Pharmaceuticals, Lafayette, Indiana) and 120 mL of diatrizoate meglumine and diatrizoate sodium (Gastrografin, Bracco Diagnostics, Princeton, New Jersey) has been administered in divided doses [52]. The patient typically ingests the oral contrast in addition to the

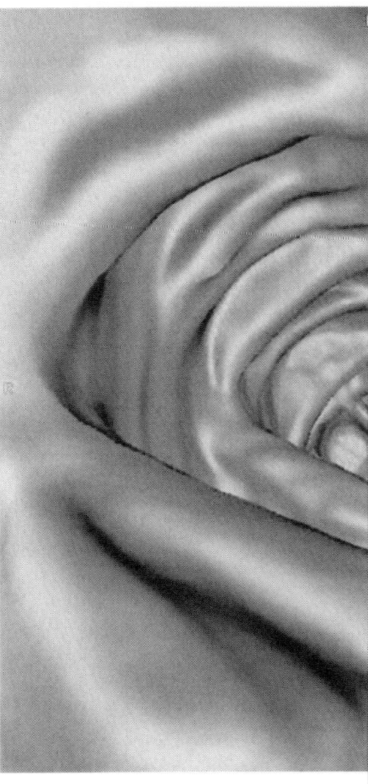

Fig. 3. Three-dimensional endoluminal fly-thro
a well-prepared colon.

intensive, and costly than two-dimens
dimensional flythrough is performed l
supine and prone studies.

Three-dimensional image processir
Recent technologic advances have i
rendering and automated navigation c
dimensional systems consequently tak
Until recently two-dimensional mul
used for polyp detection and the thr
problem solving of abnormalities de
[62–64,66–69]. The two- and three-c
have complimentary roles with both
three-dimensional endoluminal view
tant with further advances in co
delineated and folds more easily ide
the two-dimensional view.

## Radiologic interpretation

The colon contains six segments:
descending colon, (4) transverse colo



standard cathartics [52], but the contrast can be administered without cathartics, often during ingestion of the clear liquid diet [46,53,54]. Labeled stool has a high density, which distinguishes it from the medium, soft tissue density of colonic polyps (Fig. 2).

Without administration of oral contrast, a CT colonography that reveals a polyp or mass can be followed immediately by a colonoscopy without the need for a second colonic preparation. In contrast, a barium enema that reveals a lesion cannot be followed immediately by colonoscopy because of the presence of intraluminal contrast in the colon. Likewise, colonoscopy cannot be performed immediately after CT colonography if oral contrast is administered.

Fecal material is automatically subtracted in digital subtraction bowel cleansing [55,56]. Simple threshold techniques, in which labeled stool is identified and subtracted, fail to identify and correct volume averaging artifacts at stool-air interfaces within the colonic lumen [55]. Sophisticated postimaging techniques address these partial volume effects and subtract labeled stool without artifacts [54]. Digital subtraction techniques have been used successfully either with [52] or without [56] cathartics. These techniques are not yet widely used, but could improve the accuracy of CT colonography and possibly eliminate the need for cathartics.

In contrast-enhanced CT colonography, intravenous contrast is injected 15 seconds before the CT scanning. Polyps, but not stool, enhance with intravenous contrast [46]. This technique may help identify medium-sized polyps in a suboptimally prepared colon and improve delineation of the bowel wall [57]. Contrast-enhanced CT colonography can accurately distinguish colon cancers from benign strictures on the basis of contrast enhancement [58]. Intravenous contrast is unlikely to be used routinely

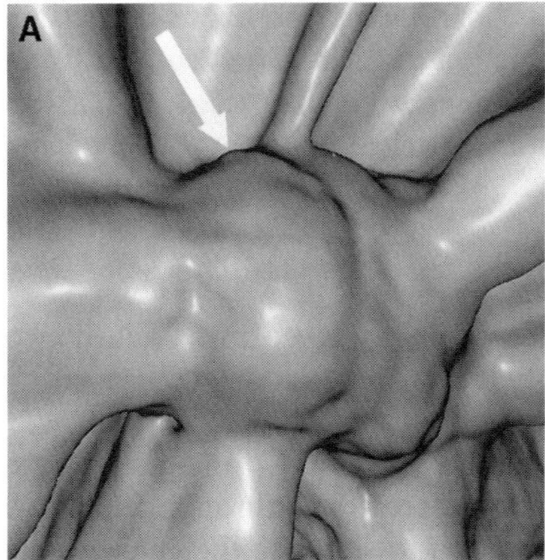


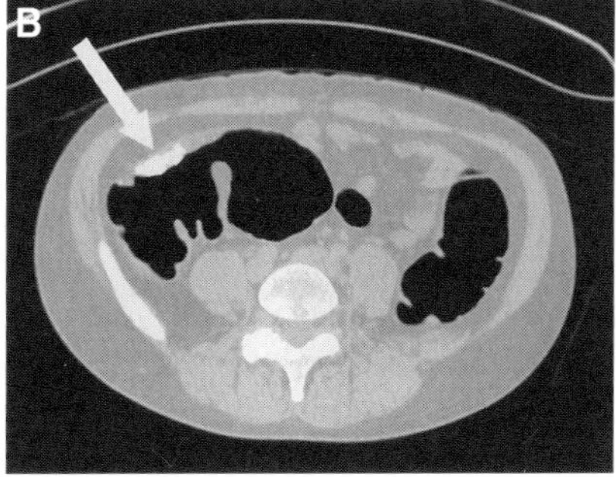


Fig. 2. (*A*) Endoluminal fly-through (three-dimensional) view demonstrates a questionable lobular endoluminal filling defect. (*B*) Prone two-dimensional axial view demonstrates that the filling defect is caused by labeled fecal material layering anteriorly.

The rectum is generally well distended and contains three distinct folds (valves of Houston). The sigmoid colon is best distended in the prone position. The sigmoid colon is frequently tortuous and inadequately distended because of mural spasm and can be difficult to evaluate, especially in patients with diverticular disease. Polyps may be missed when the sigmoid colon is poorly distended. The descending and ascending colon are relatively featureless and contain gracile folds. The transverse colon is triangular in cross-section and has prominent, rounded, triangular intrahaustral folds. The cecum is usually well distended and contains the ileocecal valve and appendix. The ileocecal valve appears as a filling defect in the cecum, most commonly medially, but occasionally laterally [70]. This valve is usually easily distinguished from a polyp or mass on two-dimensional images by following the terminal ileum directly into the valve [68].

An intraluminal filling defect should be carefully analyzed in both the supine and prone views in both the two-dimensional and three-dimensional images. The differential of an intraluminal filling defect includes residual fecal material, bulbous or irregular interhaustral folds, lipomas, extrinsic compression defects, diverticula, foreign bodies, and colonic polyps [39,64,68,70,71]. Radiologic characteristics that help differentiate between these findings are listed in Table 2. Colonic polyps, whether sessile or

Table 2
Differentiation of true polyps from other filling defects by CT colonography

| Filling defect | Appearance on CT colonography |
|---|---|
| Fecal matter | Stool moves because of the effects of gravity when the patient changes from the supine to prone position. Polyps relatively immobile. Stool may contain low-density air or high-density food particles. Best differentiated by fecal tagging. |
| Bulbous or irregular haustral folds | Usually occur in the hepatic or splenic flexures, and typically prominent in incompletely distended colonic segment. Endoluminal view typically demonstrates the linear shape of the filling defect, compared with the globular nature of a polyp. |
| Lipomas | Attenuation characteristics of fat on abdominal soft tissue CT window settings. |
| Extrinsic compression defects | Extrinsic nature of lesion usually easily discerned by two-dimensional CT imaging. |
| Diverticulum | Characteristically has a completely dark ring corresponding to the air-filled diverticular orifice on three-dimensional view; contains air or stool and projects beyond the lumen on two-dimensional imaging; inverted diverticulum may contain pericolic fat best seen on two-dimensional images at abdominal soft tissue window settings. |
| Bulbous ileocecal valve | This filling defect in the cecum is distinguished from a true polyp by following the terminal ileum into the ileocecal valve on two-dimensional images. |

pedunculated, appear as immobile bulbous, and cap-like, round, oval, or lobulated structures in prone or supine views on two-dimensional or three-dimensional images (Figs. 4–6). Polyps can appear to move, particularly when they have a long stalk, because the colon rotates when the patient rotates. Careful analysis of both supine and prone images usually demonstrates the immobility of polyps. The location, size, and morphology of colonic polyps are assessed. Polyp size is measured with electronic calipers. Morphologic characteristics include whether the polyp is flat or elevated, sessile or pedunculated, and multilobular or unilobular, and whether the polyp surface is smooth or ulcerated. Polyps generally are homogeneous in attenuation and have a smooth surface, but may have an irregular, ulcerated surface when large.

Adenomas are occasionally nonpolypoid and flat. Adenomas may be more aggressive when flat than polypoid [72–74]. A flat adenoma may appear as a small flat protuberance or as subtle soft tissue thickening, but may be undetectable by CT colonography when truly flat [75]. This lesion is also often difficult to detect by conventional colonoscopy and may require chromoendoscopy, with vital staining of colonic mucosa using indigocarmine or methylene blue, for detection [76,77].

## Sensitivity and specificity for colonic polyps and colon cancer

The accuracy of CT colonography for the detection of colonic polyps and neoplasms has been frequently analyzed (Table 3) [41,57,62,78–91]. The first blinded prospective study reported a sensitivity of 75% for lesions 10 mm or

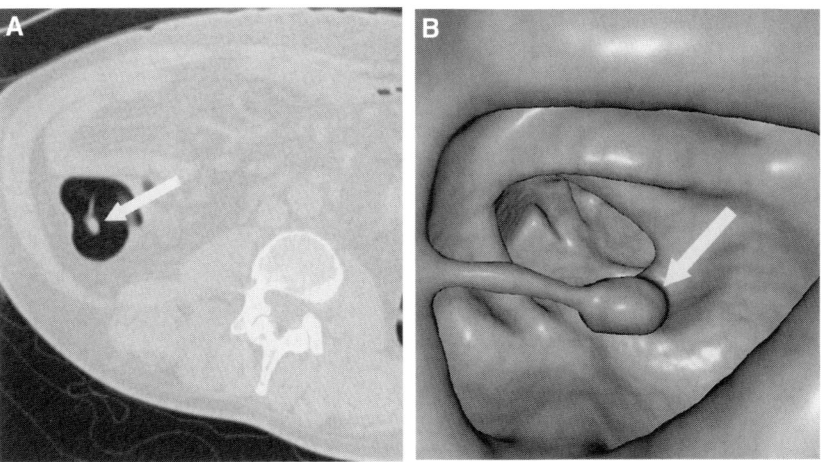


Fig. 4. (*A*) Two-dimensional axial image demonstrates an endoluminal filling defect (*arrow*) in the ascending colon. (*B*) Three-dimensional endoluminal fly-through view demonstrates a conspicuous pedunculated polyp (*arrow*) on a long and narrow stalk.

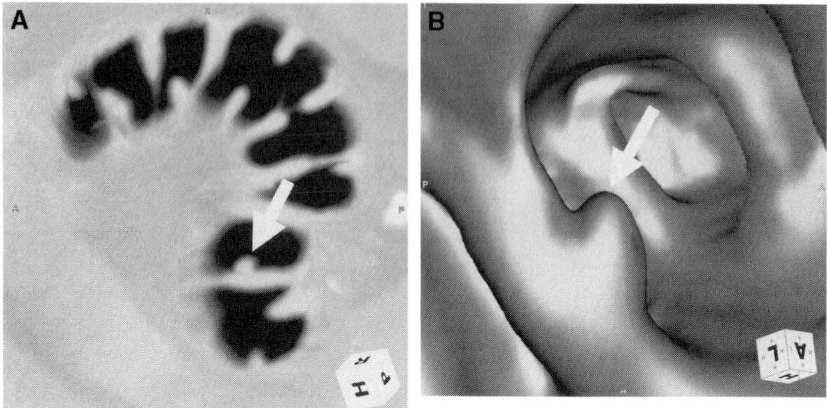

Fig. 5. (*A*) Two-dimensional axial image of the sigmoid colon demonstrates a filling defect in the sigmoid colon associated with a fold (*arrow*). (*B*) Three-dimensional endoluminal fly-through view of the sigmoid colon shows the filling defect is caused by a sessile polyp (*arrow*) arising from a fold.

larger, 66% for 5 to 10 mm lesions, and 45% for lesions less than 5 mm using only supine position CT colonography [41]. Higher sensitivity has been subsequently reported in parallel with improving technology. In 2001, Yee et al [45] reported a sensitivity of 90% for detection of polyps 10 mm or larger, 80% for polyps 5 to 9.9 mm, and 59% for polyps smaller than 5 mm.

In 2003, Pickhardt et al [43] reported a sensitivity of 93.8% for polyps at least 10 mm in diameter, 93.9% for polyps at least 8 mm in diameter, and 88.7% for polyps at least 6 mm in diameter. Moreover, the specificity of CT

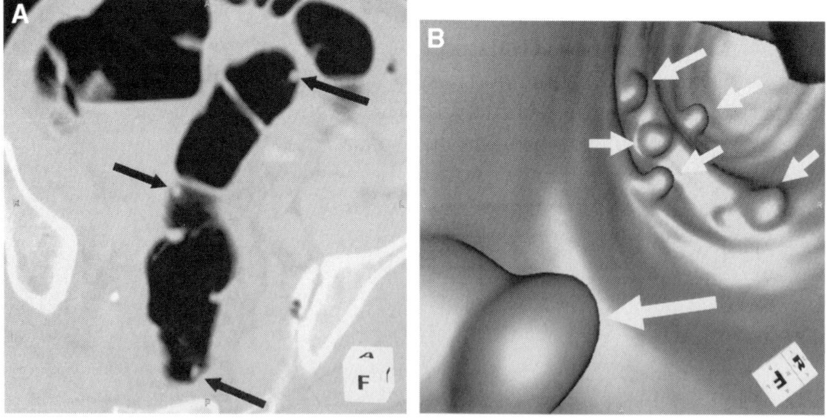

Fig. 6. (*A*) Two-dimensional axial image of the rectosigmoid in a patient with familial polyposis coli demonstrates several small filling defects in the sigmoid colon (*arrows*). (*B*) Three-dimensional endoluminal fly-through view demonstrates numerous sessile polyps both in the foreground and background of the same area (*arrows*).

Table 3
Sensitivity of virtual colonoscopy with conventional colonoscopy used as the gold standard in selected clinical studies

| Study authors, year | No. of study patients | Sensitivity for polyps (%) <6 mm in diameter | 6–10 mm in diameter | >10 mm in diameter |
|---|---|---|---|---|
| Hara et al, 1999 [41] | 70 | 45 | 66 | 75 |
| Fenlon et al, 1999 [95] | 87 | 55 | 82 | 91 |
| Yee et al, 2001 [45] | 300 | 59 | 80 | 90 |
| Pickhardt et al, 2003 [43] | 1233 | — | 88.7 | 93.8 |
| Cotton et al, 2004 [44] | 308 | 14 | 30 | 55 |
| Macari et al, 2004 [85] | 68 | 11.5 | 52.9 | 100 |
| Edwards et al, 2004 [78] | 184 | 37 | 70 | 100 |

colonography in this study for polyp detection was 96% for polyps at least 10 mm, 92.2% for polyps at least 8 mm, and 79.6% for polyps at least 6 mm in diameter [43]. In this study, the sensitivity of conventional colonoscopy was 87.5%, 91.5%, and 92.3%, respectively, for these three categories of polyp size [43]. An interesting phenomenon reported in this study was that CT colonography occasionally detected polyps that were missed by colonoscopy. Colonoscopy may miss polyps at sharp turns (flexures); behind folds; in areas with stool or fluid; and in areas of colonic spasm. Colonoscopy may also miss diminutive polyps or flat adenomas. This study used highly trained expert radiologists for image interpretation, advanced CT technology, and dual fecal tagging with digital subtraction.

In a study by Cotton et al [44], 600 patients underwent both CT colonography and colonoscopy. The sensitivity of CT colonography was only 39% for lesions sized less than 6 mm, and 55% for lesions sized more than 10 mm. These two recent studies report diametrically opposite results. In the study by Pickhardt et al [43] virtual colonoscopy was an excellent screening test with a very high sensitivity and specificity that rivals that for colonoscopy, whereas in the study by Cotton et al [44] virtual colonoscopy was so poorly sensitive and specific as not to be useful as a screening test [92]. It is important to analyze potential reasons for this discrepancy (Box 1), to identify correctable deficiencies, and to improve virtual colonoscopy as a screening test.

The sensitivity of CT colonography depends on lesion size [41,43,45,62, 66,79,81,88,90]. It is more sensitive at detecting colon cancer than benign polyps because cancer tends to be much larger (Fig. 7). Nearly 100% sensitivity has been reported for colon cancer [43,45,79,89]. Fenlon et al [79] reported that CT colonography identified all three cancers in their study. Yee et al [45] reported that all eight carcinomas were detected in their study. Royster et al [89] reported that two-dimensional CT colonography detected 20 of 20 mass lesions greater than 2 cm in diameter, and three-dimensional virtual colonoscopy detected 19 of the 20 masses. In Pickhardt's et al [43]

**Box 1. Potential reasons for discrepancies in the reported sensitivity of CT colonography**

*Professional proficiency*

- Well-trained CT technologist to obtain better images
- Inexperienced versus trained radiologist (learning curve)
- General radiologist versus expert in CT interpretation
- Insufficient versus sufficient time for interpretation of CT colonographic images

*Elimination of stool*

- Education of patient about technique and importance of cathartic administration
- Compliant patients (properly take the colonic preparation)
- Intense versus casual bowel preparation
- Electronic subtraction of stool and residual colonic liquid
- Use versus avoidance of oral contrast versus use of a dual label of contrast to tag stool

*Colonic distention*

- Antispasmodic administration to promote colonic distention (eg, glucagon)
- Poor colonic distention because of mural spasm (especially in sigmoid)
- Improved colonic distention by patient-controlled air insufflation
- Patient toleration of colonic distention (healthy patients)

*Imaging technique*

- Intravenous contrast administration during CT colonography
- Decreased resolution caused by scanning with low-dose radiation
- Two- and three-dimensional imaging versus only two-dimensional imaging
- Use of supine only versus supine and prone views
- 16- versus 4-slice CT scanners
- Variable quality of flythrough software for virtual colonoscopy

study of 1233 asymptomatic adults, two patients had malignant polyps. Both were detected on virtual colonoscopy, but one was missed by conventional colonoscopy [43].

## Other CT colonographic findings

CT colonography may reveal unexpected colonic pathology other than polyps or cancers. For example, Serracino-Inglott et al [48] in a study of 100

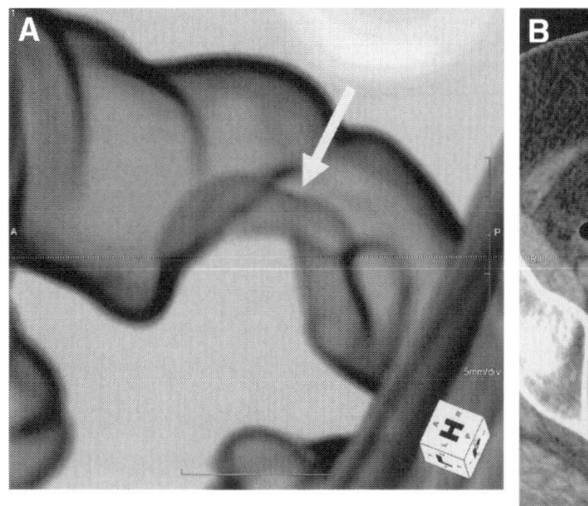

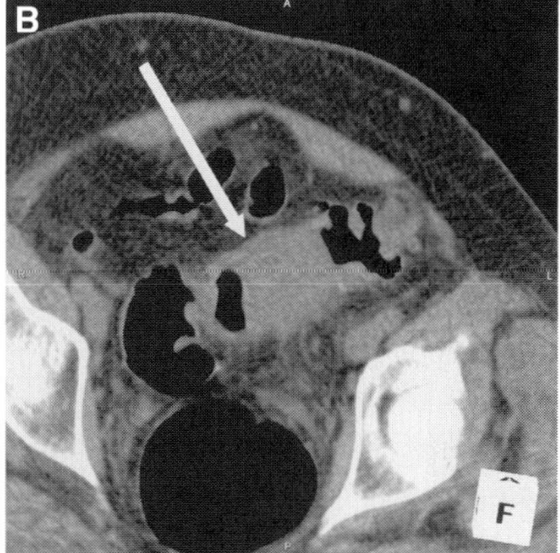

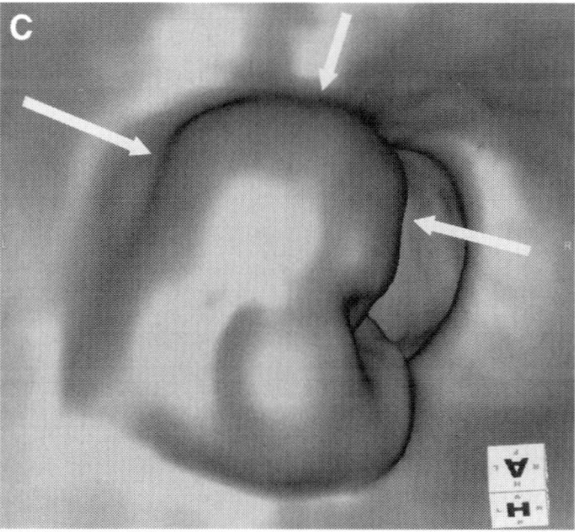

Fig. 7. Large, bulky sigmoid colon carcinoma (*arrows*) as demonstrated on a cone-down scout view of the sigmoid colon (*A*), two-dimensional axial view (*B*), and three-dimensional endoluminal fly-through view (*C*).

patients found clinically unsuspected Crohn's disease in one patient, an appendiceal abscess in one, and an appendiceal fecalith in one. Additionally 36% of the patients had colonic diverticulosis.

Unlike conventional colonoscopy, CT colonography allows visualization of extracolonic organs and detection of significant extracolonic abnormalities, such as malignancies or aneurysms, potentially resulting in earlier and improved therapy (Fig. 8). Hara et al [83] reported that 11% of patients had highly important extracolonic findings detected at CT colonography, including indeterminate adrenal or pulmonary lesions, indeterminate masses at least 1 cm in diameter in a solid organ (kidney, liver, or spleen), likely malignant masses, and other lesions requiring prompt medical or surgical treatment, such as abdominal aortic aneurysm, hernia containing bowel, and pneumothorax. Pickhardt et al [43] reported significant extracolonic findings in 4.5%, including 0.4% with extracolonic cancer and 0.2% with an

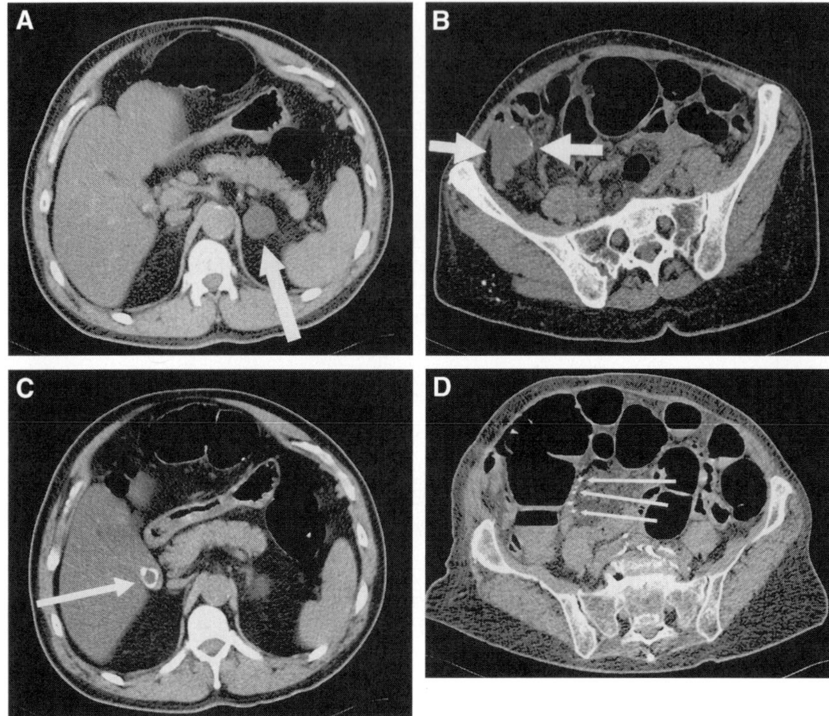


Fig. 8. Extracolonic abnormalities detected on axial CT images obtained for virtual colonoscopy. (*A*) Adrenal adenoma (*arrow*). (*B*) Mucocele of the appendix (*arrows*). (*C*) Gallstone (*arrow*). (*D*) Multiple appendecoliths (*arrows*).

abdominal aortic aneurysm requiring surgery. Mildly significant extracolonic findings included nephrolithiasis in 7.9% and cholelithiasis in 5.6%. Serracino-Inglott et al [48] reported that 8% of patients had extracolonic malignancy diagnosed by CT colonography. Hellstrom et al [84] reported that 23% of patients had potentially important extracolonic findings and another 62% had minor incidental extracolonic findings. Detection of incidental and insignificant extracolonic findings may sometimes result in unnecessary additional examinations and increased costs [83]. Ironically, CT colonography may identify more clinically important extracolonic than colonic disease because the prevalence of colonic polyps greater than 1 cm is only about 5% in the average-risk population [68].

## Advantages, disadvantages, and current role

The advantages and disadvantages of CT colonography are summarized in Box 2. CT colonography is extremely helpful to evaluate the colon proximal to an obstructing colonic lesion or after failed colonoscopy [93–96]. Indeed, it seems to be better than a barium enema, with a higher sensitivity

**Box 2. Advantages and disadvantages of virtual colonoscopy**

*Advantages*

- Does not require sedation and analgesia or an anesthesiologist
- Less time off from work for patient than for colonoscopy (no anesthesia recovery time)
- Generally performed within 10 to 15 minutes
- Less invasive and safer than alternative tests of sigmoidoscopy or colonoscopy
- Detects synchronous lesions proximal to an obstructing colonic lesion not reachable by conventional colonoscopy
- Can replace colonoscopy when colonoscopy is dangerous (eg, severe diverticulosis)
- Provides an accessible road map of intraluminal findings (lesions accurately localized)
- Detects extracolonic abnormalities
- Less expensive than conventional colonoscopy
- Generally well tolerated and accepted by patients
- Can identify polyps missed at colonoscopic blind spots (eg, behind a fold)
- Can be performed with some stool present in the colon using digital subtraction technology
- Can diagnose and stage colon cancer in one examination

*Disadvantages*

- Radiation exposure
- Resolution limited by colonic spasm or incomplete colonic distention
- Requires bowel preparation
- Lesions not pathologically characterized; follow-up conventional colonoscopy needed for tissue diagnosis
- Not therapeutic: requires subsequent colonoscopic polypectomy for identified polyps
- Sensitivity of detecting polyps less well studied than that of colonoscopy
- Currently limited availability compared with colonoscopy
- Discomfort from insertion of a rectal tube and colonic insufflation without sedation

and specificity, for these indications. Fenlon et al [95] found 2 (7%) of 29 patients with an occluding colorectal cancer had a synchronous proximal lesion detected by CT colonography. CT colonography can diagnose and stage colon cancer at one examination. Morrin et al [96] reported that CT colonography could correctly stage 81% of colorectal cancers. Patient acceptance of CT colonography is high [43,97], and possibly higher than that for conventional colonoscopy [98]. Adequate colonic preparation is critical to maintain the high sensitivity of polyp detection. The colonic preparation is unpleasant for most patients, however, and is a major obstacle to patient compliance [99]. Dual supine-prone patient positioning, fecal tagging, and electronic fluid cleansing software improve the accuracy of virtual colonoscopy. The current indications and relative contraindications for virtual colonoscopy are summarized in Box 3.

CT colonography is extremely safe [39,68,100]. Pickhardt et al [43] reported no complications among 1233 patients undergoing this test. An extremely rare serious complication is colonic perforation from overinflation

**Box 3. Indications and relative contraindications for virtual colonoscopy**

*Indications*

- Failed conventional colonoscopy
- Evaluation of the colon proximal to an obstructing lesion or stricture inaccessible to conventional colonoscopy
- Elderly or frail patients who cannot tolerate conventional colonoscopy
- Anticipated difficult or dangerous colonoscopy (eg, acute colitis, very recent myocardial infarction, or tight colonic stricture)
- Patients who cannot tolerate sedation
- Patients who refuse conventional colonoscopy for any other reason
- Colon cancer screening???

*Relative contraindications*

- Severe allergy to administered contrast (can be performed without contrast)
- Suspected colonic perforation or peritonitis
- Highly clinically unstable patient
- Acute lower gastrointestinal bleeding
- Lack of trained personnel to interpret the test
- Pregnancy (radiation teratogenicity)
- Inability to tolerate pneumocolon
- Abnormal anorectal anatomy (eg, imperforate anus, tight anal stricture, painful rectal fissure)
- Toxic colitis, toxic megacolon, massive dilatation from colonic pseudo-obstruction
- Complete mechanical colonic obstruction
- Inability to tolerate colonic preparation (eg, congestive heart failure, severe electrolyte imbalances)

of the colon [101]. Minor complications include abdominal pain from colonic insufflation, nausea with abdominal distention, diaphoresis and flushing during the CT scan, and dizziness or dehydration from the colonic preparation [78].

A potential drawback of CT colonography is radiation exposure. The radiation exposure from CT colonography is similar to that from a barium enema [48]. Several techniques may reduce radiation exposure without compromising test sensitivity [75,102]. Iannaccone et al [103] reported that lower-dose multidetector CT colonography maintained excellent sensitivity in detecting polyps while significantly reducing radiation exposure compared with standard dose tests. Use of MRI instead of CT could eliminate radiation exposure during CT colonography [104].

CT colonography may miss polyps at or near the anorectal junction (dentate line) because of an inability to insufflate this area [85]. Digital rectal examination should be performed to exclude a polyp in this location for comprehensive colorectal cancer screening.

## Future role

Conventional colonoscopy is currently the gold standard for the detection and evaluation of colonic polyps and colon cancer, but virtual colonoscopy has the potential to become important in the initial screening. Additional large prospective studies in asymptomatic patients using state-of-the-art CT machines and software are needed to compare the accuracy of virtual colonoscopy with conventional colonoscopy and to define the role of virtual colonoscopy for the initial screening for colonic polyps. If virtual colonoscopy is demonstrated to be a highly accurate screening test for colonic polyps and cancers, virtual colonoscopy could play a major role in mass screening of the population (Fig. 9). Medicare reimbursement for this indication would then be justified.

The accuracy of virtual colonoscopy is directly correlated with polyp size [42,43,45]. Polyps less than 6 mm in diameter are often clinically insignificant [105,106]. Diminutive polyps are sometimes adenomatous but rarely contain severe dysplasia or cancer. The 6- to 9-mm polyp has an indeterminate status, whereas the 10-mm or larger polyp is generally clinically significant. Large polyps detected at virtual colonoscopy require colonoscopy and colonoscopic polypectomy because large polyps are highly likely to be adenomatous and may have a focus of cancer. Whether diminutive colonic polyps detected at virtual colonoscopy require prompt colonoscopy for evaluation and removal is uncertain. A strategy of deferring colonoscopy for one to several years after detecting diminutive colonic polyps considerably reduces the total costs, but the medical justification for such a strategy requires careful clinical analysis [92]. Unambiguous and universally accepted guidelines and surveillance strategies for small (<6 mm) and intermediate sized (6–9 mm) colonic polyps must be developed.

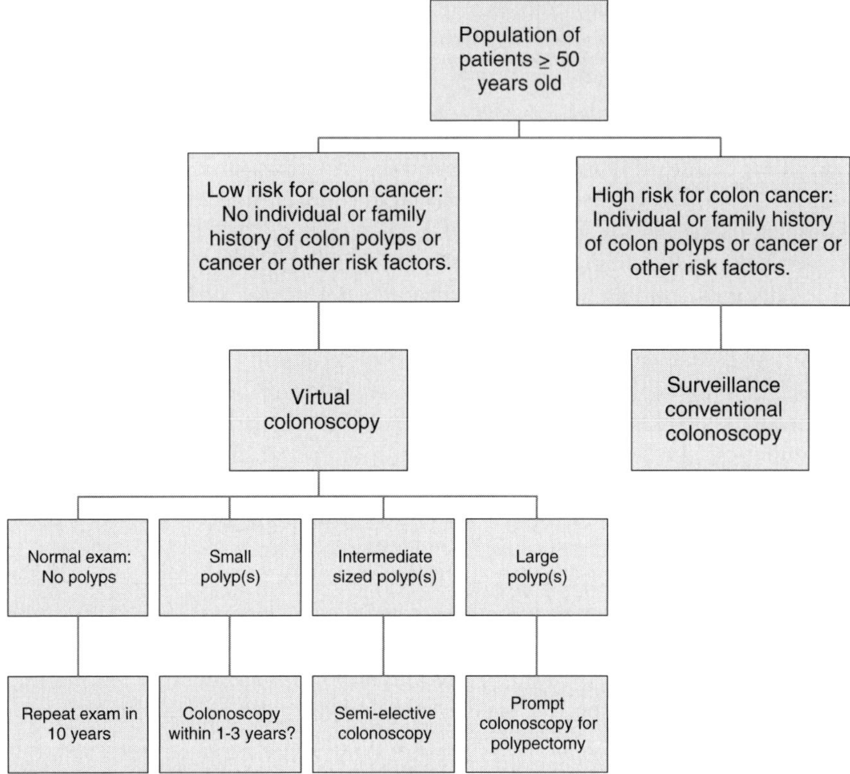


Fig. 9. A potential algorithm for screening of patients more than 50 years old for colon cancer using virtual colonoscopy. Realization of this potential requires that virtual colonoscopy is proved to be highly accurate at detecting colonic polyps and cancers. The colonoscopic management of small polyps detected at virtual colonoscopy (prompt versus delayed elective colonoscopy) is controversial.

Further technical advances, which can enhance the sensitivity and specificity of virtual colonoscopy, include computer-aided diagnosis software [107,108], enhanced electronic fluid cleansing software [52–56], and improved training protocols for radiologists [55,109]. Stool tagging might ultimately replace colonic preparation to provide patients with a highly accurate, safe, widely available, and relatively inexpensive preparation-less screening modality.

## References

[1] Winawer SJ, Zauber AG, Ho MN, O'Brien MJ, Gottlieb LS, Sternberg SS, et al. Prevention of colorectal cancer by colonoscopic polypectomy. The National Polyp Study Workgroup. N Engl J Med 1993;329:1977–81.

[2] Jemal A, Tiwari RC, Murray T, Ghafoor A, Samuels A, Ward E, et al. Cancer statistics, 2004. CA Cancer J Clin 2004;54:8–29.

[3] Nelson DE, Bolen J, Marcus S, Wells HE, Meissner H. Cancer screening estimates for US metropolitan areas. Am J Prev Med 2003;24:301–9.
[4] Harewood GC, Lieberman DA. Colonoscopy practice patterns since introduction of Medicare coverage for average-risk screening. Clin Gastroenterol Hepatol 2004;2:72–7.
[5] Kolata G. 50 and ready for a colonoscopy? Doctors say there is often a wait. New York Times. December 8, 2003, pages A1, A23.
[6] Dukes C. Simple tumours of the large intestine and their relation to cancer. Br J Surg 1924-5;13:720–33.
[7] Dukes CF. The classification of rectal cancer. J Pathol Bacteriol 1932;35:323–32.
[8] Morson BC. Polyps in cancer of the large bowel. In: Yardley JH, Morson BC, Abell MR, editors. The gastrointestinal tract. Baltimore: Williams and Wilkins; 1977. p. 101.
[9] Enterline HT. Polyps and cancer of the large bowel. Curr Top Pathol 1976;63:95–141.
[10] Wolff WI, Shinya H. Colonofiberoscopy. JAMA 1971;217:1509–12.
[11] Cappell MS, Waye JD, Farrar JT, Sleisenger MH. Fifty landmark discoveries in gastroenterology during the past 50 years: a brief history of modern gastroenterology at the millennium. Part I. Gastrointestinal procedures and upper gastrointestinal disorders. Gastroenterol Clin North Am 2000;29:223–63.
[12] Gilbertsen VA. Proctosigmoidoscopy and polypectomy in reducing the incidence of rectal cancer. Cancer 1974;34(suppl):936–9.
[13] Boas I. Die lehre von den okkulten blutungen. Leipzig: Georg Thieme; 1914.
[14] Macrae FA, St. John DJ. Relationship between patterns of bleeding and Hemoccult sensitivity in patients with colorectal cancers or adenomas. Gastroenterology 1982;82: 891–8.
[15] Greegor DH. Diagnosis of large-bowel cancer in the asymptomatic patient. JAMA 1967; 201:943–5.
[16] Greegor DH. A progress report: detection of colorectal cancer using guaiac slides. CA Cancer J Clin 1972;22:360–3.
[17] Mandel JS, Bond JH, Church TR, Snover DC, Bradley GM, Schuman LM, et al. Reducing mortality from colorectal cancer by screening for fecal occult blood. Minnesota Colon Cancer Control Study. N Engl J Med 1993;328:1365–71.
[18] Macrae FA, St. John DJ, Caligiore P, Taylor LS, Legge JW. Optimal dietary conditions for Hemoccult testing. Gastroenterology 1982;82:899–903.
[19] Reilly JM, Ballantyne GH, Fleming FX, Zucker KA, Modlin IM. Evaluation of the occult blood test in screening for colorectal neoplasms: a prospective study using flexible endoscopy. Am Surg 1990;56:119–23.
[20] Hardcastle JD, Armitage NC, Chamberlain J, Amar SS, James PD, Balfour TW. Fecal occult blood screening for colorectal cancer in the general population: results of a controlled trial. Cancer 1986;58:397–403.
[21] Selby JV, Friedman GD, Quesenberry CP Jr, Weiss NS. A case-control study of screening sigmoidoscopy and mortality from colorectal cancer. N Engl J Med 1992;326:653–7.
[22] Rex DK, Chak A, Vasudeva R, Gross T, Lieberman D, Bhattacharya I, et al. Prospective determination of distal colon findings in average-risk patients with proximal colon cancer. Gastrointest Endosc 1999;49:727–30.
[23] Imperiale TF, Wagner DR, Lin CY, Larkin GN, Rogge JD, Ransohoff DF. Risk of advanced proximal neoplasms in asymptomatic adults according to the distal colorectal findings. N Engl J Med 2000;343:169–74.
[24] Levin TR. Flexible sigmoidoscopy for colorectal cancer screening: valid approach or short sighted? Gastroenterol Clin North Am 2002;31:1015–29.
[25] Lieberman DA, Smith FW. Screening for colon malignancy with colonoscopy. Am J Gastroenterol 1991;86:946–51.
[26] Winawer SJ, Stewart ET, Zauber AG, Bond JH, Ansel H, Waye JD, et al. A comparison of colonoscopy and double-contrast barium enema for surveillance after polypectomy. National Polyp Study Work Group. N Engl J Med 2000;342:1766–72.

[27] Rex DK, Cutler CS, Lemmel GT, Rahmani EY, Clark DW, Helper DJ, et al. Colonoscopic miss rates of adenomas determined by back-to-back colonoscopies. Gastroenterology 1997;112:24–8.

[28] Citarda F, Tomaselli G, Capocaccia R, Barcherini S, Crespi M; Italian Multicentre Study Group. Efficacy in standard clinical practice of colonoscopic polypectomy in reducing colorectal cancer incidence. Gut 2001;48:812–5.

[29] Lieberman DA, Weiss DG, Bond JH, Ahnen DJ, Garewal H, Chejfec G. Use of colonoscopy to screen asymptomatic adults for colorectal cancer: Veterans Affairs Cooperative Study Group 380. N Engl J Med 2000;343:162–8.

[30] Nelson DB, McQuaid KR, Bond JH, Lieberman DA, Weiss DG, Johnston TK. Procedural success and complications of large-scale screening colonoscopy. Gastrointest Endosc 2002; 55:307–14.

[31] Winawer SJ, Fletcher RH, Miller L, Godlee F, Stolar MH, Mulrow CD, et al. Colorectal cancer screening: clinical guidelines and rationale. Gastroenterology 1997;112:594–642.

[32] Byers T, Levin B, Rothenberger D, Dodd GD, Smith RA. American Cancer Society guidelines for screening and surveillance for early detection of colorectal polyps and cancer: update 1997-American Cancer Society Detection and Treatment Advisory Group on Colorectal Cancer. CA Cancer J Clin 1997;47:154–60.

[33] Bond JH. Polyp guideline: diagnosis, treatment, and surveillance for patients with colorectal polyps. Practice Parameters Committee of the American College of Gastroenterology. Am J Gastroenterol 2000;95:3053–63.

[34] American Society for Gastrointestinal Endoscopy. Guidelines for colorectal screening and surveillance. Gastrointest Endosc 2000;51:777–82.

[35] Winawer S, Fletcher R, Rex D, Bond J, Burt R, Ferrucci J, et al. Colorectal cancer screening and surveillance: clinical guidelines and rationale – update based on new evidence. Gastroenterology 2003;124:544–60.

[36] Smith RA, Cokkinides V, Eyre H. American Cancer Society guidelines for the early detection of cancer, 2004. CA Cancer J Clin 2004;54:41–52.

[37] Cappell MS, Friedel D. The role of sigmoidoscopy and colonoscopy in the diagnosis and management of lower gastrointestinal disorders: technique, indications, and contraindications. Med Clin North Am 2002;86:1217–52.

[38] Johnson DA, Gurney MS, Volpe RJ, Jones DM, VanNess MM, Chobanian SJ, et al. A prospective study of the prevalence of colonic neoplasms in asymptomatic patients with an age-related risk. Am J Gastroenterol 1990;85:969–74.

[39] Vining DJ. Virtual colonoscopy: the inside story. In: Dachman A, editor. Atlas of virtual colonoscopy. New York: Springer-Verlag; 2003. p. 3–4.

[40] Durkalski VL, Palesch YY, Pineau BC, Vining DJ, Cotton PB. The virtual colonoscopy study: a large multicenter clinical trial designed to compare two diagnostic screening procedures. Control Clin Trials 2002;23:570–83.

[41] Hara AK, Johnson CD, Reed JE, Ahlquist DA, Nelson H, MacCarty RL, et al. Detection of colorectal polyps with CT colography: initial assessment of sensitivity and specificity. Radiology 1997;205:59–65.

[42] Johnson CD, Harmsen WS, Wilson LA, MacCarty RL, Welch TJ, Ilstrup DM, et al. Prospective blinded evaluation of computed tomographic colonography for screen detection of colorectal polyps. Gastroenterology 2003;125:311–9.

[43] Pickhardt PJ, Choi JR, Hwang I, Butler JA, Puckett ML, Hildebrandt HA, et al. Computed tomographic virtual colonoscopy to screen for colorectal neoplasia in asymptomatic adults. N Engl J Med 2003;349:2191–200.

[44] Cotton PB, Durkalski VL, Pineau BC, Palesch YY, Mauldin PD, Hofman B, et al. Computed tomographic colonography (virtual colonoscopy): a multicenter comparison with standard colonoscopy for detection of colorectal neoplasia. JAMA 2004; 291:1713–8.

[45] Yee J, Akerkar GA, Hung RK, Steinauer-Gebauer AM, Wall SD, McQuaid KR. Colorectal neoplasia: performance characteristics of CT colonography for detection in 300 patients. Radiology 2001;219:685–92.
[46] Yee J. CT colonography: examination prerequisites. Abdom Imaging 2002;27:244–52.
[47] Fass R, Do S, Hixson LJ. Fatal hyperphosphatemia following Fleet phosphosoda in a patient with colonic ileus. Am J Gastroenterol 1993;88:929–32.
[48] Serracino-Inglott F, Atkinson HDE, Jha P, Parker I, Anderson DN. Early experiences with computed axial tomography colonography. Am J Surg 2004;187:511–4.
[49] Bessette JR, Maglinte DD. Double-contrast barium enema study: simple conversion to $CO_2$. Radiology 1987;162:274–5.
[50] Chernish SM, Maglinte DD. Glucagon: common untoward reactions – review and recommendations. Radiology 1990;177:145–6.
[51] Yee J, Hung RK, Akerkar GA, Wall SD. The usefulness of glucagon hydrochloride in CT colonography. AJR Am J Roentgenol 1999;173:1–4.
[52] Pickhardt PJ, Choi JH. Electronic cleansing and stool tagging in CT colonography: advantages and pitfalls with primary three-dimensional evaluation. AJR Am J Roentgenol 2003;181:799–805.
[53] Callstrom MR, Johnson CD, Fletcher JG, Reed JE, Ahlquist DA, Harmsen WS, et al. CT colonography without cathartic preparation: feasibility study. Radiology 2001;219:693–8.
[54] Zalis ME, Perumpillichira J, Del Frate, Hahn PF. CT colonography: digital subtraction bowel cleansing with mucosal reconstruction: initial observations. Radiology 2003;226: 911–7.
[55] Fletcher JG. Future directions in CT colonography. Abdom Imaging 2002;27:301–8.
[56] Zalis ME, Hahn PF. Digital subtraction bowel cleansing in CT colonography. AJR Am J Roentgenol 2001;176:646–8.
[57] Morrin MM, Farrell RJ, Kruskal JB, Reynolds K, McGee JB, Raptopoulos V. Utility of intravenously administered contrast material at CT colonography. Radiology 2000;217: 765–71.
[58] Harvey CJ, Amin Z, Hare CM, Gillams AR, Novelli MR, Boulos PB, et al. Helical CT pneumocolon to assess colonic tumors: radiologic-pathologic correlation. AJR Am J Roentgenol 1998;170:1439–43.
[59] Chu KJ. Angiography. In: Yamada T, Alpers DH, Kaplowitz N, et al, editors. Textbook of gastroenterology. 4th edition. Philadelphia: Lippincott Williams & Wilkins; 2003. p. 3229–47.
[60] Witten DM, Hirsch FD, Hartman GW. Acute reactions to urographic contrast medium: incidence, clinical characteristics and relationship to history of hypersensitivity states. AJR Am J Roentgenol 1973;119:832.
[61] McCollough CH. Optimization of multidetector array CT acquisition parameters for CT colonography. Abdom Imaging 2002;27:253–9.
[62] Macari M, Milano A, Lavelle M, Berman P, Megibow AJ. Comparison of time-efficient CT colonography with two- and three-dimensional colonic evaluation for detecting colorectal polyps. AJR Am J Roentgenol 2000;174:1543–9.
[63] Macari M, Megibow AJ. Pitfalls of using three-dimensional CT colonography with two-dimensional imaging correlation. AJR Am J Roentgenol 2001;176:137–43.
[64] McFarland EG. Reader strategies for CT colonography. Abdom Imaging 2002;27: 275–83.
[65] Pickhardt PJ. Three-dimensional endoluminal CT colonography (virtual colonoscopy): comparison of three commercially available systems. AJR Am J Roentgenol 2003;181: 1599–606.
[66] Dachman AH, Kuniyoshi JK, Boyle CM, Samara Y, Hoffmann KR, Rubin DT, et al. CT colonography with three-dimensional problem solving for detection of colonic polyps. AJR Am J Roentgenol 1998;171:989–95.

[67] McFarland EG, Brink JA, Pilgram TK, Heiken JP, Balfe DM, Hirselj DA, et al. Spiral CT colonography: reader agreement and diagnostic performance with two- and three-dimensional image-display techniques. Radiology 2001;218:375–83.
[68] Johnson CD, Dachman AH. CT colonography: the next screening examination? Radiology 2000;216:331–41.
[69] Ferrucci JT. Colon cancer screening with virtual colonoscopy: promise, polyps, politics. AJR Am J Roentgenol 2001;177:975–88.
[70] Fenlon HM. CT colonography: pitfalls and interpretation. Abdom Imaging 2002;27:284–91.
[71] Macari M, Bini EJ, Jacobs SL, Lange N, Lui YW. Filling defects at CT colonography: pseudo and diminutive lesions (the good), polyps (the bad), flat lesions, masses, and carcinomas (the ugly). Radiographics 2003;23:1073–91.
[72] Fidler JL, Johnson CD, MacCarty RL, Welch TJ, Hara AK, Harmsen WS. Detection of flat lesions in the colon with CT colonography. Abdom Imaging 2002;27:292–300.
[73] Rembacken BJ, Fujii T, Cairns A, Dixon MF, Yoshida S, Chalmers DM, et al. Flat and depressed colonic neoplasms: a prospective study of 1000 colonoscopies in the UK. Lancet 2000;355:1211–4.
[74] Wolber RA, Owen DA. Flat adenomas of the colon. Hum Pathol 1991;22:70–4.
[75] Macari M, Bini EJ, Xue X, Milano A, Katz SS, Resnick D, et al. Colorectal neoplasms: prospective comparison of thin-section low-dose multi-detector row CT colonography and conventional colonoscopy for detection. Radiology 2002;224:383–92.
[76] Kiesslich R, Fritsch J, Holtmann M, Koehler HH, Stolte M, Kanzler S, et al. Methylene blue-aided chromoendoscopy for the detection of intraepithelial neoplasia and colon cancer in ulcerative colitis. Gastroenterology 2003;124:880–8.
[77] Lee JH, Kim JW, Cho YK, Sohn CI, Jeon WK, Kim BI, et al. Detection of colorectal adenomas by routine chromoendoscopy with indigocarmine. Am J Gastroenterol 2003;98: 1284–8.
[78] Edwards JT, Mendelson RM, Fritschi L, Foster NM, Wood C, Murray D, et al. Colorectal neoplasia screening with CT colonography in average-risk asymptomatic subjects: community-based study. Radiology 2004;230:459–64.
[79] Fenlon HM, Nunes DP, Schroy PC III, Barish MA, Clark PD, Ferrucci JT. A comparison of virtual and conventional colonoscopy for the detection of colorectal polyps. N Engl J Med 1999;341:1496–503.
[80] Fletcher JG, Johnson CD, Welch TJ, MacCarty RL, Ahlquist DA, Reed JE, et al. Optimization of CT colonography technique: prospective trial in 180 patients. Radiology 2000;216:704–11.
[81] Glueckner T, Dorta G, Keller W, Jomod P, Meuli R, Schnyder P. Performance of multidetector computed tomography compared with conventional colonoscopy. Gut 2002; 51:207–11.
[82] Hara AK, Johnson CD, MacCarty RL, Welch TJ, McCollough CH, Hamsen WS. CT colonography: single-versus multi-detector row imaging. Radiology 2001;219:461–5.
[83] Hara AK, Johnson CD, MacCarty RL, Welch TJ. Incidental extracolonic findings at CT colonography. Radiology 2000;215:353–7.
[84] Hellstrom M, Svensson MH, Lasson A. Extracolonic and incidental findings on CT colonography (virtual colonoscopy). AJR Am J Roentgenol 2004;182:631–8.
[85] Macari M, Bini EJ, Jacobs SL, Naik S, Lui YW, Milano A, et al. Colorectal polyps and cancers in asymptomatic average-risk patients: evaluation with CT colonography. Radiology 2004;230:629–36.
[86] Mendelson RM, Foster NM, Edwards JT, Meuli R, Pantoflickova D, Duvoisin B, et al. Virtual colonoscopy compared with conventional colonoscopy: a developing technology. Med J Aust 2000;173:472–5.
[87] Pescatore P, Glucker T, Delari J, Meuli R, Pantoflickova D, Duvoisin B, et al. Diagnostic accuracy and interobserver agreement of CT colonography (virtual colonoscopy). Gut 2000;47:126–30.

[88] Rex DK, Vining D, Kopecky KK. An initial experience with screening for colon polyps using spiral CT with and without colography (virtual colonoscopy). Gastrointest Endosc 1999;50:309–13.
[89] Royster AP, Fenlon HM, Clarke PD, Nunes DP, Ferrucci JT. CT colonoscopy of colorectal neoplasms: two-dimensional and three-dimensional virtual-reality techniques with colonoscopic correlation. AJR Am J Roentgenol 1997;169:1237–42.
[90] Sosna J, Morrin MM, Kruskal JB, Lavin PT, Rosen MP, Raptopoulos V. CT colonography of colorectal polyps: a meta-analysis. AJR Am J Roentgenol 2003;181: 1593–8.
[91] Spinzi G, Belloni G, Martegani A, Sangiovanni A, Del Favero C, Minoli G. Computed tomographic colonography and conventional colonoscopy for colon diseases: a prospective, blinded study. Am J Gastroenterol 2001;96:394–400.
[92] Ransohoff DF. Virtual colonoscopy: what it can do vs. what it will do [editorial]. JAMA 2004;291:1772–4.
[93] Macari M, Berman P, Dicker M, Milano A, Megibow AJ. Usefulness of CT colonography in patients with incomplete colonography. AJR Am J Roentgenol 1999;173:561–4.
[94] Morrin MM, Kruskal JB, Farrell RJ, Goldberg SN, McGee JB, Raptopoulos V. Endoluminal CT colonography after an incomplete endoscopic colonoscopy. AJR Am J Roentgenol 1999;172:913–8.
[95] Fenlon HM, McAneny DB, Nunes DP, Clarke PD, Ferrucci JT. Occlusive colon carcinoma: virtual colonoscopy in the preoperative evaluation of the proximal colon. Radiology 1999;210:423–8.
[96] Morrin MM, Farrell RJ, Raptopoulos V, McGee JB, Bleday R, Kruskal JB. Role of virtual computed tomographic colonography in patients with colorectal cancers and obstructing colorectal lesions. Dis Colon Rectum 2000;43:303–11.
[97] Taylor SA, Halligan S, Saunders BP, Bassett P, Vance M, Bartram CI. Acceptance by patients of multidetector CT colonography compared with barium enema examinations, flexible sigmoidoscopy, and colonoscopy. AJR Am J Roentgenol 2003;181:913–21.
[98] Svensson MH, Svensson E, Lasson A, Hellstrom M. Patient acceptance of CT colonography and conventional colonoscopy: prospective comparative study in patients with or suspected of having colorectal disease. Radiology 2002;222:337–45.
[99] Weitzman ER, Zapka J, Estabrook B, Goins KV. Risk and reluctance: understanding impediments to colorectal cancer screening. Prev Med 2001;32:502–13.
[100] Ji H, Rolnick JA, Haker S, Barish MA. Multislice CT colonography: current status and limitations. Eur J Radiol 2003;47:123–4.
[101] Kamar M, Portnoy O, Bar-Dayan A, Amitai M, Munz Y, Ayalon A, et al. Actual colonic perforation in virtual colonoscopy: report of a case. Dis Colon Rectum 2004;47: 1242–6.
[102] van Gelder RE, Venema HW, Serlie IW, Nio CY, Determann RM, Tipker CA, et al. CT colonography at different radiation dose levels: feasibility of dose reduction. Radiology 2002;224:25–33.
[103] Iannaccone R, Laghi A, Catalano C, Brink JA, Mangiapane F, Trenna S, et al. Detection of colorectal lesions: lower-dose multi-detector row helical CT colonography compared with conventional colonoscopy. Radiology 2003;229:775–81.
[104] Schreyer AG, Golder S, Seitz J, Harfarth H. New diagnostic avenues in inflammatory bowel diseases: capsule endoscopy, magnetic resonance imaging and virtual enteroscopy. Dig Dis 2002;21:129–37.
[105] Bond JH. Clinical relevance of the small colorectal polyp. Endoscopy 2001;33:454–7.
[106] Kulling D, Christ AD, Karaaslan N, Fried M, Bauerfeind P. Is histological investigation of polyps always necessary? Endoscopy 2001;33:428–32.
[107] Summers RM. Challenges for computer-aided diagnosis for CT colonography. Abdom Imaging 2002;27:268–74.

[108] Summers RM, Beaulieu CF, Pusanik LM, Malley JD, Jeffrey RB Jr, Glazer DI, et al. Automated polyp detector for CT colonography: feasibility study. Radiology 2000;216: 284–90.
[109] McFarland EG, Pilgram TK, Brink JA, McDermott RA, Santillan CV, Brady PW, et al. CT colonography: multiobserver diagnostic performance. Radiology 2002;225:380–90.

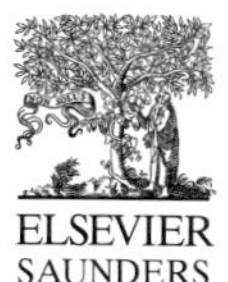

ELSEVIER
SAUNDERS

Med Clin N Am 89 (2005) 139–158

THE MEDICAL CLINICS OF NORTH AMERICA

# Endoscopic ultrasound in the diagnosis, staging, and management of gastrointestinal and adjacent malignancies

Radha Tamerisa, MD[a], Atsushi Irisawa, MD, PhD[b], Manoop S. Bhutani, MD, FACG, FACP[a,*]

[a]*Department of Medicine, University of Texas Medical Branch, 301 University Boulevard, Route 0764, Galveston, TX 77555–0764, USA*

[b]*Fukushima University School of Medicine, 1 Kanayasawa, Fukushima 960-1296, Japan*

Endoscopic ultrasound (EUS) was initially developed in the early 1980s primarily to overcome the limitations of transabdominal ultrasound in imaging the pancreas. In EUS, a small high-frequency ultrasound transducer is incorporated into the tip of a flexible endoscope. EUS is now recognized as the best modality for local staging of esophageal, gastric, and rectal cancer, with T staging accuracy near 90%, and for identification of pancreatic tumors with a sensitivity of over 95% [1–6]. In interventional endosonography, linear array echoendoscopes permit real-time EUS-guided puncture of target lesions for cytologic evaluation of such lesions.

## Technique

Radial scanning echoendoscopes were initially most frequently used for EUS. The ultrasound transducer rotates to provide a 360-degree cross-sectional image (Fig. 1). Viewing frequencies between 5 and 20 MHz are used. A balloon with water-filling capacity encases the ultrasound transducer at the tip of the endoscope. The water in the balloon helps overcome the difficulty of imaging in an air-filled lumen. Solid-state radial EUS instruments, without rotating parts, have been recently introduced. Linear array echoendoscopes provide ultrasound images along the long axis of the

* Corresponding author.
*E-mail address:* msbhutan@utmb.edu (M.S. Bhutani).


doi:10.1016/j.mcna.2004.08.010

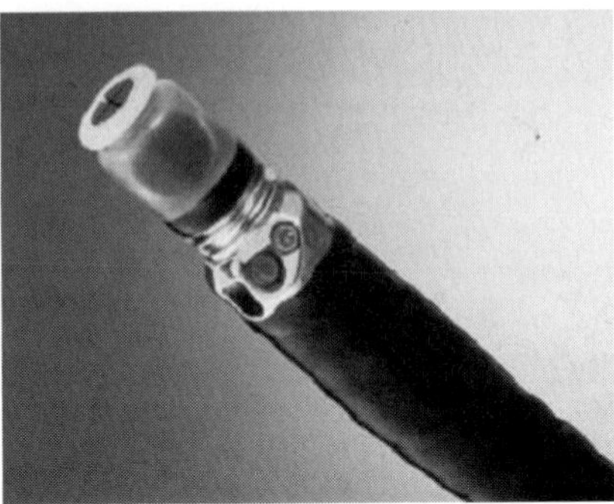

Fig. 1. Tip of a radial echoendoscope showing the ultrasound transducer that provides a 360-degree circular scan perpendicular to the long axis of the instrument. (Courtesy of Olympus Corporation, Melville, NY; with permission.)

echoendoscope. This type of echoendoscope provides a linear array view along the axis of the needle as is required for interventional EUS (Fig. 2).

Endoscopic ultrasound provides a detailed view of the gastrointestinal wall layers, which appear as alternating bright and dark bands [7]. These layers include (1) superficial mucosa (hyperechoic); (2) deep mucosa (hypoechoic); (3) submucosa (hyperechoic); (4) muscularis propria (hypoechoic); and (5) serosa (hyperechoic) (Fig. 3).

In high-frequency ultrasound probe sonography, or miniprobe EUS, a catheter, which is inserted through a standard endoscopic channel, contains a small rotating ultrasound transducer at the tip. High-frequency ultrasound probe sonography is helpful to evaluate small mucosal lesions or intramural lesions because the probe can be placed directly over the lesion. The gastrointestinal tract is imaged in detail at frequencies of 12 and

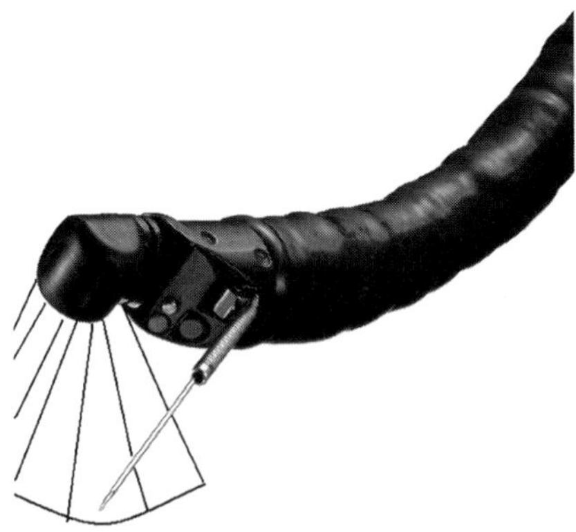

Fig. 2. Tip of a linear echoendoscope that provides a linear array view along the length of a needle for interventional procedures under real-time endosonographic guidance. (Courtesy of Pentax Corporation, Montvale, NJ; with permission.)

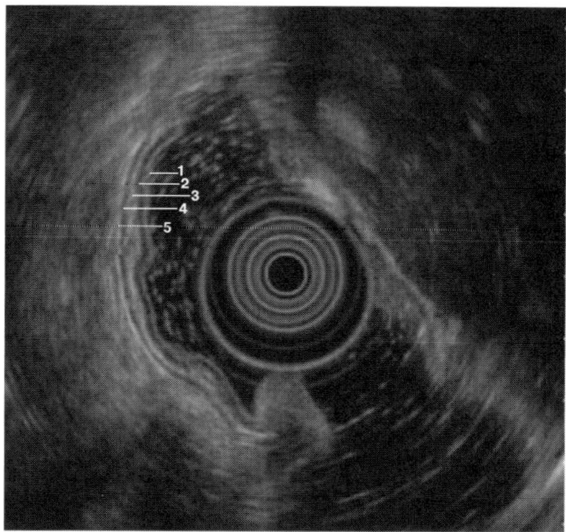


Fig. 3. Endosonography showing the typical five-layer echo pattern of the normal gastric wall that correlates with histology. Superficial mucosa or border echo (*1*), deep mucosa (*2*), submucosa (*3*), muscularis propria (*4*), and serosa (*5*).

30 MHz. The higher operating frequencies afford better resolution of the wall layers, with definition of up to nine layers, and improve the assessment of depth of lesion penetration [8]. Other advantages of the miniprobe include better imaging of small 1- to 2-cm, flat lesions, which are sometimes difficult to locate with a standard echoendoscope; visualization of esophageal varices without variceal compression; and colonic imaging during routine colonoscopy. Akahoshi et al [8] demonstrated that the accuracy in staging of gastric cancer with the miniprobe was 84% for lesions less than 10 mm deep, but declined to only 42% for lesions more than 30 mm deep. The miniprobe is relatively inaccurate in detecting lymph node metastases because of depth of penetration.

## General indications for diagnostic ultrasound evaluation of cancer

### *Staging of gastrointestinal luminal cancers*

EUS is useful for TNM (tumor, node, metastases) staging of esophageal, gastric, duodenal, and colorectal cancer. T signifies the local extent of tumor. Tumors that involve the mucosa or submucosa but do not invade the muscularis propria are classified as T1. Extension into the muscularis propria but not beyond is T2. Extension beyond the muscularis propria signifies a T3 lesion. T4 denotes local invasion from advanced cancer of surrounding structures or important vessels. N staging is reported as N0, N1, N2, and so forth in sequence to signify progressively greater lymph node involvement.

*Submucosal masses*

Diagnosis of submucosal lesions is often challenging. Endoscopic biopsies are usually nondiagnostic. The differential diagnosis of a submucosal gastrointestinal mass is broad and includes lipoma, carcinoid tumor, granular cell tumor, pancreatic rest, lymphoma, metastasis, and gastrointestinal stromal cell tumor versus extrinsic compression from a normal adjacent organ or pathologic process in the abdomen or thorax. EUS reliably distinguishes between the layers of the gastrointestinal tract and is useful in the diagnosis of submucosal lesions. For example, a lipoma appears as a hyperechogenic, homogeneous lesion arising in the submucosa (layer 3). A gastrointestinal stromal cell tumor, which arises from intestinal pacemaker cells, the interstitial cells of Cajal located in the myenteric plexus, may appear as a hypoechoic lesion arising in the muscularis propria (layer 4). Up to 70% of gastrointestinal stromal cell tumors arise in the stomach; 20% to 30% in the small intestine; and up to 10% in the esophagus, colon, or rectum [9,10]. Although EUS imaging alone does not conclusively distinguish benign from malignant lesions, some echofeatures are suggestive. Large tumor size (>4 cm), irregular borders, echogenic foci, and cystic spaces are suggestive of malignancy. Lack of these features favors a benign lesion [11,12]. EUS-guided real-time fine-needle aspiration (FNA) of submucosal lesions permits a cytologic diagnosis. The sensitivity of EUS-guided FNA cytology for submucosal tumors was approximately 60% in earlier studies [13,14]. In a prospective multicenter cohort study, Nickl et al [15] reported that approximately 75% of resected hypoechoic submucosal tumors were gastrointestinal stromal tumors. The interstitial cells of Cajal normally regulate gut peristalsis [16–18], and express CD 117, a product of a c-*kit* proto-oncogene that regulates cellular proliferation of gastrointestinal stromal cell tumors. In virtually all gastrointestinal stromal cell tumors, the c-*kit* oncogene is mutated and exhibits consistent expression of c-*kit*, a pathognomonic characteristic [16–18]. The sensitivity of EUS-guided FNA seems to be improving over the initial sensitivity of 60% because of identification of specific markers, such as CD 117, in cytologic material and use of larger-bore needles in selected circumstances.

*Extramural masses*

Extramural masses can compress and indent the wall of the gastrointestinal tract and resemble submucosal lesions. EUS can reliably distinguish between submucosal lesions and extrinsic compression. Extramural masses detected by EUS include extrinsic tumors, pancreatic pseudocysts, or lymphadenopathy. A normal liver, spleen, gallbladder, or splenic artery may also produce extrinsic compression.

*Evaluation of lymph nodes*

EUS is the most accurate modality for local (T staging) of gastrointestinal tumors, but has only 60% to 80% accuracy for N staging [19].

Echofeatures of lymph nodes including size greater than 1 cm, round shape, hypoechogenicity, and distinct margins have been proposed as highly predictive of malignant invasion, but these features may be inconclusive because of interobserver variability and overlap in the echofeatures between benign and malignant lymph nodes [20]. EUS-guided FNA of lymph nodes has improved the ability to detect malignant lymph node invasion. EUS-guided FNA is possible for subcarinal, aortopulmonary window, para-aortic, paratracheal, celiac axis, and peripancreatic lymph nodes [20]. EUS-guided FNA has a sensitivity of about 80% and a specificity of about 94% for the diagnosis of malignant lymph node invasion [21].

## Indications for evaluation of specific gastrointestinal cancers

### *Early esophageal cancer*

EUS is the most accurate locoregional staging modality for early and advanced esophageal carcinoma [22–25]. Early esophageal cancers, limited to the mucosa (T1m) or submucosa (T1sm), have a good prognosis after treatment (Fig. 4). Endoscopic mucosal resection may be considered in patients with small lesions (<2 cm in diameter or < one third of circumference involved) [26–28]. A high-frequency EUS probe introduced through the standard endoscope may more accurately differentiate between a T2m and T1sm lesion than a standard EUS probe. EUS is generally

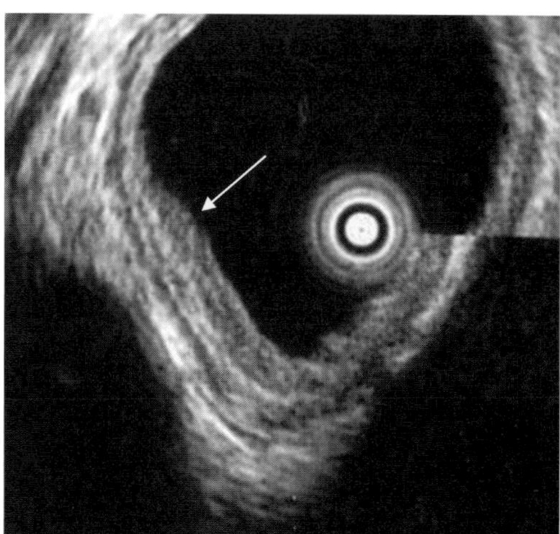

Fig. 4. Early squamous cell esophageal carcinoma as imaged by a high-frequency EUS miniprobe. The lesion appears as a hypoechoic lesion (*arrow*) in the first and second echo layers of the esophagus (superficial and deep mucosa). Because of the high resolution of the miniprobe, the muscularis propria is separated into three layers (internal circular muscle, border echo, outer longitudinal muscle) and a total of seven layers are visualized instead of five.

a prerequisite for endoscopic mucosal resection of early esophageal carcinoma.

Scotiniotis et al [29] evaluated the accuracy of EUS using 7.5- or 12.5-MHz echoendoscopes in 22 patients with a diagnosis of high-grade dysplasia or intramucosal carcinoma diagnosed by conventional methods. EUS detected all five patients with submucosal invasion and the one patient with lymph node involvement proved by surgical and pathologic evaluation. Preoperative EUS carries a sensitivity of 100%, specificity of 81% and a negative predictive value of 100% for detection of submucosal invasion. EUS seems to be a useful tool when nonsurgical management is contemplated.

### *Advanced esophageal cancer*

Appropriate staging is essential for advanced squamous cell or adenocarcinoma of the esophagus (Fig. 5), because the prognosis correlates with T and N staging and the presence of celiac lymph node invasion [30]. T4 cancers that may not benefit from surgery are more reliably identified by EUS than CT scan. EUS staging helps in decisions regarding neoadjuvant therapy in patients with locally advanced cancer.

CT is useful in detecting distant metastases, but EUS provides better locoregional staging. Tio et al [31] reported 50% accuracy for T and N staging by CT compared with 85% for T staging and 75% for N staging by EUS [22,32]. Celiac lymph node invasion, classified as stage M1, may render

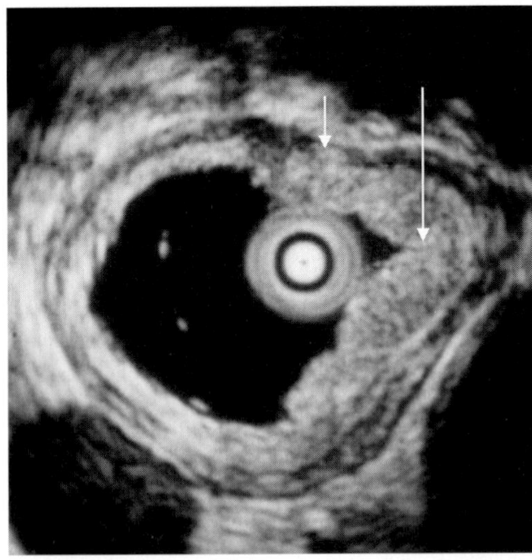

Fig. 5. A T2 esophageal cancer seen as a hypoechoic mass by EUS (*long arrow*) in the esophageal wall, infiltrating into the musclaris propria (*short arrow*).

the lesion unresectable. It is associated with a poor prognosis. Eloubeidi et al [33] reported 77% sensitivity and 85% specificity for celiac lymph node detection by EUS, with 98% accuracy for FNA [33]. EUS and EUS-FNA seem to be less costly than CT-guided FNA [34].

### *Early gastric adenocarcinoma*

Early gastric cancer, confined to the mucosa (T1m) or the submucosa (T1sm), has a 95% 5-year survival rate following resection. T1m cancers have a 5% risk of lymph node metastases and are potentially endoscopically resectable. T1sm cancers have a 10% to 20% risk of metastases and require surgery [35,36]. EUS imaging is critical to identify patients with early gastric cancer. High-frequency miniprobes (20 MHz) better visualize early lesions, especially those under 2 cm in diameter, and improve the accuracy of staging [37].

### *Advanced gastric adenocarcinoma*

EUS staging helps assess the resectability and prognosis of advanced gastric cancer, and the need for multimodal therapy (Fig. 6). EUS has 80% accuracy in T staging of gastric cancers [38–44]. EUS is more accurate than CT in the T staging (92% versus 48%) [39]. CT is, however, the best test to detect distant metastases and is part of the standard evaluation of gastric cancer. EUS alters the surgical management in approximately 30% of patients with gastric cancer. EUS has an accuracy of 85% in predicting resectability by demonstrating no invasion into adjacent structures.

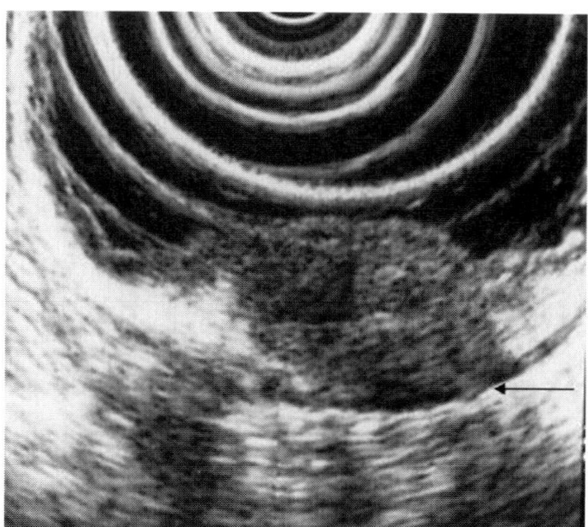

Fig. 6. Gastric carcinoma appears as a large hypoechoic intramural mass by EUS. EUS revealed that the mass had infiltrated into the musclaris propria (*arrow*) but had not penetrated through it because the margin of the tumor was still well defined.

### *Gastric lymphoma including mucosa-associated lymphoid tissue lymphoma*

Primary gastric lymphoma is rare, but is increasing in incidence. These tumors are believed mostly to arise in the mucosa or submucosa from mucosa-associated lymphoid tissue, usually in the setting of chronic inflammation induced by *Helicobacter pylori* infection [45–48]. Some gastric lymphomas are non–mucosa-associated lymphoid tissue type. EUS can help determine the depth of invasion, horizontal tumor extension, and perigastric lymph node invasion [49–53]. Infiltrative carcinomas tend to grow transmurally, whereas lymphomas tend to extend horizontally [54,55]. Mucosa-associated lymphoid tissue may regress after *H pylori* therapy and eradication. EUS detects regression as normalization of wall thickness [53,56–58]. Surveillance of patients with mucosa-associated lymphoid tissue lymphomas should include extensive gastric sampling with biopsies of the gastric antrum and body [59].

### *Anastomotic recurrence*

EUS helps in assessing anastomotic recurrence after surgery for gastric cancer. Early gastric cancers are associated with 15% recurrence as opposed to 77% recurrence in stage T3 and T4 cancers [60]. EUS has a sensitivity of 95% and specificity of 80% in postoperative staging. Anastomotic recurrence is identified by mural thickening and nodularity and irregularity of the outer margin. Lymph node invasion is also assessed by EUS.

### *Pancreatic cancer*

EUS is the most accurate diagnostic imaging modality for pancreatic cancer. EUS is estimated to have an accuracy of 93% to 100% compared with 53% to 90% for CT, MRI, endoscopic retrograde cholangiopancreatography (ERCP), or angiography [61–68]. Legmann et al [61] reported that both dual-phase CT and EUS had 100% sensitivity for pancreatic cancers greater than 15 mm, but CT was much less sensitive than EUS for cancers less than 15 mm (67% versus 100%). EUS seems to provide better assessment of small pancreatic lesions. The addition of EUS-guided FNA increases the sensitivity of diagnosing malignancy to 85% to 95% and the specificity to near 100% [61,69–72]. T and N staging of pancreatic cancer by EUS has an accuracy of 85% and 70%, respectively. T staging is technically difficult with pancreatitis because inflammation can mimic the typical echofeatures of malignancy, including hypoechogenicity and irregular borders.

Resectability of pancreatic cancer is directly influenced by the presence of vascular invasion. EUS detects venous invasion better than arterial invasion, and invasion into the portal vein and splenic confluence better than invasion of the superior mesenteric vein and artery [73]. Echofeatures of vascular invasion include visualization of tumor in the lumen, presence of collaterals because of vascular obstruction, and complete vascular obstruction. Ahmad et al [74] reported EUS had a sensitivity of 61% and a positive predictive value of 69% in predicting resectability compared with a sensitivity of 73% and a positive predictive value of 71% for MRI. These recent data show a lower accuracy of EUS for pancreatic cancer staging than earlier studies. With technical improvements in helical CT and MRI, they should be the initial imaging techniques for diagnosis and staging, with EUS reserved for pancreatic cancers that have equivocal criteria for resectability, equivocal findings of a pancreatic mass, or for suspected small tumors (<2 cm) not detectable by CT or MRI.

## *Periampullary cancer*

Periampullary tumors arise from or near the ampulla. They include ampullary, distal choledochal, pancreatic head, and duodenal tumors. Periampullary cancer has a 40% 5-year survival rate. Accurate preoperative staging can prevent unnecessarily radical resection. In a study of 21 patients, Chen et al [75] reported EUS was superior to CT and ultrasound in detecting ampullary tumors, but was equal to ERCP in sensitivity (EUS 95%, ERCP 95%, CT 19%, ultrasound 5%). EUS was superior to CT and ultrasound in T staging (EUS 75%, CT 5%, ultrasound 0%) and in detecting lymph node metastasis (EUS 50%, CT 33%, ultrasound 0%) of ampullary cancers. Endobiliary stents may adversely affect the accuracy of T and N staging of ampullary tumors by EUS (with stents: T 71%, N 75%; without stents: T 83%, N 100%), but the difference was not statistically significant. Intraductal ultrasound seems to be more accurate than conventional EUS for periampullary tumors less than 3 cm in diameter [76,77].

## *Neuroendocrine pancreatic tumors*

Patients with neuroendocrine tumors typically present with symptoms caused by secretory products of the tumor, but these tumors are nonfunctional in 15% to 30% of cases. Twenty percent of functional tumors are accurately localized by conventional CT or transabdominal ultrasound [78,79]. More invasive procedures, such as selective arteriography or somatostatin receptor scintigraphy with single positron emission CT, often localize tumors and detect metastases, with a reported sensitivity of 90%. Gastrinomas and insulinomas, however, are poorly identified by somatostatin receptor scintigraphy, with sensitivity less than 60%. EUS is accurate for preoperative localization of pancreatic neuroendocrine tumors and often replaces more invasive diagnostic procedures [66,67]. EUS is much more sensitive (63%) than spiral CT (17%) for insulinomas [80]. EUS has a sensitivity of 70% for pancreatic insulinomas and 50% for extrapancreatic insulinomas. Combined EUS and somatostatin receptor scintigraphy have greater sensitivity than either test alone. EUS is an important imaging modality for neuroendocrine tumors [81–83].

*Pancreatic cystic neoplasms*

EUS aids in the diagnosis and management of patients with cystic pancreatic lesions, including pseudocysts and cystic pancreatic neoplasms. EUS helps differentiate between these two cystic lesions. Echofeatures that suggest benignity include uniloculated, simple, and well-defined cysts, whereas complex, thick-walled, septated, and internally inhomogeneous cysts are likely to be malignant [84]. These criteria are greater than 90% accurate [84], although some investigators have reported some overlap between EUS features of neoplastic and benign cysts. EUS imaging, along with EUS-guided FNA cytology in selected cases, can assist in managing diagnostically equivocal cystic pancreatic lesions [85]. The accuracy of EUS-guided FNA in diagnosing a cystic neoplasm may be as high as 83%. Cyst fluid analysis for tumor markers, including CA 19-9, CA 72-4, CA 15.3, carcinoembryonic antigen, and mucin, may increase the accuracy of diagnosis of neoplasia to 86% [86]. Some initial studies of EUS-guided FNA reported that infectious complications were more common during aspiration of cystic (14%) than solid (0.5%) pancreatic lesions [87]. Antibiotic prophylaxis is recommended for EUS-guided FNA of cystic pancreatic lesions to prevent infectious complications. EUS-guided FNA should be considered on a case-by-case basis for suspected cystic pancreatic neoplasms [88].

*Rectal cancer*

EUS is the most accurate imaging modality for T and N staging of rectal cancer. Endosonography helps evaluate the depth of tumor invasion and presence of sphincter involvement to help determine the treatment approach (eg, transanal excision versus more invasive surgery, abdominoperineal resection versus preoperative neoadjuvant chemoradiation). The accuracy is better than 85% in T staging and 75% in N staging [89]. The impact of EUS-guided FNA of perirectal lymph nodes is less clear. Harewood et al [90] prospectively studied the effect of staging evaluation with CT scan, EUS, and EUS-FNA of visualized perirectal lymph nodes on management decisions in 80 patients with rectal cancer. EUS staging changed the surgeon's original treatment plan based on CT, resulting in preoperative adjuvant treatment in one third of the patients. Addition of EUS-guided FNA changed the therapy in only one patient. EUS-FNA seems to change management in only selected patients with early T stage cancers by detecting unrecognized nodal metastases or excluding cancer in imaged lymph nodes.

### Colon cancer

Most of the data on EUS of the lower gastrointestinal tract involve rectal and anal canal lesions. Matsumoto et al [91] reported that catheter EUS probes had an accuracy of 92% compared with an accuracy of 63% for magnifying colonoscopy. The accuracy for detecting lymph node metastasis was 24% for catheter ultrasound probes and 72% for magnifying colonoscopy. Tseng et al [92] reported an overall accuracy of catheter ultrasound probes for T staging of 85% and for N staging of 73%. EUS application in colon cancer proximal to the rectum may be limited because most patients without distant metastases undergo surgery. With increasing popularity of minimally invasive laparoscopic colon cancer resection, accurate determination of local T and N staging may become more important in the future.

## Indications for evaluation of possible cancers adjacent to the gastrointestinal tract

### Mediastinal lymphadenopathy

EUS-FNA is useful to evaluate mediastinal lymphadenopathy in patients with lung cancer. Nodes in the posterior mediastinum, aortopulmonary window, and subcarina can be sampled by EUS-FNA to evaluate for malignant spread with 90% sensitivity and 83% to 100% specificity [93–95]. Gress et al [96] reported that unnecessary surgery was avoided in 58% of patients with non–small cell lung cancer by malignant cytology detected by EUS-FNA. EUS-FNA is also useful in patients with mediastinal lymphadenopathy without a history of lung cancer. For example, the diagnostic accuracy of EUS-FNA was 84%, with a false-negative rate of 20%, in a study of 59 patients with mediastinal lymphadenopathy [97]. In another study, EUS-FNA established a diagnosis in 56 of the 62 patients with mediastinal lymphadenopathy of unknown etiology and influenced the subsequent evaluation and therapy in 87% of the patients [98].

## Training and availability issues

EUS has become standard practice in the diagnosis and staging of gastrointestinal malignancies. Parada et al [99] found that the current EUS resources are insufficient to meet the current demand in the United States. Future efforts should be focused on increasing the number of endoscopy units with EUS capability and expertise, the capacity of individual endoscopy units, and the number of training programs.

Endoscopic ultrasound requires substantial training. In 1994, the Tenth World Congress of Gastroenterology recommended that a minimum of 50 examinations for esophageal carcinoma staging by EUS was necessary to master the technique [100]. Fockens et al [101], however, reported that novice endosonographers had 58% accuracy for staging esophageal cancer by EUS, a level equivalent to that of CT scanning. Acceptable accuracy rates were achieved only after performing 100 examinations. These authors believed that endoscopic skill, especially with side-viewing endoscopes, is also important. Training in transabdominal ultrasonography is an advantage. Study of textbooks, atlases, laser disks, and videotapes, although important, cannot replace supervised, hands-on endosonographic training.

## Therapeutic and interventional endoscopic ultrasound

EUS-guided FNA biopsy is useful for lesions too small to be visualized or accessed percutaneously. Minimally invasive aspiration biopsies are performed in real time by passing a 22-gauge needle through the channel of a linear echoendoscope. The entire length of the needle is visualized in real time to monitor sonographically the depth of penetration. A cytopathologist can examine the aspirate at the bedside for a preliminary diagnosis during the procedure. FNA is generally a safe procedure, with rare complications. The complication rate ranges from 0.3% to 2% [71,102–104]. Complications include perforation, pancreatitis, hemorrhage, and infection. Antibiotics are recommended before cyst aspiration. Lesions sampled by EUS include mediastinal, intra-abdominal, and perirectal lymph nodes; pancreatic masses; submucosal gastrointestinal lesions; perirectal masses; retroperitoneal masses; and cholangiocarcinomas. EUS-guided FNA of small lesions in the liver, adrenal masses, gallbladder lesions, and renal neoplasms have also been reported.

### *Celiac plexus neurolysis*

In patients experiencing significant abdominal pain from unresectable pancreatic cancer, EUS-guided celiac plexus neurolysis can be performed because the celiac axis is near the gastric wall (Fig. 7). The risk of paraplegia is theoretically less for this technique than for the conventional posterior approach under CT or ultrasound guidance [105,106]. This procedure often effectively palliates the pain. A mixture of a local anesthetic and alcohol is injected by a transgastric approach close to the origin of the celiac artery using a linear echoendoscope for guidance. Gunaratnam et al [107] showed a significant (78%) reduction in pain in patients with pancreatic cancer 24 weeks postprocedure. There were some minor complications of postural hypotension and diarrhea.

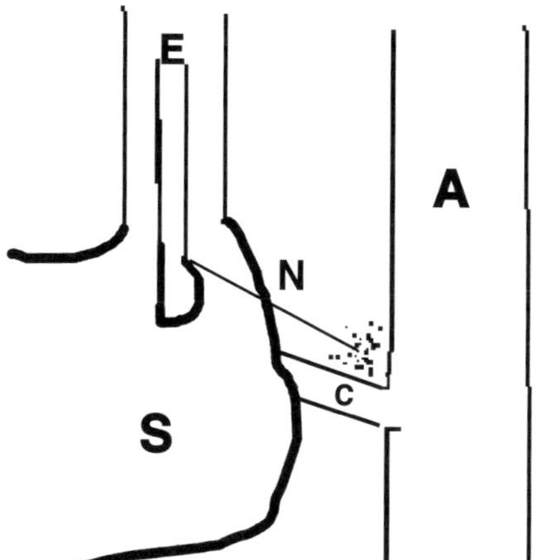


Fig. 7. A cartoon depicting the technique of EUS-guided celiac plexus neurolysis. S, stomach; E, linear echoendoscope in the stomach near the gastroesophageal junction; A, aorta; C, celiac artery; N, needle passed under EUS guidance into the angle between the celiac artery and the aorta to perform the neurolysis.

## New and experimental or controversial applications and trends of endoscopic ultrasound[1]

### *Endoscopic ultrasound–guided radiofrequency ablation*

Goldberg et al [108] analyzed the effects of radiofrequency thermal ablation of the pancreas using a 19-guage needle in 13 pigs. At necropsy, radiofrequency thermal ablation was shown to cause a 1-cm round area of necrosis immediately postprocedure. One of the pigs developed pancreatitis with an elevated lipase and a fluid collection. Radiofrequency thermal ablation may become useful to palliate unresectable pancreatic tumors and treat neuroendocrine tumors, where serum hormonal levels could be monitored to suggest a complete cure.

### *Endoscopic ultrasound–guided fine-needle injection of chemotherapy*

EUS can provide minimally invasive targeted delivery of specific therapies to tumors. EUS-guided FNA of a local immunotherapy (Cytoimplant) in patients with advanced pancreatic carcinoma resulted in a median survival of 13.2 months, with no procedure- related complications [109]. Injection of a modified adenovirus into pancreatic adenocarcinomas under EUS guidance produced up to 47% tumor regression, with five patients experiencing disease progression. Two patients had 57% or 75% reduction

[1] These applications are experimental and not yet established for routine clinical use.

in tumor size with subsequent injection of gemcitabine [110]. Significant side effects included sepsis, cystic fluid collection, and duodenal perforation from the echoendoscope.

*High-intensity focused ultrasound*

Ultrasound has thermal, mechanical, and chemical effects on tumors. Tumor cells are more vulnerable to thermal injury than normal cells. Strong mechanical push-pull forces lead to cellular defects. Ultrasound therapy also leads to easier diffusion of macromolecules [111]. High-intensity focused ultrasound is produced by focusing ultrasound waves in a very narrow focal zone. High-intensity focused ultrasound can be applied successfully with small transducers placed at the tip of an endoscope to cause coagulation necrosis of well-defined lesions in animal models. Prat et al [112] attempted high-intensity focused ultrasound in 10 human subjects during ERCP for treatment of biliary tree and ampullary carcinomas. Three patients had a good response, four had a partial response, and three had no response. More studies are needed to assess the clinical role of high-intensity focused ultrasound.

*Endoscopic ultrasound–guided radiation therapy*

Lohnert et al [113] developed a specially designed applicator permeable to sound waves to apply radiation directly by needles under ultrasound guidance for anal cancer. In a study of 18 patients with anal cancer EUS-guided chemotherapy produced complete initial remission in all patients with 13.9% recurrence at mean follow-up of 44 months [114]. The authors concluded that this method allows them to reach a high rate of cure, with a low complication rate.

## Summary

EUS has become an extremely useful modality for numerous imaging and interventional applications in gastrointestinal cancer [115]. EUS has many promising potential applications in cancer diagnosis and treatment that are currently experimental but may become the standard of care in the future.

## References

[1] Rosch T, Lightdale CJ, Botet JF, Boyce GA, Sivak MV Jr, Yasuda K, et al. Localization of pancreatic endocrine tumors by endoscopic ultrasonography. N Engl J Med 1992;326: 1721–6.

[2] Rosch T, Lorenz R, Braig C, Feuerbach S, Siewart JR, Schusdziarra V, et al. Endoscopic ultrasound in pancreatic tumor diagnosis. Gastrointest Endosc 1991;37:347–52.

[3] Rosch T, Braig C, Gain T, Feuerbach S, Siewart JR, Schusdzierra V, et al. Staging of pancreatic and ampullary carcinoma by endoscopic ultrasonography: comparison with

conventional sonography, computed tomography, and angiography. Gastroenterology 1992;102:188–99.
[4] Rice TW, Boyce GA, Sivak MV, Adelstein DJ, Kirby TJ. Esophageal carcinoma: esophageal ultrasound assessment of preoperative chemotherapy. Ann Thorac Surg 1992; 53:972–7.
[5] Akahoshi K, Misawa T, Fujishima H, Chijiiwa Y, Maruoka A, Ohkubo A, et al. Preoperative evaluation of gastric cancer by endoscopic ultrasound. Gut 1991;32:479–82.
[6] Boyce GA, Sivak MV Jr, Lavery IC, Fazio VW, Church JM, Milsom J, et al. Endoscopic ultrasound in the pre-operative staging of rectal carcinoma. Gastrointest Endosc 1992;38: 468–71.
[7] Kimmey MB, Martin RW, Haggitt RC, Wang KY, Franklin DW, Silverstein FE. Histologic correlates of gastrointestinal ultrasound images. Gastroenterology 1989;96: 433–41.
[8] Akahoshi K, Chijiiwa Y, Hamada S, Sasaki I, Nawata H, Kabemura T, et al. Pretreatment staging of endoscopically early gastric cancer with a 15 MHz ultrasound catheter probe. Gastrointest Endosc 1998;48:470–6.
[9] Miettinen M, Sarlomo-Rikala M, Lasota J. Gastrointestinal stromal tumors: recent advances in understanding of their biology. Hum Pathol 1999;30:1213–20.
[10] Greenson JK. Gastrointestinal stromal tumors and other mesenchymal lesions of the gut. Mod Pathol 2003;16:366–75.
[11] Chak A, Canto MI, Rosch T, Dittler HJ, Hawes RH, Tio TL, et al. Endosonographic differentiation of benign and malignant stromal cell tumors. Gastrointest Endosc 1997;45: 468–73.
[12] Palazzo L, Landi B, Cellier C, Cuillerier E, Roseau G, Barbier JP. Endosonographic features predictive of benign and malignant gastrointestinal stromal cell tumours. Gut 2000;46:88–92.
[13] Giovannini M, Seitz JF, Monges G, Perrier H, Rabbia I. Fine-needle aspiration cytology guided by endoscopic ultrasonography: results in 141 patients. Endoscopy 1995;27:171–7.
[14] Chang KJ, Durbin TE, Katz KD, et al. The clinical value of endoscopic (EUS)-guided fine-needle aspiration (FNA) in gastrointestinal and pulmonary malignancies [abstract]. Am J Gastroenterol 1994;89:1704.
[15] Nickl N, Gress F, McClave SA, et al. Hypoechoic intramural tumor study: final report. Gastrointest Endosc 2002;55:AB252.
[16] Kindblom LG, Remotti HE, Aldenborg F, Meis-Kindblom JM. Gastrointestinal pacemaker cell tumor (GIPACT): gastrointestinal stromal tumors show phenotypic characteristics of the interstitial cells of Cajal. Am J Pathol 1998;152:1259–69.
[17] Sircar K, Hewlett BR, Huizinga JD, Chorneyko K, Berezin I, Riddell RH. Interstitial cells of Cajal as precursors of gastrointestinal stromal tumors. Am J Surg Pathol 1999;23: 377–89.
[18] Sarlomo-Rikala M, Kovatich AJ, Barusevicius A, Miettinen M. CD117: a sensitive marker for gastrointestinal stromal tumors that is more specific than CD34. Mod Pathol 1998;11: 728–34.
[19] Caletti G, Odegard S, Rosch T, Sivak MV, Tio TL, Yasuda K. Endoscopic ultrasonography (EUS): a summary of the conclusions of the Working Party for the Tenth World Congress of Gastroenterology Los Angeles, California October, 1994. The Working Group on Endoscopic Ultrasonography. Am J Gastroenterol 1994;89(Suppl 8): S138–43.
[20] Bhutani MS, Hawes RH, Hoffman BJ. A comparison of the accuracy of echo features during endoscopic ultrasound (EUS) and EUS-guided fine-needle aspiration for diagnosis of malignant lymph node invasion. Gastrointest Endosc 1997;45:474–9.
[21] Harada N, Wiersema M, Wiersema L. Endosonography guided fine-needle aspiration biopsy (EUS FNA) in the evaluation of lymphadenopathy: staging accuracy of EUS FNA versus EUS alone [abstract]. Gastrointest Endosc 1997;45:AB31.

[22] Botet JF, Lightdale CJ, Zauber AG, Gerdes H, Urmacher C, Brennan MF. Preoperative staging of esophageal cancer: comparison of endoscopic US and dynamic CT. Radiology 1991;181:419–25.
[23] Lightdale CJ, Botet JF. Staging of esophageal cancer. Endoscopy 1993;25:655–9.
[24] Hasegawa N, Niwa Y, Arisawa T, Hase S, Goto H, Hayakawa T. Preoperative staging of superficial esophageal carcinoma: comparison of an ultrasonic probe and standard endoscopic ultrasonography. Gastrointest Endosc 1996;44:388–93.
[25] Murata Y, Suzuki S, Ohta M, Mitsunaga A, Hayashi K, Yoshida K, et al. Small ultrasonic probes for determination of the depth of superficial esophageal cancer. Gastrointest Endosc 1996;44:23–8.
[26] Ell C, May A, Gossner L, Pech O, Gunter E, Mayer G, et al. Endoscopic mucosal resection of early cancer and high-grade dysplasia in Barrett's esophagus. Gastroenterology 2000; 118:670–7.
[27] Nijhawan PK, Wang KK. Endoscopic mucosal resection for lesions with endoscopic features suggestive of malignancy and high-grade dysplasia within Barrett's esophagus. Gastrointest Endosc 2000;52:328–32.
[28] Takeshita K, Tani M, Inoue H, Saeki I, Hayashi S, Honda T, et al. Endoscopic treatment of early oesophageal or gastric cancer. Gut 1997;40:123–7.
[29] Scotiniotis IA, Kochman ML, Lewis JD, Furth EE, Rosato EF, Ginsberg GG. Accuracy of EUS in the evaluation of Barrett's esophagus and high-grade dysplasia or intramucosal carcinoma. Gastrointest Endosc 2001;54:689–96.
[30] Pfau PR, Ginsberg GG, Lew RJ, Brensinger CM, Kochman ML. EUS predictors of long-term survival in esophageal carcinoma. Gastrointest Endosc 2001;53:463–9.
[31] Tio TL, Cohen P, Coene PP, Udding J, den Hartog Jager FE, Tytgat GN. Endosonography and computed tomography of esophageal carcinoma: preoperative classification compared to the new (1987) TNM system. Gastroenterology 1989;96:1478–86.
[32] Rosch T. Endosonographic staging of esophageal cancer: a review of literature results. Gastrointest Endosc Clin N Am 1995;5:537–47.
[33] Eloubeidi MA, Wallace MB, Reed CE, Hadzijahic N, Lewin DN, Van Velse A, et al. The utility of EUS and EUS guided fine needle aspiration in detecting celiac lymph node metastasis in patients with esophageal cancer: a single-center experience. Gastrointest Endosc 2001;54:714–9.
[34] Harewood GC, Wiersema MJ. A cost analysis of endoscopic ultrasound in the evaluation of esophageal cancer. Am J Gastroenterol 2002;97:452–8.
[35] Kodama Y, Inokuchi K, Soejima K, Matsusaka T, Okamura T. Growth patterns and prognosis in early gastric carcinoma: superficially spreading and penetrating growth types. Cancer 1983;51:320–6.
[36] Yasuda K. Endoscopic ultrasonic probes and mucosectomy for early gastric carcinoma. Gastrointest Endosc 1996;43:S29–31.
[37] Yanai H, Matsumoto Y, Harada T, Nishiaki M, Tokiyama H, Shigemitsu T, et al. Endoscopic ultrasonography and endoscopy for staging depth of invasion in early gastric cancer: a pilot study. Gastrointest Endosc 1997;46:212–6.
[38] Akahoshi K, Misawa T, Fujishima H, Chijiiwa Y, Maruoka A, Ohkubo A, et al. Preoperative evaluation of gastric cancer by endoscopic ultrasound. Gut 1991;32: 479–82.
[39] Botet JF, Lightdale CJ, Zauber AG, Koch J, Gerdes H, Winawer SJ, Urmacher C, et al. Preoperative staging of gastric cancer: comparison of endoscopic US and dynamic CT. Radiology 1991;181:426–32.
[40] Dittler HJ, Siewert JR. Role of endoscopic ultrasonography in gastric carcinoma. Endoscopy 1993;25:162–6.
[41] Grimm H, Binmoeller KF, Hamper K, Koch J, Henne-Bruns D, Soehendra N. Endosonography for preoperative locoregional staging of esophageal and gastric cancer. Endoscopy 1993;25:224–30.

[42] Murata Y, Suzuki S, Hashimoto H. Endoscopic ultrasonography of the upper gastrointestinal tract. Surg Endosc 1988;2:180–3.
[43] Rosch T, Lorenz R, Zenker K, von Wichert A, Dancygier H, Hofler H, et al. Local staging and assessment of resectability in carcinoma of the esophagus, stomach, and duodenum by endoscopic ultrasonography. Gastrointest Endosc 1992;38:460–7.
[44] Tio TL, Schouwink MH, Cikot RJ, Tytgat GN. Preoperative TNM classification of gastric carcinoma by endosonography in comparison with the pathological TNM system: a prospective study of 72 cases. Hepatogastroenterology 1989;36:51–6.
[45] Radaszkiewicz T, Dragosics B, Bauer P. Gastrointestinal malignant lymphomas of the mucosa-associated lymphoid tissue: factors relevant to prognosis. Gastroenterology 1992; 102:1628–38.
[46] Parsonnet J, Hansen S, Rodriguez L, Gelb AB, Warnke RA, Jellum E, et al. *Helicobacter pylori* infection and gastric lymphoma. N Engl J Med 1994;330:1267–71.
[47] Stolte M. *Helicobacter pylori* gastritis and gastric MALT lymphoma. Lancet 1992;339: 745–6.
[48] Isaacson P, Wright DH. Extranodal malignant lymphoma arising from mucosa associated lymphoid tissue. Cancer 1984;53:2515–24.
[49] Wotherspoon AC, Ortiz-Hidalgo C, Falzon MR, Isaccson PG. *Helicobacter pylori*-associated gastritis and primary B-cell gastric lymphoma. Lancet 1991;338:1175–6.
[50] Bayerdorffer E, Neubauer A, Rudolph B, Thiede C, Lehn N, Edit S, et al. Regression of primary gastric lymphoma of mucosa-associated lymphoid tissue type after cure of *Helicobacter pylori* infection. MALT Lymphoma Study Group. Lancet 1995;345: 1591–4.
[51] Roggero E, Zucca E, Pinotti G, Pascarella A, Capella C, Savio A, et al. Eradication of *Helicobacter pylori* infection in primary low-grade gastric lymphoma of mucosa-associated lymphoid tissue. Ann Intern Med 1995;122:767–9.
[52] Steinbach G, Ford R, Glober G, Sample D, Hagemeister FB, Lynch PM, et al. Antibiotic treatment of gastric lymphoma of mucosa-associated lymphoid tissue: an uncontrolled trial. Ann Intern Med 1999;131:88–95.
[53] Weston AP, Banerjee SK, Horvat RT, Zoubine MN, Campbell DR, Cherian R. Prospective long-term endoscopic and histologic follow-up of gastric lymphoproliferative disease of early stage IE low-grade B-cell mucosa-associated lymphoid tissue type following *Helicobacter pylori* eradication treatment. Int J Oncol 1999;15:899–907.
[54] Yucel C, Ozdemir H, Isik S. Role of endosonography in the evaluation of gastric malignancy. J Ultrasound Med 1999;18:283–8.
[55] Caletti G, Fusaroli P, Togliani T, Bocus P, Roda E. Endosonography in gastric lymphoma and large gastric folds. Eur J Ultrasound 2000;11:31–40.
[56] Levy M, Hammel P, Lamarque D, Marty O, Chaumette MT, Haioun C, et al. Endoscopic ultrasonography for the initial staging and follow-up in patients with low-grade gastric lymphoma of mucosa-associated lymphoid tissue treated medically. Gastrointest Endosc 1997;46:328–33.
[57] Nobre-Leitao C, Lage P, Cravo M, Cabecadas J, Chaves P, Alberto-Santos A, et al. Treatment of gastric MALT lymphoma by *Helicobacter pylori* eradication: a study controlled by endoscopic ultrasonography. Am J Gastroenterol 1998;93:732–6.
[58] Sackmann M, Morgner A, Rudolph B, Neubauer A, Thiede C, Schulz H, et al. Regression of gastric MALT lymphoma after eradication of *Helicobacter pylori* is predicted by endosonographic staging. MALT Lymphoma Study Group. Gastroenterology 1997;113: 1087–90.
[59] Genta RM, Lew GM, Graham DY. Changes in the gastric mucosa following eradication of *Helicobacter pylori*. Mod Pathol 1993;6:281–9.
[60] Smith JW, Brennan MF, Botet JF, Gerdes H, Lightdale CJ. Preoperative endoscopic ultrasound can predict the risk of recurrence after operation for gastric carcinoma. J Clin Oncol 1993;11:2380–5.

[61] Legmann P, Vignaux O, Dousset B, Baraza AJ, Palazzo L, Dumontier I, et al. Pancreatic tumors: comparison of dual-phase helical CT and endoscopic sonography. AJR Am J Roentgenol 1998;170:1315–22.
[62] Mertz HR, Sechopoulos P, Delbeke D, Leach SD. EUS, PET, and CT scanning for evaluation of pancreatic adenocarcinoma. Gastrointest Endosc 2000;52:367–71.
[63] Midwinter MJ, Beveridge CJ, Wilsdon JB, Bennett MK, Baudouin CJ, Charnley RM. Correlation between spiral computed tomography, endoscopic ultrasonography and findings at operation in pancreatic and ampullary tumours. Br J Surg 1999;86: 189–93.
[64] Muller MF, Meyenberger C, Bertschinger P, Schaer R, Marincek B. Pancreatic tumors: evaluation with endoscopic US, CT, and MR imaging. Radiology 1994;190:745–51.
[65] Nakaizumi A, Uehara H, Iishi H, Tatsuta M, Kitamura T, Kuroda C, et al. Endoscopic ultrasonography in diagnosis and staging of pancreatic cancer. Dig Dis Sci 1995;40: 696–700.
[66] Palazzo L, Roseau G, Gayet B, Vilgrain V, Belghiti J, Fekete F, et al. Endoscopic ultrasonography in the diagnosis and staging of pancreatic adenocarcinoma: results of a prospective study with comparison to ultrasonography and CT scan. Endoscopy 1993;25: 143–50.
[67] Snady H, Cooperman A, Siegel J. Endoscopic ultrasonography compared with computed tomography with ERCP in patients with obstructive jaundice or small peri-pancreatic mass. Gastrointest Endosc 1992;38:27–34.
[68] Yasuda K, Mukai H, Nakajima M, Kawai K. Staging of pancreatic carcinoma by endoscopic ultrasonography. Endoscopy 1993;25:151–5.
[69] Bhutani MS, Hawes RH, Baron PL, Sanders-Cliette A, van Velse A, Osborne JF. Endoscopic ultrasound guided fine needle aspiration of malignant pancreatic lesions. Endoscopy 1997;29:854–8.
[70] Gress F, Savides T, Cummings O, Sherman S, Lehman G, Zaidi S, et al. Radial scanning and linear array endosonography for staging pancreatic cancer: a prospective randomized comparison. Gastrointest Endosc 1997;45:138–42.
[71] Gress FG, Hawes RH, Savides TJ, Ikenberry SO, Lehman GA. Endoscopic ultrasound-guided fine-needle aspiration biopsy using linear array and radial scanning endosonography. Gastrointest Endosc 1997;45:243–50.
[72] Tio TL, Sie LH, Kallimanis G, Luiken GJ, Kimmings AN, Huibregtse K, et al. Staging of ampullary and pancreatic carcinoma: comparison between endosonography and surgery. Gastrointest Endosc 1996;44:706–13.
[73] Brugge WR, Lee MJ, Kelsey PB, Schapiro RH, Warshaw AL. The use of EUS to diagnose malignant portal venous system invasion by pancreatic cancer. Gastrointest Endosc 1996; 43:561–7.
[74] Ahmad NA, Lewis JD, Ginsberg GG, Rosato EF, Morris JB, Kochman MI. EUS in preoperative staging of pancreatic cancer. Gastrointest Endosc 2000;52:463–8.
[75] Chen CH, Tseng LJ, Yang CC, Yeh YH. Preoperative evaluation of periampullary tumors by endoscopic sonography, transabdominal sonography, and computed tomography. J Clin Ultrasound 2001;29:313–21.
[76] Itoh A, Goto H, Naitoh Y, Hirooka Y, Furukawa T, Hayakawa T. Intraductal ultrasonography in diagnosing tumor extension of cancer of the papilla of Vater. Gastrointest Endosc 1997;45:251–60.
[77] Menzel J, Hoepffner N, Sulkowski U, Reimer P, Heinecke A, Poremba C, et al. Polypoid tumors of the major duodenal papilla: preoperative staging with intraductal US, EUS, and CT. A prospective, histopathologically controlled study. Gastrointest Endosc 1999;49: 349–57.
[78] Pälvansalo M, Mäkäräinen H, Siniluoto T, Stahlberg M, Jalovaara P. Ultrasound compared with computed tomography and pancreatic arteriography in the detection of endocrine tumours of the pancreas. Eur J Radiol 1989;9:173–8.

[79] Roche A, Raisonnier A, Gillon-Savouret MC. Pancreatic venous sampling and arteriography in localizing insulinomas and gastrinomas: procedure and results in 55 cases. Radiology 1982;145:621–7.

[80] Ardengh JC, Rosenbaum P, Ganc AJ, Goldenberg A, Lobo EJ, Malheiros CA, et al. Role of EUS in the preoperative localization of insulinomas compared with spiral CT. Gastrointest Endosc 2000;51:552–5.

[81] Glover JR, Shorvon PJ, Lees WR. Endoscopic ultrasound for localisation of islet cell tumours. Gut 1992;33:108–10.

[82] Thompson NW, Czako PF, Fritts LL, Bude R, Bansal R, Nostrant TT, et al. Role of endoscopic ultrasonography in the localization of insulinomas and gastrinomas. Surgery 1994;116:1131–8.

[83] Zimmer T, Scherubl H, Faiss S, Stolzel U, Reicken EO, Wiedenmann B. Endoscopic ultrasonography of neuroendocrine tumours. Digestion 2000;62:45–50.

[84] Koito K, Namieno T, Nagakawa T, Shyonai T, Hirokawa N, Morita K. Solitary cystic tumor of the pancreas: EUS-pathologic correlation. Gastrointest Endosc 1997;45:268–76.

[85] Hernandez LV, Mishra G, Forsmark C, Draganov PV, Petersen JM, Hochwald SN, et al. Role of endoscopic ultrasound (EUS) and EUS-guided fine needle aspiration in the diagnosis and treatment of cystic lesions of the pancreas. Pancreas 2002;25:222–8.

[86] Mallery S, Quirk D, Lewandrowski K, et al. EUS-guided FNA with cyst fluid analysis in pancreatic cyst lesions. Gastrointest Endosc 1998;47:AB149.

[87] Wiersema M, Vilmann P, Giovannini M, et al. Prospective multicenter evaluation of EUS-guided fine needle aspiration biopsy (FNA) diagnostic accuracy and complication assessment [abstract]. Gastrointest Endosc 1996;43:432.

[88] Hernandez LV, Bhutani MS. Endoscopic ultrasound and pancreatic cysts: a sticky situation!. Am J Gastroenterol 2001;96:3229–30.

[89] Rosch T. Endoscopic ultrasonography. Endoscopy 1994;26:148–68.

[90] Harewood GC, Wiersema MJ, Nelson H, Maccarty RI, Olson JE, Ahlquist DA, et al. A prospective, blinded assessment of the impact of preoperative staging on the management of rectal cancer. Gastroenterology 2002;123:24–32.

[91] Matsumoto T, Hizawa K, Esaki K, Kurahara K, Mizuno M, Hirakawa K, et al. Comparison of EUS and magnifying colonoscopy for assessment of small colorectal cancers. Gastrointest Endosc 2002;56:354–60.

[92] Tseng LJ, Jao YT, Mo LR. Preoperative staging of colorectal cancer with a balloon-sheathed miniprobe. Endoscopy 2002;34:564–8.

[93] Fritscher-Ravens A, Petrasch S, Reinacher-Schick A, Graeven U, Konig M, Schmiegel W. Diagnostic value of endoscopic ultrasonography-guided fine-needle aspiration cytology of mediastinal masses in patients with intrapulmonary lesions and nondiagnostic bronchoscopy. Respiration 1999;66:150–5.

[94] Hunerbein M, Ghadimi BM, Haensch W, Schlag PM. Transesophageal biopsy of mediastinal and pulmonary tumors by means of endoscopic ultrasound guidance. J Thorac Cardiovasc Surg 1998;116:554–9.

[95] Silvestri GA, Hoffman BJ, Bhutani MS, et al. Endoscopic ultrasound with fine-needle aspiration in the diagnosis and staging of lung cancer. Ann Thorac Surg 1996;61:1441–5.

[96] Gress FG, Savides TJ, Sandler A, Kesler K, Conces D, Cummings O, et al. Endoscopic ultrasonography, fine-needle aspiration biopsy guided by endoscopic ultrasonography, and computed tomography in the preoperative staging of non-small-cell lung cancer: a comparison study. Ann Intern Med 1997;127:604–12.

[97] Hernandez LV, Mishra G, George S, Bhutani MS. A descriptive analysis of EUS-FNA for mediastinal lymphadenopathy: an emphasis on clinical impact and false negative results. Am J Gastroenterol 2004;99:249–54.

[98] Catalano MF, Nayar R, Gress F, Scheiman J, Wassef W, Rosenblatt ML, et al. EUS-guided fine needle aspiration in mediastinal lymphadenopathy of unknown etiology. Gastrointest Endosc 2002;55:863–9.

[99] Parada KS, Peng R, Erickson RA, Hawes R, Sahai AV, Ziogas A, et al. A resource utilization projection study of EUS. Gastrointest Endosc 2002;55:328–34.
[100] Caletti G, Odegaard S, Rösch T, Sivak MV, Tio TL, Yasuda K. Endoscopic ultrasonography (EUS): a summary of the conclusions of the working party for the Tenth World Congress of Gastroenterology, Los Angeles, California October 2–7, 1994. Am J Gastroenterol 1994;89:5138–43.
[101] Fockens P, Van den Brande JH, van Dullemen HM, van Lanschot JJ, Tytgat GN. Endosonographic T-staging of esophageal carcinoma: a learning curve. Gastrointest Endosc 1996;44:58–62.
[102] O'Toole D, Palazzo L, Arotcarena R, Dancour A, Aubert A, Hammel P, et al. Assessment of complications of EUS-guided fine-needle aspiration. Gastrointest Endosc 2001;53: 470–4.
[103] Wiersema MJ, Vilmann P, Giovannini M, Chang KJ, Wiersema LM. Endosonography-guided fine-needle aspiration biopsy: diagnostic accuracy and complication assessment. Gastroenterology 1997;112:1087–95.
[104] Williams DB, Sahai AV, Aabakken L, Penman ID, van Velse A, Webb J, et al. Endoscopic ultrasound guided fine needle aspiration biopsy: a large single centre experience. Gut 1999; 44:720–6.
[105] Eisenberg E, Carr DB, Chalmers TC. Neurolytic celiac plexus block for treatment of cancer pain: a meta-analysis. Anesth Analg 1995;80:290–5.
[106] Wiersema MJ, Wiersema LM. Endosonography-guided celiac plexus neurolysis. Gastrointest Endosc 1996;44:656–62.
[107] Gunaratnam NT, Sarma AV, Norton ID, Wiersema MJ. A prospective study of EUS-guided celiac plexus neurolysis for pancreatic cancer pain. Gastrointest Endosc 2001;54: 316–24.
[108] Goldberg SN, Mallery S, Gazelle GS, Brugge WR. EUS-guided radiofrequency ablation in the pancreas: results in a porcine model. Gastrointest Endosc 1999;50:392–401.
[109] Chang KJ, Nguyen PT, Thompson JA, et al. Phase I clinical trial of local immunotherapy (Cytoimplant) delivered by endoscopic ultrasound (EUS) -guided fine needle injection (FNI) in patients with advanced pancreatic carcinoma [abstract]. Gastrointest Endosc 1998;47:AB144.
[110] Bedford RA, Hecht JR, Lahoti S, et al. Tolerability and efficacy of direct injection of pancreatic adenocarcinomas with ONYX-015 under endoscopic ultrasound (EUS) guidance. Gastrointest Endosc 2000;51:AB97.
[111] Lubbe AS, Bergemann C. Ultrasound therapy for malignant tumors: a conceptual assessment. J Clin Ultrasound 1994;22:113–7.
[112] Prat F, Chapelon J-Y, Arefiev A, Cathignol D, Souchon R, Theilliere Y. High-intensity focused ultrasound transducers suitable for endoscopy: feasibility study in rabbits. Gastrointest Endosc 1997;46:348–51.
[113] Lohnert M, Doniec MJ, Kovacs G, Schroder J, Dohrmann P. New method of radiotherapy for anal cancer with three-dimensional tumor reconstruction based on endoanal ultrasound and ultrasound-guided afterloading therapy. Dis Colon Rectum 1998;41:169–76.
[114] Doniec MJ, Loehnert MS, Kovacs G, et al. Rectal EUS guided HDR-brachytherapy in patients with anal and peri-anal malignancies. Gastrointest Endosc 2000;51:AB106.
[115] Bhutani MS, editor. Interventional endoscopic ultrasound. Amsterdam: Harwood Academic Publishers; 1999.

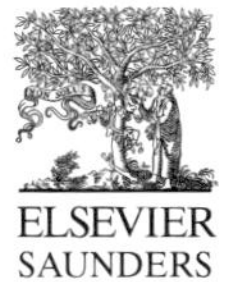
ELSEVIER
SAUNDERS

THE MEDICAL CLINICS OF NORTH AMERICA

Med Clin N Am 89 (2005) 159–186

# Novel endoscopic therapies for gastrointestinal malignancies: endoscopic mucosal resection and endoscopic ablation

Gregory J. Monkewich, MD, FRCPC[a,*], Gregory B. Haber, MD, FRCPC[b]

[a]*Gastroenterology and Therapeutic Endoscopy, 2055 York Avenue, Suite 325, Vancouver, British Columbia V6J 1E5, Canada*
[b]*Division of Gastroenterology, Lenox Hill Hospital, New York, NY 10021, USA*

Gastrointestinal (GI) malignancies are often detected at advanced stages when the prognosis is poor. Advanced GI malignancies are rarely curable with the current treatment modalities of surgery, radiation therapy, and chemotherapy. Surgical resection of early GI malignancies does not invariably lead to cure, and entails the morbidity and mortality of cancer surgery. For example, prophylactic esophagectomy for high-grade dysplasia (HGD) in Barrett's esophagus (BE) has a mortality of 3.3% and a complication rate of 20% [1]. Furthermore, many patients are inoperable or are at increased surgical risk because of significant comorbidity. Earlier cancer detection and less invasive, but effective, treatments are clinically needed.

Early detection of GI malignancies, when they are limited to the mucosa and have a low risk of metastasis, is the rationale for screening patients for BE, early gastric cancer (EGC), and colorectal cancer. Such lesions are potentially curable with endoscopic therapy. Screening guidelines that vary according to the regional disease prevalence are needed. High-resolution endoscopy, magnification endoscopy, chromoendoscopy, light autofluorescence endoscopy, and optical coherence tomography are new technologies designed to improve endoscopic detection. Once detected, lesions must be accurately staged, including depth of mucosal penetration and lymph node

* Corresponding author.
*E-mail address:* gregmonkewich@telus.net (G.J. Monkewich).

0025-7125/05/$ - see front matter 
doi:10.1016/j.mcna.2004.08.016

involvement, to determine endoscopic resectability. Endoscopic ultrasound (EUS) and EUS-guided fine-needle aspiration are essential for staging.

The next requirement is a simple, widely applicable, relatively safe, and minimally invasive alternative to surgery that is effective. Endoscopic mucosal resection (EMR) and endoscopic ablation are potentially curative for malignancies limited to the mucosa, obviating the need for surgery in these patients. EMR has rapidly evolved and is becoming technically easier. Endoscopic ablative therapies, including photodynamic therapy (PDT), laser photoablation, argon plasma coagulation (APC), and cryotherapy, are under evaluation. Ablative therapies have a disadvantage in that mucosal specimens required for complete histologic evaluation are destroyed by this therapy.

Large regional variability in the incidence of early esophageal or gastric cancers accounts in part for the variable reported international experience. The incidence of EGC in Japan is more than twice that in Western countries, yet the two regions share similar clinicopathologic features of the disease [2]. Different histopathologic diagnostic criteria for early cancer together with the mass endoscopic screening of the asymptomatic Japanese population, initiated in 1957, may account for the higher incidence of early cancers reported in Japan. Western pathologists use the term HGD for neoplastic lesions that have not penetrated through the basement membrane to the lamina propria, whereas Japanese pathologists classify these lesions as intramucosal cancer on the basis of malignant cytologic features and the potential for tissue invasion. Schlemper et al [3] found that Japanese pathologists attach great significance to cytologic and architectural features, whereas Western pathologists require invasion for the diagnosis of gastric cancer. Consensus is needed for the pathologic nomenclature of epithelial neoplasia to render comparisons between Japanese and Western early cancer more meaningful.

## Endoscopic mucosal resection

EMR removes GI lesions by resecting through the middle or deep layers of the submucosa. In contrast to ablative therapies, EMR does not destroy the resected tissue, thereby permitting the pathologist to stage the lesion by examining its deep and lateral margins. To determine whether a lesion has been adequately removed clinicians rely on data on the correlation between mucosal stage and risk of lymph node metastasis. EMR potentially cures early cancer provided that the lesion is entirely removed. Without a surgically resected specimen, can one be certain that the lesion has been correctly staged and entirely removed? How often are EMR and the pathologic specimens that it yields adequate to confirm complete resection? Can one be sure that neither synchronous lesions nor invasive disease are present? These questions are answered with outcomes data on recurrence rate and long-term survival. Studies comparing EMR with surgical outcomes are also needed.

EMR and surgery currently play complementary roles in managing early GI cancers. A shift toward EMR will likely continue as the clinical experience with this technique increases with increasing screening of asymptomatic patients to detect earlier cancers. Proper patient selection is vital to the success of EMR. The selection of endoscopic versus surgical therapy is guided by weighing the pros and cons of each therapy. The initial diagnosis obtained by pathologic analysis of endoscopic biopsies may change as a result of the pathologic analysis of the EMR specimens resulting in up-staging and the need for surgical evaluation. Selection of EMR involves regular follow-up with endoscopic surveillance to detect metachronous neoplasia or local recurrence.

*History of endoscopic mucosal resection*

Rosenberg et al [4] introduced saline-assisted polypectomy in 1955 in the era of rigid sigmoidoscopy to reduce the risk of colorectal perforation. In 1973, 8 years after the introduction of flexible fiberoptic colonoscopy, Deyhle et al [5] reported saline-assisted polypectomy for sessile colonic polyps in the proximal colon. In 1976, Martin et al [6] introduced the grasping and snaring method in which a lesion is first retracted with a grasper, and then snared and excised with electrocautery.

Over the past 30 years Japanese endoscopists introduced several EMR techniques to treat the large number of early esophageal and gastric cancers in Japan. In 1983, Tada et al [7] reported on the treatment of EGC by endoscopic submucosal injection followed by snaring. Elements of the injection and snaring and grasping and snaring techniques were integrated and popularized as the strip biopsy method.

EMR of esophageal lesions began in 1989 when Makuuchi et al [8] and Monma et al [9] used the strip biopsy technique. Inoue and Endo [10] developed an EMR tube to permit larger resection of esophageal mucosa. Makuuchi [11] also developed an EMR tube, and Kawano et al [12] modified the Makuuchi tube with a lateral window to serve as the suction trap.

Simpler techniques have superseded the EMR tube techniques. The EMR cap technique (EMRC), pioneered by Inoue et al [13], is a refinement of the EMR tube allowing safe and effective EMR for most of the upper or lower GI tracts. EMR with variceal ligation (EMRL) was first reported in 1994 and was promoted for lesions within the reach of a gastroscopy [14,15]. It is a popular technique because of its simplicity and low cost. In 1997, Soehendra et al [16] introduced a simple EMR technique in the esophagus using a steel monofilament snare without prior submucosal injection.

Piecemeal resection of large lesions limits the ability to assess resection margins accurately, and results in high recurrence rates because of incomplete resection. This problem provided the impetus for developing en bloc resection. In 1988, Hirao et al [17] introduced a method to remove large EGCs en bloc, termed "injection, precutting, and snaring." A needle-knife was used to create a circumferential cut in the mucosa around the lesion. The lesion was then removed in one piece with a snare. The high rate of perforation with this technique led, in 1994, to the introduction of the insulated-tip diathermic knife by Ohkuwa et al [18]. Ono et al [19] successfully resected 96% (471 out of 488) of lesions in one piece using this instrument. In 1998, Yamamoto et al [20] introduced sodium hyaluronate as an injectate to prolong the mucosal lift achieved with submucosal injection to facilitate the insulated-tip diathermic knife EMR technique.

Endoscopic submucosal dissection was developed to resect large EGCs en bloc (Fig. 1). Yamamoto et al [21] introduced submucosal dissection using a cap and needle knife for very large EGCs. A new triangle-tipped needle knife has been evaluated by Inoue et al [22] with good results.

### *Classification of early cancers*

The American Joint Committee on Cancer and the International Union Against Cancer recently published the sixth edition of the TNM staging system. Classifications for esophageal and gastric cancers are listed in Tables 1–4. Early and superficial cancers are synonymous and refer to T1 lesions (ie, lesions limited to the mucosa and submucosa; Fig. 2). Intramucosal cancers are subclassified as follows: m1, intraepithelial cancer; m2, cancer limited to the lamina propria; and m3, cancer close to or infiltrating the muscularis mucosa. Submucosal cancers are subclassified into thirds based on depth of penetration: sm1, first third, closest to the lamina propria; sm2, middle third; and sm3, deepest third (Fig. 3).

### *Pretreatment staging with endoscopic ultrasound*

EUS improves the application of EMR by permitting more accurate staging of early esophageal and gastric cancers. EUS can also provide

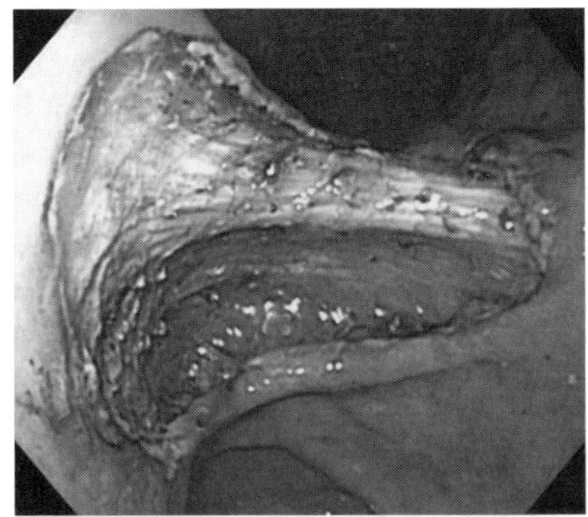

Fig. 1. A large gastric ulcer crater following en bloc EMR using the TT-knife. (Courtesy of Haruhiro Inoue, MD, Yokohama, Japan.)

Table 1
American Joint Committee on Cancer 6th edition Tumor–Node–Metastasis system for staging esophageal cancer

| Type of esophageal cancer | Staging |
|---|---|
| *Primary tumor (T)* | |
| Primary tumor cannot be assessed | TX |
| No evidence of primary tumor | T0 |
| Carcinoma in situ | Tis |
| Tumor invades lamina propria or submucosa | T1 |
| Tumor invades muscularis propria | T2 |
| Tumor invades adventitia | T3 |
| Tumor invades adjacent structures | T4 |
| *Regional lymph nodes (N)* | |
| Regional lymph nodes cannot be assessed | NX |
| No regional lymph node metastasis | N0 |
| Regional lymph node metastasis | N1 |
| *Distant metastasis (M)* | |
| Distant metastasis cannot be assessed | MX |
| No distant metastasis | M0 |
| Distant metastasis | M1 |
| Tumors of the lower thoracic esophagus | |
| M1a: Metastasis in celiac lymph nodes | |
| M1b: Other distant metastases | |
| Tumors of the midthoracic esophagus | |
| M1a: Not applicable | |
| M1b: Nonregional lymph nodes and/or other distant metastasis | |
| Tumors of the upper thoracic esophagus | |
| M1a: Metastasis in cervical nodes | |
| M1b: Other distant metastasis | |

*Data from* Greene FL, Page DL, Fleming ID, Fritz A, Balch CM, Haller DG, et al. Esophagus. In: AJCC cancer staging manual. 6th edition. New York: Springer; 2002. p. 91–8.

prognostic information, as demonstrated recently in patients with esophageal cancer in whom survival was related to T- and N-staging by EUS [23].

### *Conventional endoscopic ultrasound*

Low-frequency (7.5–12 MHz) echoendoscopes permit the visualization of regional lymph nodes. Murata et al [24] have used EUS since 1983 to determine the depth of cancer invasion and the presence of lymph node metastasis. Among 78 patients with esophageal cancer who underwent esophagectomy, the extent of cancer invasion was correctly determined preoperatively in 84%. Diagnostic criteria for lymph node metastasis included a spherical shape, a distinct border, and heterogeneous echoic foci within the nodes. These criteria yielded a sensitivity of 87%, a specificity of 90%, and an overall accuracy of 89%, according to the histologic examination of subsequently resected lymph nodes.

Meining et al [25] demonstrated a low accuracy of EUS for staging upper GI cancers and high interobserver variability when experienced endosonographers reviewed EUS videotapes and were blinded to the clinical

Table 2
American Joint Committee on Cancer 6th edition stage groupings for esophageal cancer

| Stage | TNM pathology | | |
|---|---|---|---|
| 0 | Tis | N0 | M0 |
| I | T1 | N0 | M0 |
| IIA | T2 | N0 | M0 |
| | T3 | N0 | M0 |
| IIB | T1 | N1 | M0 |
| | T2 | N1 | M0 |
| III | T3 | N1 | M0 |
| | T4 | Any N | M0 |
| IV | Any T | Any N | M1 |
| IVA | Any T | Any N | M1a |
| IVB | Any T | Any N | M1b |

*Data from* Greene FL, Page DL, Fleming ID, Fritz A, Balch CM, Haller DG, et al. Esophagus. In: AJCC cancer staging manual. 6th edition. New York: Springer; 2002. p. 91–8.

information. With histopathology as the reference, the accuracy of EUS in T staging was 73% under normal examination conditions, 53% for the blinded evaluation, and 62% for an unblinded evaluation of videotapes [26]. Blinded analysis of videotapes significantly reduced the accuracy, but the accuracy improved when clinical information was added.

Table 3
American Joint Committee on Cancer 6th edition Tumor–Node–Metastasis system for staging gastric cancer

| Type of gastric cancer | Staging |
|---|---|
| *Primary tumor (T)* | |
| Primary tumor cannot be assessed | TX |
| No evidence of primary tumor | T0 |
| Carcinoma in situ: intraepithelial tumor without invasion of lamina propria | Tis |
| Tumor invades lamina propria or submucosa | T1 |
| Tumor invades the muscularis propria or the subserosa | T2 |
| Tumor invades muscularis propria | T2a |
| Tumor invades the subserosa | T2b |
| Tumor penetrates the serosa without invading adjacent structures | T3 |
| Tumor invades adjacent structures | T4 |
| *Regional lymph nodes (N)* | |
| Regional lymph nodes cannot be assessed | NX |
| No regional lymph node metastasis | N0 |
| Metastasis to 1-6 regional lymph nodes | N1 |
| Metastasis to 7-15 regional lymph nodes | N2 |
| Metastasis to more than 15 regional lymph nodes | N3 |
| *Distant metastasis (M)* | |
| Distant metastasis cannot be assessed | MX |
| No distant metastasis | M0 |
| Distant metastasis | M1 |

*Data from* Greene FL, Page DL, Fleming ID, Fritz A, Balch CM, Haller DG, et al. Stomach. In: AJCC cancer staging manual. 6th edition. New York: Springer; 2002. p. 99–106.

Table 4
American Joint Committee on Cancer 6th edition stage groupings for stomach cancer

| Stage | Tumor | Node | Metastasis |
|---|---|---|---|
| 0 | Tis | N0 | M0 |
| IA | T1 | N0 | M0 |
| IB | T1 | N1 | M0 |
| | T2a | N0 | M0 |
| | T2b | N0 | M0 |
| II | T1 | N1 | M0 |
| | T2a | N1 | M0 |
| | T2b | N1 | M0 |
| | T3 | N0 | M0 |
| IIIA | T2a | N2 | M0 |
| | T2b | N2 | M0 |
| | T3 | N1 | M0 |
| | T4 | N0 | M0 |
| IIIB | T3 | N2 | M0 |
| IV | T4 | N1 | M0 |
| | T4 | N2 | M0 |
| | T4 | N3 | M0 |
| | T1 | N3 | M0 |
| | T2 | N3 | M0 |
| | T3 | N3 | M0 |
| | Any T | Any N | M1 |

*Data from* Greene FL, Page DL, Fleming ID, Fritz A, Balch CM, Haller DG, et al. Stomach. In: AJCC cancer staging manual. 6th edition. New York: Springer; 2002. p. 99–106.

Sampling lymph nodes for histologic analysis may improve the staging of upper GI cancers. EUS fine-needle aspiration of lymph nodes is possible with curved linear array echoendoscopes. Malignant lymph nodes are greater than 5 to 10 mm in diameter, have a distinct border, a hypoechoic internal echo, and a round shape. EUS fine-needle aspiration for malignant lymph nodes has a sensitivity of 81% to 97%, specificity of 83% to 100%, and accuracy of 83% to 97%. EUS fine-needle aspiration provided diagnostic information that altered the clinical management in 13% of esophageal and 14% of gastric cancers [27].

*High-frequency endoscopic ultrasound probes*

High-frequency EUS probes (20–30 MHz), introduced in 1989 by Silverstein et al [28], provide high-resolution images of the layers of GI mucosa allowing better definition of the depth of invasion of superficial tumors. These probes may be applied under endoscopic vision in a targeted fashion without compressing the lesion. Murata et al [29], using 15- and 20-MHz probes, reported an overall accuracy compared with histology of 75% (40 out of 53). The accuracy in distinguishing mucosal from submucosal esophageal cancers was 94% (46 out of 49). Precise delineation is sometimes obscured by the presence of glandular components, inflammation, or scarring. A disadvantage of high-frequency EUS probes is the relatively

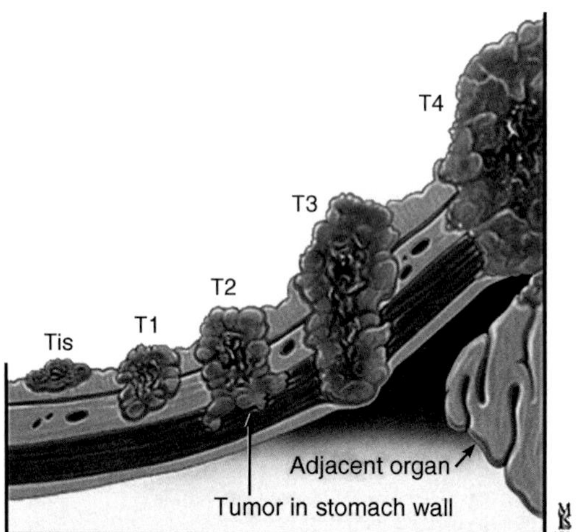


Fig. 2. T-stage subclassifications for gastric cancer.

limited depth of tissue penetration such that the entire margins of large tumors are not always clearly delineated.

May et al [30] reported a diagnostic accuracy compared with histology of 80% (74 out of 93) for the 20-MHz probe in patients with early esophageal cancer. The sensitivity was 91% (62 out of 68) for mucosal tumors and was 48% (12 out of 25) for submucosal tumors. Results were better for the tubular esophagus than for the gastroesophageal junction, and results were better for tumors infiltrating the second and third submucosal layers (sm2, sm3) than for tumors with slight infiltration of the upper submucosal layer (sm1). They concluded that the technique is not yet satisfactory for

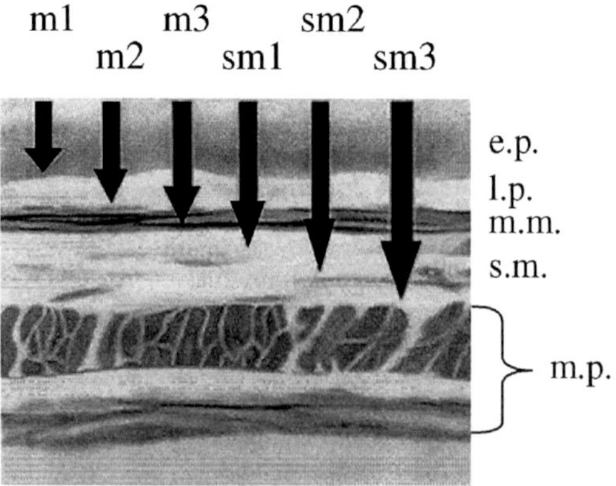


Fig. 3. Subdivision of mucosal cancer according to depth of invasion. (*From* Soetikno RM, Gotoda T, Nakanishi Y, Soehendra N. Endoscopic mucosal resection [review]. Gastrointest Endosc 2003;57:567–79; with permission.)

submucosal tumors located at the gastroesophageal junction or for tumor infiltrating the upper third of the submucosa (sm1).

### *Preparation for endoscopic mucosal resection*

#### *Chromoendoscopy*

Chromoendoscopy with Lugol's solution (2% potassium iodide) can improve the detection of squamous dysplasia and early squamous cell cancer (SCC). Normal mucosa stains dark brown, whereas dysplasia, neoplasia, inflamed tissue, and BE do not stain. Neoplastic mucosa loses its glycogen granules and appears as yellow unstained areas adjacent to the brown iodine-stained normal mucosa. The sensitivity and specificity of Lugol's solution for the detection of squamous dysplasia or SCC was 96% and 63%, respectively, in a large study in Linxian, China [31]. The sensitivity and specificity of endoscopically visible lesions for identifying HGD or invasive cancer before staining in this study was 62% and 79%, respectively.

Indigo carmine (indigotindisulfonate sodium 0.1%–0.4%) enhances mucosal contrast in the stomach. The solution pools in mucosal crevices and depressions highlighting a lesion's borders, and enhancing visualization of surface irregularities [32].

#### *Marking lesion margins*

Marking the margins of a lesion before EMR is essential because the margins often become blurred after submucosal injection. Markings are made 5 to 10 mm away from the lesion using coagulation current (20 W) with a needle knife or the tip of a snare. APC may also be used for marking. The completeness of resection is assessed by whether all the marks were removed during resection. The markings also may help to orient specimens resected piecemeal (Fig. 4). Marking is usually unnecessary in the colon because the margins are more clearly demarcated.

#### *Submucosal injection*

EMR techniques generally use submucosal injection under the lesion to lift it and reduce the risk of perforation during resection. The wall of the GI tract is less than 4 mm thick. Saline injection into the submucosal layer is the most effective technique to avoid muscle entrapment in the snare and perforation. It may be performed in any part of the GI tract. Inoue et al [12] recommend injecting a minimum of 10 mL of normal saline before each resection. Lifting is achieved by injecting into the submucosa with the needle at a 45-degree angle to the bowel wall. Injection is most easily performed by targeting the distal site of the lesion first and then proceeding proximally.

A lesion that can be raised above the level of the surrounding mucosa is likely to be superficial and amenable to complete resection by EMR. The nonlifting sign refers to the absence of such lifting. Lesions may fail to lift because of invasive carcinoma, desmoplastic reaction, ulceration, or

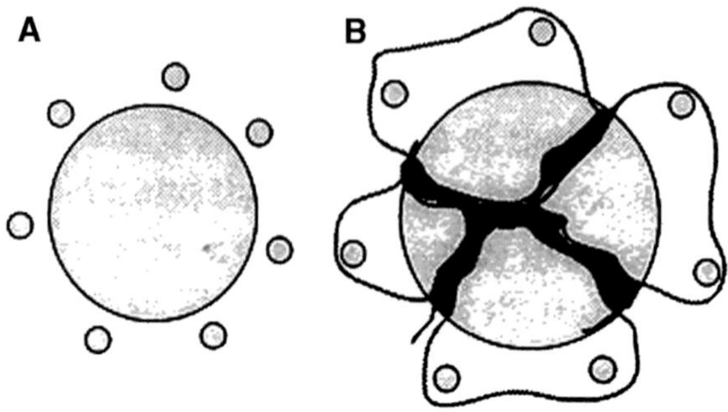


Fig. 4. Preparation of the specimen after piecemeal EMR in the endoscopy room. (*A*) Before resection, the margins are marked with seven dots made using the electrocautery at a distance from the target neoplastic lesion. (*B*) After resection, the complete shape of the lesion can be reconstituted on a board by stretching each of the resected fragments. (*From* Lambert R. Treatment of esophagogastric tumors [review]. Endoscopy 2003;35:118–26; with permission.)

submucosal fibrosis from a previous biopsy or cautery [32]. The lifting sign was reported to have a sensitivity of 100%, specificity of 99%, and positive predictive value of 83% as a predictor of invasive colorectal cancer [33]. Kato et al [34] studied EMR in early colorectal cancer and found that almost all completely lifting lesions were mucosal, whereas incompletely lifting lesions included stages sm1 to sm3, and nonlifting lesions were almost always deeper than sm3. Ishiguro et al [35] determined that 94% (29 out of 31) of sm1 colorectal cancers lift, whereas 100% (6 out of 6) of sm3 cancers do not.

Yamamoto et al [20,21,36,37] introduced sodium hyaluronate injection to prolong the mucosal elevation to resect large EGCs. The mixture is 0.5% sodium hyaluronate, 1:100,000 epinephrine, and 0.004% indigo carmine. Sodium hyaluronate 0.5% is made by mixing 1% sodium hyaluronate (Artz 1%, Kaken Pharmaceutical, Tokyo, Japan) with an equal volume of normal saline. Epinephrine reduces the risk of immediate hemorrhage. A 23-gauge needle and a 5-mL syringe minimize the resistance to injection of this viscous solution. Unlike hypertonic solutions, such as 50% glucose, this solution is isotonic and does not injure surrounding tissue.

### *Specific endoscopic mucosal resection techniques*

The most commonly used EMR techniques are described next. The techniques are classified according to whether snaring or submucosal dissection is used.

#### *Snaring techniques*

The strip biopsy technique requires a two-channel endoscope and two assistants. The periphery of the lesion is marked and the submucosa is injected in the standard fashion. A snare and a grasping forceps are then advanced through the two channels and positioned near the lesion. The snare is opened to capture the forceps and then closed around the forceps; the center of the lesion is grasped by the forceps and the snare is opened around the lesion; and the forceps is pulled gently while the snare is advanced slightly before it is closed at the base of the lesion for electrocautery and resection [32].

EMRC requires a special transparent plastic cap fitted onto the tip of a standard diagnostic or therapeutic endoscope (Fig. 5). Different sized caps are available with either straight or oblique distal ends. A hard oblique cap with a diameter of 16 mm is commonly used. A soft oblique 18-mm diameter cap is designed for en bloc resection of large lesions. After marking the periphery of the lesion, the submucosa is injected. A soft crescent-shaped snare is prelooped inside an inner groove at the distal end of the cap. Prelooping is performed by lightly pressing against normal mucosa away from the lesion to seal the cap outlet. Gentle suction is performed and the snare is opened and forced to rest along the inner groove of the cap. The suction is then released and the scope tip is returned to the site of the lesion. The lesion, in whole or in part, is suctioned into the cap and the snare is quickly closed by the assistant. The suction is then released and blended current is used to resect the lesion. The resected specimen may be suctioned into the cap for safe removal from the GI tract. Several snares are typically needed for multiple piecemeal resections at one EMRC session, significantly adding to the procedure cost.

EMRL uses a standard endoscopic variceal ligation device fitted onto the tip of a regular single-channel endoscope (Fig. 6). The lesion, in whole or in part, is suctioned into the cap and a band is deployed to create a polypoid target. Using a standard polypectomy snare, the polypoid target is snared at its base above or below the rubber band and resected by electrocautery. EMRL and EMRC are similar in terms of their maximum diameters of resection. Both techniques have low complication rates [38]. With EMRL, lifting is not needed and marking the periphery of the lesion is usually unnecessary. EMRL eliminates two steps required for EMRC, but EMRL requires two endoscopes, one for ligation and one for snaring. Each ligated specimen is usually resected immediately after ligation because of the difficulty in placing bands next to an existing band without leaving an island of residual tissue between them. Removing ligated lesions individually allows for more precise placement of the next band to maintain a clear resection line. When deploying the bands, it is important not to suction the submucosa from an adjacent crater into the cap to avoid perforation. Using the current apparatus, EMRL requires alternating removal and introduction of the ligation and snaring endoscopes, adding complexity and time to the procedure. New ligation devices will soon be available that permit the snare to be passed through the endoscopic channel with the ligation device in place at the endoscopic tip so that only one endoscope is required. This will render EMRL a simple technique for EMR.

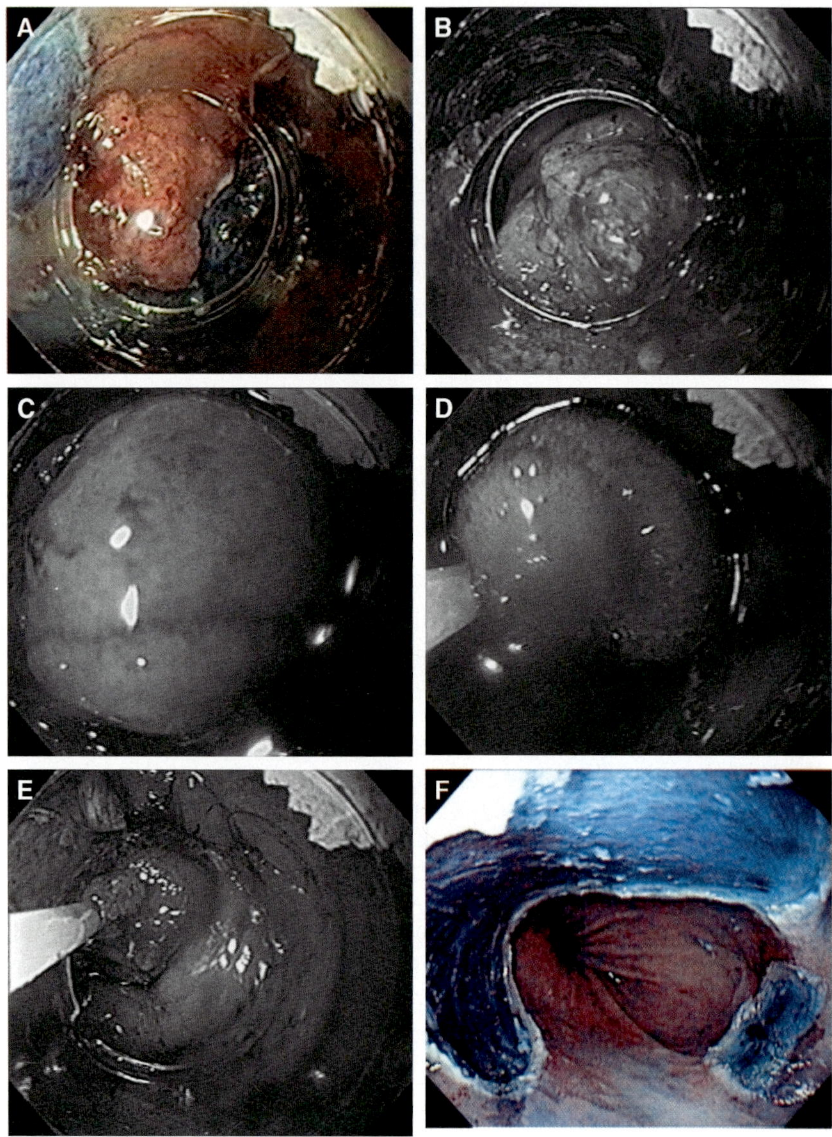


Fig. 5. EMRC technique. (*A*) Mucosal island between craters (note injectate contained methylene blue to stain the submucosa). (*B*) Snare in position inside the inner groove of the cap. (*C*) Lesion is suctioned into the cap. (*D*) Snare is tightened around the lesion. (*E*) The lesion is cauterized. (*F*) Ulcer crater with submucosa stained blue. (*A–F*, courtesy of Norman Marcon, MD, Toronto, Canada.)

Soehendra et al [16] described the use of a polypectomy snare made of 0.4-mm monofilament steel wire for small early esophageal cancers. A therapeutic dual-channel endoscope is used to allow adequate suction while the snare is in one channel. The snare is positioned around the lesion and

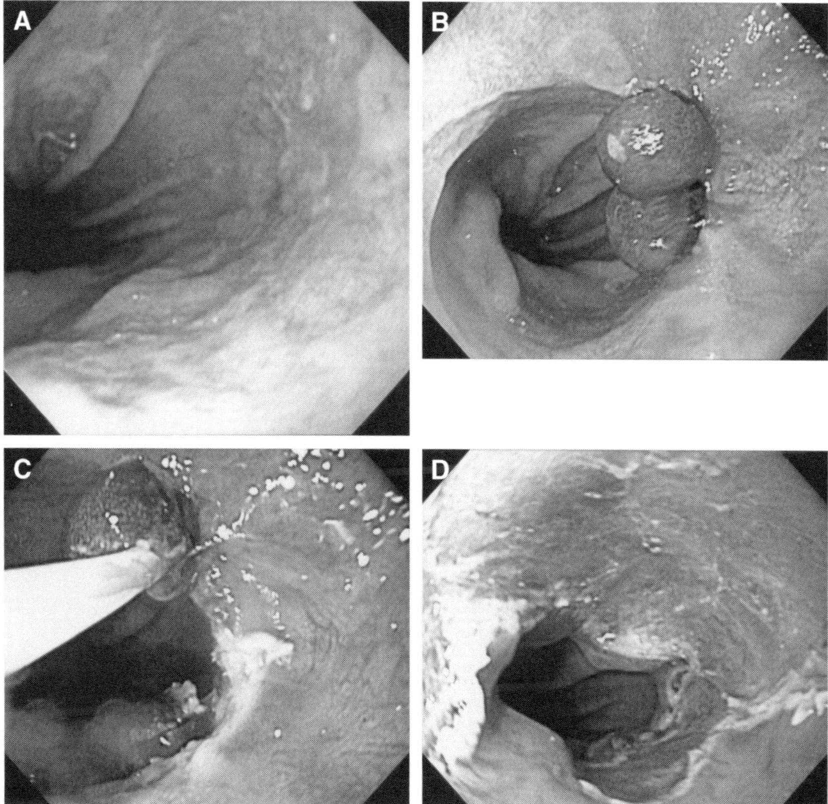


Fig. 6. EMRL technique. (*A*) Barrett's esophagus with HGD before EMRL. (*B*) Two EMRL bands applied. (*C*) First band removed, second band in process of being removed with snare and electrocautery. (*D*) The esophageal crater following six EMRL band resections. (*A–D*, courtesy of Norman Marcon, MD, Toronto, Canada.)

pressed against the mucosa while suction is applied to draw the lesion into the snare, and the snare is then closed. Pure coagulation current is used for resection. A piecemeal technique is used, if necessary, for complete lesion removal. Seven patients with early esophageal cancer as defined by EUS (3 cm or less in size, limited to the submucosal layer) were treated. Complete removal was achieved in one session in all seven patients. No complications were observed. Two patients subsequently underwent radical surgery with no tumor remnant or metastatic lymph node in the resected specimen. This method has also been used for circumferential EMR of BE [39].

Circumferential mucosal incision using a needle-knife followed by en bloc snaring was developed in Japan to remove large (> 20 mm) EGCs. At first, a standard needle-knife was used to create a circumferential trench but this technique was associated with high rates of bleeding and perforation [17].

Ohkuwa et al [40] later introduced the insulated-tip diathermic knife to decrease the risk of these complications. Insulated-tip diathermic knife EMR made it possible to perform en bloc resections of large EGCs safely with a reduced recurrence rate [7,18,41,42]. A single-channel endoscope is used. The periphery of the lesion is marked in the usual manner. Saline or hyaluronate is injected just outside the marks. A 2-mm incision is made in the mucosa with a conventional needle-knife for insertion of the insulated-tip diathermic knife into the submucosal layer. The incision is extended along the outside of the marks using 50-W blended current, adding submucosal saline injection when necessary. Once the trench is complete, saline is injected into the submucosal layer in the center of and adjacent to the lesion. The raised lesion is then removed using a standard polypectomy snare with blended current [18,19]. Snaring lesions greater than 20 mm is difficult using this technique [18,36]; the en bloc resection rate decreases to 48% for lesions exceeding 20 mm. Newer methods, such as endoscopic submucosal dissection, are needed. Bleeding is a frequent complication. Yamamoto et al [36] increased the en bloc resection rate by using sodium hyaluronate as the submucosal injectate. They observed lower rates of perforation, bleeding, and local recurrence.

*Endoscopic submucosal dissection*

Some experts believe that local recurrence is often caused by inappropriate assessment of the multiple fragments in resected specimens. A higher rate of local recurrence has been reported with piecemeal than with en bloc resection [43]. Accurate rearrangement of the multiple pieces of the specimen is usually impossible. En bloc EMR is better whenever possible.

Yamamoto et al [21] introduced a cap-assisted needle-knife method, with a needle knife and a transparent hood with a small-caliber tip. After sufficient marking (forced coagulation, 15 W) and mucosal elevation with hyaluronate, a circumferential incision is made around the lesion with the needle knife (Endo-cut, maximum 120 W). A transparent hood with a soft tapered small-caliber tip is then attached the end of the endoscope and inserted into the incision line to visualize the submucosal layer. A regular needle knife is used (pure coagulation, 30 W), protected by the plastic cap, to dissect the submucosa until the lesion is removed en bloc.

Inoue et al [22] use a new device, the TT-knife, for submucosal dissection of large lesions (Fig. 7). In 66 cases of GI neoplasms, 64 en bloc resections were performed and histologically confirmed. Perforation occurred in two cases of T1 cancer in the upper body of the stomach, but these perforations were easily closed using a clipping device. It was concluded that any T1 lesion can be resected safely with this method.

*Managing immediate complications*

The most important immediate complications of EMR are bleeding and perforation. Injection, cauterization, or APC may be used to control

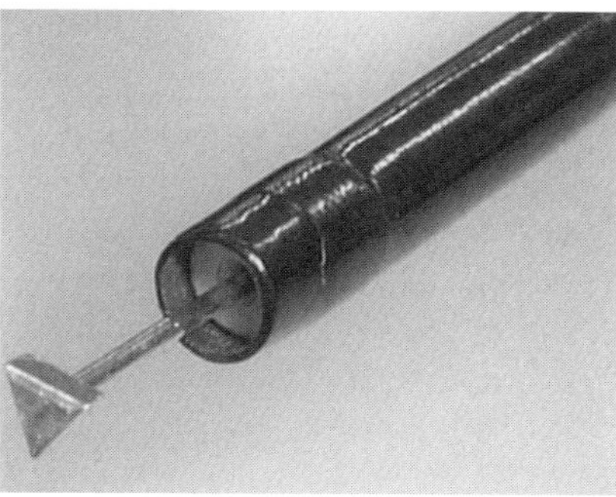

Fig. 7. The triangle-tip knife. The triangular-shaped metal plate is attached onto the tip of needle knife. The outer diameter of the plate is 1.8 mm, whereas the width is 0.6 mm. (Courtesy of Haruhiro Inoue, MD, Yokohama, Japan.)

bleeding. Epinephrine and hemoclips are useful to control spurting bleeding from the ulcer bed, as more commonly required in the stomach.

Small perforations may be managed endoscopically with clips followed by admission to the hospital and conservative management with nasogastric suction, decompression of pneumoperitoneum, and antibiotics [19]. Medium or large perforations that do not close with clipping usually require immediate surgery.

### *Healing following uncomplicated endoscopic mucosal resection*

EMR is usually performed on an outpatient basis. Following an uncomplicated procedure, the patient may drink cold water. They may eat a soft diet on the following day and eat a full diet on the second day. In the esophagus, the artificial ulcer is covered by a white exudate 3 days after EMR and has mostly disappeared with a thin normal squamous epithelium 12 days after EMR. A proton-pump inhibitor is usually prescribed for several weeks after EMR to promote ulcer healing, although no studies have so far examined the healing rates with this empiric therapy. Antibiotics are generally not prescribed. In a study of 38 patients who underwent EMRC of the upper GI tract, Lee et al [44] found that bacteremia was infrequent and transient.

### *Specimen retrieval*

Piecemeal specimens may be retrieved individually as they are resected or together at the end of the procedure with a net. The former is suitable for the EMRC and EMRL techniques. Large en bloc specimens are usually retrieved with a net.

### *Preparation of the specimen*

All resected specimens should be flattened and fixed onto cork or Styrofoam plates using fine needles and then completely submersed in formalin. Piecemeal resections should be reconstituted into the complete lesion from the multiple fragments, but this is often difficult. One method for reconstitution suggested by Lambert [45] involves outward alignment of the coagulation markings.

The Japanese Classification of Gastric Cancer [46] recommends sectioning of en bloc gastric EMR specimens in 2-mm slices parallel to a line that includes the closest resection margin, or perpendicular to the long axis of the specimen when the resection margin is unclear (Fig. 8). All sections are numbered for accurate assessment of tumor margins. A schematic diagram is made of the size and shape of the tumor within the resected specimen. If identified, the proximal end of the specimen is marked with an arrow. A complete resection with negative margins is defined as the absence of neoplasia in the first and last slices of the specimen.

### *Disease-specific considerations*

For analyzing the efficacy of EMR, the following outcome measures are important: complete resection rate (negative margin); en bloc resection rate (stratified according to lesion size); major complications (perforation and bleeding); local recurrence rate; and incorrect staging (need for surgery). The criteria for safe resection are based on retrospective data from large surgical series with histopathologic confirmation. Important data are surfacing from prospective studies on the long-term outcome after EMR.

#### *Esophagus*

Squamous and glandular epithelial neoplasia exhibit different rates of progression. EMR has established indications for SCC of the esophagus (see

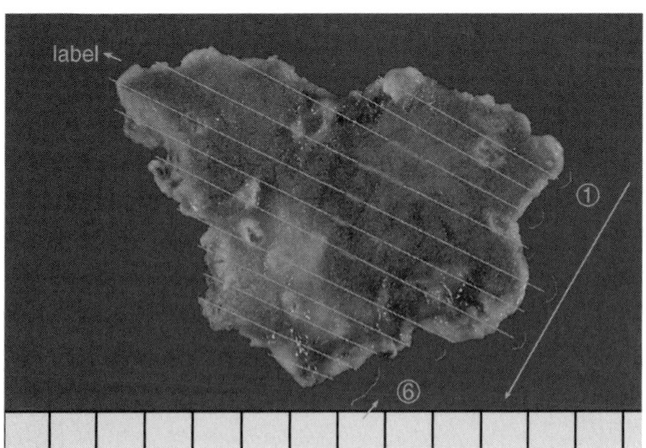


Fig. 8. En bloc resection specimen of EGC. (Courtesy of Haruhiro Inoue, MD, Yokohama, Japan.)

next), but is not yet established for the treatment of early adenocarcinoma arising from BE.

*Squamous cell cancer of the esophagus.* The normal esophageal mucosa has a smooth, pale pink, lustrous appearance at endoscopy. SCC of the esophagus appears red and matted with rough surfaces and margins. Detecting early stage SCC is difficult but may be enhanced with Lugol's solution. The accepted criteria for EMR of SCC of the esophagus include (1) well- or moderately well-differentiated SCC; (2) stage m1 or m2 with no venous or lymphatic invasion; (3) diameter less than 20 mm; and (4) endoscopic subtypes 0-IIa, 0-IIb, and 0-IIc.

EMR is indicated for well- or moderately well-differentiated SCC. The esophagus has widespread lymphatics in the submucosal layer that could permit early cancers to metastasize [47]. When venous or lymphatic invasion is observed histopathologically the risk of metastatic invasion is high, EMR is unlikely to be curative, and surgical evaluation is indicated. Estimates of the metastatic risk of early SCC vary. Most studies report no risk for lesions confined to the lamina propria (m1 and m2). The risk in the Japanese National Survey of surgically resected specimens, which contains over 10,000 cases, is 4%. The incidence of lymphatic invasion or lymph node metastases increases markedly as cancer infiltrates to the muscularis mucosa. Cancers with submucosal invasion (sm1 and deeper) have a 35% chance of lymph node metastasis; EMR is not curative in these cases. When invasion of the submucosa involves the deeper one third (sm3), the risk is 45%. In these circumstances, patients who refuse esophagectomy or who are poor surgical candidates may be offered EMR with a limited curative potential. In the study by Kodama and Kakegawa [48], most cases with 0-I or 0-III components were submucosal cancer and not acceptable for EMR. In general, the cancer should involve less than one half of the circumference of the esophageal wall to avoid post-EMR esophageal stricture, although this criterion has been recently challenged by Seewald et al [39]. Ablative therapies, such as PDT and APC, have been tried as adjuncts to EMR for large lesions, although data for combination therapies are limited.

Inoue et al [49,50] have treated more than 250 patients with early esophageal cancer. For the 72% who met all the criteria for EMR, the overall 5-year survival was 95%. Narahara et al [51] removed 25 superficial esophageal cancers in 21 patients using the strip biopsy method (72% en bloc, 28% piecemeal) and found no recurrence during a mean 2-year follow-up interval. Shimizu et al [52] found metachronous esophageal carcinoma in 14.6% (12 out of 82) of patients during a mean 38 months of follow-up and concluded that careful long-term endoscopic observation is required for patients who undergo EMR for SCC of the esophagus. Nomura et al [53] followed 51 patients with a total of 57 superficial esophageal cancers treated by EMR at the National Cancer Center Hospital East with surveillance endoscopy with iodine staining and biopsy repeated every 3 to 6 months.

Local recurrence was detected in 40% (two out of five) of patients with multiple esophageal cancers, compared with 4% (2 out of 46) of patients with solitary cancer ($P < .05$). It was concluded that multiplicity of cancer is a risk factor for local recurrence.

Pech et al [54] followed 39 patients after EMR for early esophageal carcinoma in 29, and for carcinoma in situ in 10. Ninety percent of the patients with carcinoma in situ, 100% of those with mucosal cancer, and 80% of those with submucosal cancer demonstrated a complete response during a mean follow-up interval of 29.7 months. No major complications, such as perforation or bleeding requiring blood transfusion, occurred.

There is recent evidence that EMR is as effective as esophagectomy in small m3 and sm1 SCC of the esophagus. Shimizu et al [55] compared the long-term outcome of 26 patients with m3 and sm1 superficial SCC with a mean diameter of 2.2 cm who underwent EMR with the results of 44 patients with cancer with a mean diameter of 2.9 cm with the same degree of invasion and no preoperative evidence of positive nodes who underwent esophagectomy. The overall 5-year survival rate did not differ significantly between the two groups and the disease-specific survival rate was equivalent, suggesting that small m3 or sm1 SCC lesions are potential indications for EMR. More data are needed before specific recommendations can be made.

*Barrett's esophagus and early adenocarcinoma.* The use of EMR for the treatment of early adenocarcinoma in Barrett's mucosa is less well established than for SCC of the esophagus. The incidence of esophageal adenocarcinoma is increasing in Western countries, most notably in white men. The estimated risk of developing adenocarcinoma from BE is 1% per annum. Most patients with BE do not develop cancer. HGD in BE signifies an increased risk of developing adenocarcinoma. The metaplasia-dysplasia-carcinoma sequence [56] is the rationale for obtaining endoscopic surveillance biopsies. Endoscopic surveillance results in the detection of a greater proportion of early adenocarcinoma [57].

Patients in whom either HGD or early adenocarcinoma is identified should be considered for EMR, endoscopic ablative therapies, and surgery. Often HGD or early cancer is multifocal or lacks an endoscopically visible lesion. The challenge with long-segment BE is where and how extensively to direct the therapy. Ablative therapies, particularly PDT, have been studied in these circumstances [58]. Seewald et al [39] investigated circumferential EMR in patients with BE containing multifocal HGD or intramucosal cancer (N = 5) and in patients with early stage malignant mucosal changes incidentally detected in random biopsy specimens that were not grossly visible at endoscopy (N = 7). Neither BE nor malignancy recurred during a median follow-up period of 9 months. The segments of BE were circumferential (median length of 5 cm) and completely removed in a median of 2.5 sessions. Two patients (17%) developed esophageal strictures successfully managed with bougienage. Minor bleeding occurred in 13%

(4 out of 31) of the EMR sessions. This strategy seems to be effective and safe, but more and longer follow-up data are needed in terms of recurrence rates.

Short-segment BE also has malignant potential. The prevalence of HGD in short-segment BE is 8%, whereas the prevalence of adenocarcinoma is 2% [59]. Inoue and Endo [60] first reported EMR for early adenocarcinoma in short-segment BE in 1990 using EMR tube. May et al [61] prospectively followed 28 patients who underwent EMRL for either HGD or early adenocarcinoma (all stage N0 by EUS) arising from short-segment BE. One patient was referred to surgery because of submucosal tumor infiltration. During follow-up two local recurrences and four metachronous lesions occurred, which were successfully managed with further endoscopic therapy (EMRL plus APC). After a mean of 43 months of follow-up no further recurrences or metachronous lesions occurred.

*Stomach*

Most patients in the West with gastric cancer present with either stage III or IV disease (see Table 3), although the percentage of patients with stage IV disease may be declining. The 5-year survival rate for patients without lymph node involvement is about 40%, but is only 10% for those with metastatic disease. These figures are unchanged over the past several decades despite improvements in medical and surgical therapies. Japan has experienced a continual decrease in the incidence of gastric cancer during the last 35 years, possibly because of changes in dietary habits and *Helicobacter pylori* eradication [62].

*H pylori* infection seems to be prerequisite to the development of gastric cancer. People with severe gastric atrophy, corpus-predominant gastritis, and intestinal metaplasia may also have a higher risk. Whether or not *H pylori* eradication in asymptomatic infected individuals and surveillance of patients with severe intestinal metaplasia is beneficial in terms of reducing the risk of gastric cancer remains to be determined [63].

The risk of low-grade dysplasia (LGD) progressing to HGD or noninvasive carcinoma is controversial. Over a 6-year mean of follow-up, Yamada et al [64] found that LGD has a low risk of progressing to HGD or noninvasive carcinoma and no risk of progressing to invasive carcinoma. In contrast, HGD is highly predictive of invasive carcinoma, which either coexists or appears within a short time after the biopsy. These patients should be considered for EMR.

Established criteria help determine whether or not a lesion is safely amenable to EMR. Endoscopic and histopathologic parameters are assessed and are used to predict the risk of lymph node metastasis, which should be nil. The Japanese classification of superficial (T1) neoplastic lesions is used at endoscopy (Fig. 9). Well- or moderately well-differentiated histopathology is necessary because poorly differentiated lesions, even when small, carry a significant risk of lymph node metastasis. The criteria are validated

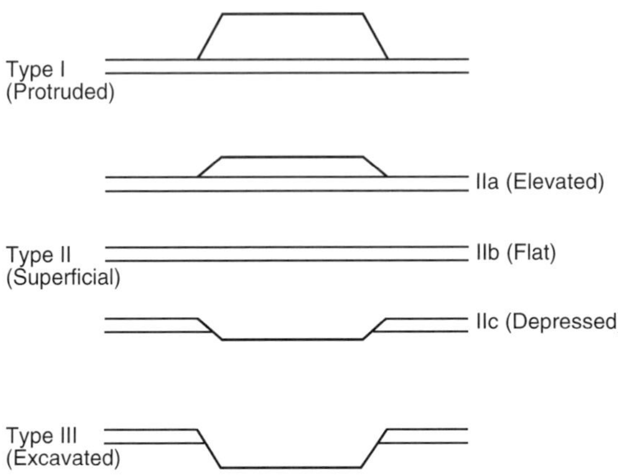


Fig. 9. Endoscopic subclassification of type 0 EGC according to the Japanese Research Society for gastric cancer. The elevation in IIa is less than twice the thickness of the adjacent mucosa. In type IIc the depression is only erosion. (*From* Lambert R. Treatment of esophagogastric tumors [review]. Endoscopy 2003;35:118–26; with permission.)

by data from several surgical series, including the retrospective review by Shimada et al [65] of 1051 patients with EGC undergoing gastrectomy. Tumors affecting the submucosa had statistically significantly more lymph node metastases (19.8%) than tumors limited to the mucosa (2.3%).

The depth of invasion can, however, sometimes be determined only post hoc from a specimen obtained at EMR, especially in 0 to IIa lesions. When the histopathology reveals submucosal invasion or vessel involvement or when the resection margins are unclear, surgical evaluation is indicated. The accepted criteria for EMR of EGC include (1) type 0 to IIa lesions less than 20 mm in diameter, (2) type 0 to IIb or 0 to IIc and less than 10 mm in diameter, and (3) well- or moderately well-differentiated histopathology.

Inoue [66] reported no local or distant metastases during a 9-year follow-up period of 102 EGCs satisfying the previously mentioned criteria and resected by EMR. Can lesions that do not satisfy all these criteria be safely removed by EMR? In general, large lesions less than 30 mm have a risk of lymph node metastasis of 29% and should be excluded [67]. Amano et al [68], however, suggest that the criteria could be extended to include well-differentiated lesions less than 30 mm without an ulcer or ulcer scar, lesions less than 20 mm with or without an ulcer scar, and lesions less than 10 mm with poorly differentiated cancer. Yamao et al [69] estimate that the risk of lymph node metastasis with mucosal gastric cancers less than 30 mm without histologic ulceration or lymphatic permeation is extremely low (0.4%).

Ono et al [19] reported 11-year data on EMR for EGC from the National Cancer Center in Tokyo. Four hundred and seventy-nine EGCs, up to 30 mm in diameter without ulceration, were resected with EMR. Intramucosal cancer was found in 85% (405 out of 479) of the lesions, whereas submucosal invasion was found in 15% (74 out of 479). Sixty-nine percent

(278 out of 405) of the intramucosal cancers were resected completely, of which 2% (5 out of 278) developed local recurrences, each of which was subsequently treated with endoscopic therapy (EMR with or without laser), with no recurrences detected after a median of 38 months of follow-up. Of the 31% (127 out of 405) who had incomplete resections, 19% (24 out of 127) received surgery; 7% (9 out of 127) received further endoscopic therapy (EMR with or without laser); and the remaining 74% (95 out of 127) received intensive endoscopic surveillance. For the last group, the local recurrence rate was 18% (17 out of 95) after a median of 4 months of follow-up. Perforation occurred in 5% (25 out of 479), usually managed with endoscopic clipping and antibiotics.

Strip biopsy and EMRC are frequently used because of their simplicity. With these techniques the size of the specimen obtained in a one-piece resection is limited to 10 to 15 mm. Piecemeal resection of larger lesions carries a higher risk of local recurrence because it is difficult to evaluate the completeness of excision histologically, which may lead to incomplete endoscopic resection. En bloc resection seems to provide better results than piecemeal resection in terms of more complete resection and lower recurrence rates, although direct comparisons are unavailable. Ohkuwa et al [18], using insulated-tip diathermic knife EMR in 41 patients with gastric mucosal tumors, demonstrated one-piece resection rates were 82% (14 out of 17) for lesions less than or equal to 10 mm; 75% (12 out of 16) for those 11 to 20 mm; and 14% (one out of seven) for those greater than 20 mm. Severe bleeding occurred in 22% and perforation occurred in 5%. There were no local recurrences during a median follow-up period of 32 months.

Miyamoto et al [70] evaluated insulated-tip diathermic knife EMR performed for 123 gastric tumors in 120 patients. The en bloc resection rates were 82% (27 out of 33) for lesions less than or equal to 10 mm; 54% (29 out of 54) for those 11 to 20 mm; and 31% (11 out of 36) for those greater than 20 mm. Complete resection rates for en bloc resections were 78% (21 out of 27) for lesions less than or equal to 10 mm; 76% (22 out of 29) for those 11 to 20 mm; and 73% (8 out of 11) for those greater than 20 mm. There were no episodes of major bleeding, and minor bleeding occurred in 38% (47 out of 123). Perforation occurred in 0.8% (1 out of 123). Ninety intramucosal lesions followed for more than 6 months required no further treatment. The local recurrence rate for en bloc resections (2 [49%] out of 49) was significantly lower than that for piecemeal resections (7 [17%] out of 41).

EUS is useful to assess the resectability of EGC by EMR. Akahoshi et al [71] reviewed EUS evaluations in 58 patients with EGC less than 20 mm who subsequently underwent radical surgery. The patients were classified as negative for EMR if EUS showed neoplastic changes of the third layer, and as positive if such changes were not observed. The prevalence of metastatic adenopathy was 3% (2 out of 58). The sensitivity and specificity of EUS for lymph node staging was 0% (0 out of 2) and 93% (52 out of 56), respectively. The sensitivity and specificity of EUS for assessing the suitability of EMR was 93% (27 out of 29) and 86% (25 out of 29), respectively.

## Endoscopic ablative therapies

### *Photodynamic therapy*

PDT uses light of appropriate power and wavelength to activate a photosensitizer distributed in tissue to produce singlet-oxygen, which is cytotoxic to mucosa. PDT has been studied primarily in BE, but has also been studied with cholangiocarcinoma.

#### *Porfimer photodynamic therapy*

PDT with porfimer sodium as the photosensitizer has been shown to eliminate Barrett's dysplasia and to reduce the length of BE in phase I and II clinical trials. To date, no studies have compared porfimer PDT with esophagectomy, the standard of care for HGD of the esophagus. A recent large phase III trial randomized 208 patients with HGD to porfimer PDT plus omeprazole versus omeprazole alone [72]. Patients were assessed with four-quadrant biopsies every 3 months. After 24 months, 77% of patients in the porfimer PDT group showed ablation of all areas of HGD compared with 39% of patients who received only omeprazole ($P < .001$). Thirteen percent of patients in the porfimer PDT group developed cancer compared with 28% in the control group ($P = .06$). The stricture rate was high (37%) after PDT therapy, but the strictures resolved after dilatation in all but 2% of the patients.

Porfimer PDT with supplemental neodymium:yttrium-aluminum-garnet photoablation and continuous treatment with omeprazole reduces the length of Barrett's mucosa, can eradicate HGD, and may reduce the expected frequency of adenocarcinoma. Overholt et al [73] examined the long-term outcome of 103 patients with LGD, HGD, or early stage carcinoma treated with porfimer PDT. These patients also received neodymium:yttrium-aluminum-garnet photoablation of the small areas of residual or untreated BE and received omeprazole, 20 mg twice a day. For the 82 patients not lost to follow-up, the mean follow-up was 58.5 months (range 41–132 months). After PDT, the length of BE decreased by a mean of 6.9 cm (range 1–22 cm). Of 65 patients with HGD, 60 (94%) had elimination of HGD. Three (4.6%) patients developed subsquamous adenocarcinoma. Subsquamous, nondysplastic, metaplastic epithelium was found in four patients (4.9%). Strictures occurred in 18% with one session of PDT, and in 50% with two treatments, for an overall 30% rate. For the 103 patients, intention-to-treat success rates were 92.9%, 77.5%, and 44.4% for LGD, HGD, and early stage carcinoma, respectively. Additional studies are needed to confirm these results.

### *5-Aminolevulinic acid photodynamic therapy*

PDT with 5-aminolevulinic acid as the photosensitizer is associated with a high rate of persistent or subsquamous Barrett's mucosa, presumably because 5-aminolevulinic acid PDT is limited to mucosal injury. Injury to the full thickness of Barrett's mucosa may be insufficient to destroy dysplasia deep in the mucosa.

### *Argon plasma coagulation*

Patients with BE without dysplasia have a low risk of cancer. There is no evidence that ablation therapy benefits these patients [74]. A few studies have demonstrated the efficacy and safety of APC for ablation of BE with HGD or intramucosal cancer. Van Laethem et al [75] treated 10 patients with either HGD (N = 7) or in situ adenocarcinoma (N = 3) associated with BE with APC and high-dose omeprazole (40 mg daily) therapy until squamous re-epithelialization or complete eradication of the initially apparent lesions. Complete eradication of HGD and in situ adenocarcinoma was achieved after a mean number of $3.3 \pm 1.5$ APC sessions in 8 (80%) out of 10 patients. These eight patients did not show any evidence of local recurrence during a median follow-up of 24 months (range 12–36 months). One patient with initial HGD had persistence of HGD 30 months after initial diagnosis, and one patient progressed to invasive adenocarcinoma after failure of APC and PDT.

### *Laser photoablation*

Little data exist to support the use of laser for early cancer. Gossner et al [76] performed neodymium:yttrium-aluminum-garnet KTP laser photoablation in 10 patients with BE and histologically proved LGD (N = 4), HGD (N = 4), or early adenocarcinoma (N = 2). Patients also received acid-suppressive therapy of up to 80 mg omeprazole daily. A complete response with squamous re-epithelialization was obtained in all 10 patients after a mean of 2.4 sessions per patient. No complications occurred. After a mean follow-up of 10.6 months, two patients showed specialized mucosa beneath the restored squamous cell epithelial layer.

An advantage of laser photoablation is the limited depth of thermal destruction in BE with a low attendant risk of perforation or stricture formation. The cost of laser systems and the available alternative therapies, such as EMR and PDT, however, have limited the application of this modality in the treatment of dysplasia and early GI cancers.

## Summary and future directions

New devices will improve the efficacy and safety of EMR for the treatment of early GI malignancies. New endoscopes are being designed to improve access to difficult-to-reach parts of the stomach. The prototype

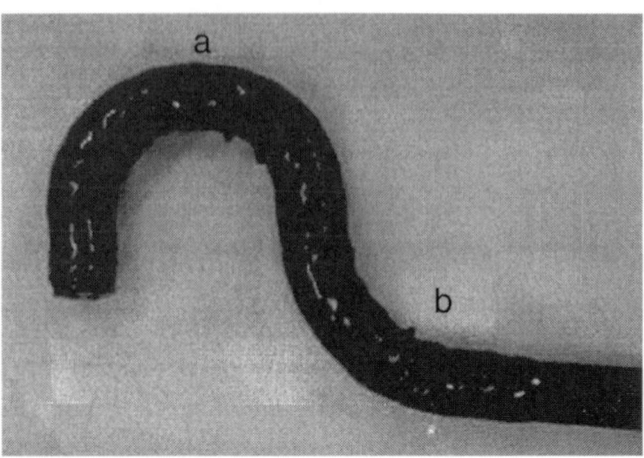


Fig. 10. The M-scope (Olympus GIF-2T240M, Olympus Optical; courtesy of Olympus Optical, Tokyo, Japan; with permission.)

two-channel multibending M-scope developed by Olympus has a distal segment that can bend in four directions and a proximal segment that can bend in two directions to permit en face views of most areas of the stomach (Fig. 10) [77]. Another prototype permits lateral movements of a needle-knife to facilitate submucosal dissection. Salameh [78] has developed a prototype capsule-shaped hood for EMR that permits direct endoscopic vision during suctioning and snaring. In animal models this resection technology yielded specimens with an average diameter of 18 mm.

Trials are needed to compare endoscopic therapy with surgical resection to establish clear criteria for EMR and ablative therapies. If mortality is similar, such outcomes as quality-of-life and cost of therapy will likely favor the less invasive endoscopic approach. Ablative therapies are important but their precise role in the management of early GI malignancies needs to be clarified. Direct comparisons with EMR may help clarify their role.

## References

[1] Heitmiller RF, Redmond M, Hamilton SR. Barrett's esophagus with high-grade dysplasia: an indication for prophylactic esophagectomy. Ann Surg 1996;224:66–71.

[2] Everett SM, Axon AT. Early gastric cancer in Europe. Gut 1997;41:142–50.

[3] Schlemper RJ, Dawsey SM, Itabashi M, Iwashita A, Kato Y, Koike M, et al. Differences in diagnostic criteria for esophageal squamous cell carcinoma between Japanese and Western pathologists. Cancer 2000;88:996–1006.

[4] Rosenberg N. Submucosal saline wheal as safety factor in fulguration or rectal and sigmoidal polypi. AMA Arch Surg 1955;70(1):120–2.

[5] Deyhle P, Jenny S, Fumagalli I. [Endoscopic polypectomy in the proximal colon: a diagnostic, therapeutic (and preventive?) intervention]. Dtsch Med Wochenschr 1973;98: 219–20 [in German].

[6] Martin TR, Onstad GR, Silvis SE, Vennes JA. Lift and cut biopsy technique for submucosal sampling. Gastrointest Endosc 1976;23:29–30.

[7] Tada M, Murakami A, Karita M, Yanai H, Okita K. Endoscopic resection of early gastric cancer. Endoscopy 1993;25:445–50.

[8] Makuuchi H, Machimura T, Sugihara T, et al. Endoscopic diagnosis and treatment of mucosal cancer of the esophagus. Endoscopia Digestiva 1990;8:175–9.
[9] Monma K, Sakaki N, Yoshida M, et al. Endoscopic mucosectomy for precise evaluation and treatment of esophageal intraepithelial cancer. Endoscopia Digestiva 1990; 2:501–6.
[10] Inoue H, Endo M. Endoscopic esophageal mucosal resection using a transparent tube. Surg Endosc 1990;4:198–201.
[11] Makuuchi H. Esophageal endoscopic mucosal resection (EEMR) tube. Surg Laparosc Endosc 1996;6:160–1.
[12] Kawano T, Miyake S, Yasuno M, et al. A new technique for endoscopic esophageal mucosectomy using a transparent overtube with intraluminal negative pressure (np-EEM). Dig Endosc 1991;3:159–67.
[13] Inoue H, Endo M, Takeshita K, Yoshino K, Muraoka Y, Yoneshima H. A new simplified technique of endoscopic esophageal mucosal resection using a cap-fitted panendoscope (EMRC). Surg Endosc 1992;6:264–5.
[14] Fleischer DE, Wang GQ, Dawsey S, Tio TL, Newsome J, Kidwell J, et al. Tissue band ligation followed by snare resection (band and snare): a new technique for tissue acquisition in the esophagus. Gastrointest Endosc 1996;44:68–72.
[15] Chaves DM, Sakai P, Mester M, Spinosa SR, Tomishige T, Ishioka S. A new endoscopic technique for the resection of flat polypoid lesions. Gastrointest Endosc 1994;40(2 Pt 1): 224–6.
[16] Soehendra N, Binmoeller KF, Bohnacker S, Seitz U, Brand B, Thonke F, et al. Endoscopic snare mucosectomy in the esophagus without any additional equipment: a simple technique for resection of flat early cancer. Endoscopy 1997;29:380–3.
[17] Hirao M, Masuda K, Asanuma T, Naka H, Noda K, Matsuura K, et al. Endoscopic resection of early gastric cancer and other tumors with local injection of hypertonic saline-epinephrine. Gastrointest Endosc 1988;34:264–9.
[18] Ohkuwa M, Hosokawa K, Boku N, Ohtu A, Tajiri H, Yoshida S. New endoscopic treatment for intramucosal gastric tumors using an insulated-tip diathermic knife. Endoscopy 2001;33: 221–6.
[19] Ono H, Kondo H, Gotoda T, Shirao K, Yamaguchi H, Saito D, et al. Endoscopic mucosal resection for treatment of early gastric cancer. Gut 2001;48:225–9.
[20] Yamamoto H, Koiwai H, Yube T, Isoda N, Sato Y, Sekine Y, et al. A successful single-step endoscopic resection of a 40 millimeter flat-elevated tumor in the rectum: endoscopic mucosal resection using sodium hyaluronate [review]. Gastrointest Endosc 1999;50:701–4.
[21] Yamamoto H, Kawata H, Sunada K, Sasaki A, Nakazawa K, Miyata T, et al. Successful en-bloc resection of large superficial tumors in the stomach and colon using sodium hyaluronate and small-caliber-tip transparent hood. Endoscopy 2003;35:690–4.
[22] Inoue H, Satoh Y, Kazawa T, et al. Endoscopic submucosal dissection using triangle tip knife. Stomach and Intestine 2004;39:53–6.
[23] Mariette C, Balon JM, Maunoury V, Taillier G, Van S, Triboulet JP. Value of endoscopic ultrasonography as a predictor of long-term survival in oesophageal carcinoma. Br J Surg 2003;90:1367–72.
[24] Murata Y, Muroi M, Yoshida M, Ide H, Hanyu F. Endoscopic ultrasonography in the diagnosis of esophageal carcinoma. Surg Endosc 1987;1:11–6.
[25] Meining A, Rosch T, Wolf A, Lorenz R, Allescher HD, Kauer W, et al. High interobserver variability in endosonographic staging of upper gastrointestinal cancers. Z Gastroenterol 2003;41:391–4.
[26] Meining A, Dittler HJ, Wolf A, Lorenz R, Schusdziarra V, Siewert JR, et al. You get what you expect? A critical appraisal of imaging methodology in endosonographic cancer staging. Gut 2002;50:599–603.

[27] Mortensen MB, Pless T, Durup J, Ainsworth AP, Plagborg GJ, Hovendal C. Clinical impact of endoscopic ultrasound-guided fine needle aspiration biopsy in patients with upper gastrointestinal tract malignancies: a prospective study. Endoscopy 2001;33:478–83.
[28] Silverstein FE, Martin RW, Kimmey MB, Jiranek GC, Franklin DW, Proctor A. Experimental evaluation of an endoscopic ultrasound probe: in vitro and in vivo canine studies. Gastroenterology 1989;96:1058–62.
[29] Murata Y, Suzuki S, Ohta M, Mitsunaga A, Hayashi K, Yoshida K, et al. Small ultrasonic probes for determination of the depth of superficial esophageal cancer. Gastrointest Endosc 1996;44:23–8.
[30] May A, Gunter E, Roth F, Gossner L, Stolte M, Vieth M, et al. Accuracy of staging in early oesophageal cancer using high resolution endoscopy and high resolution endosonography: a comparative, prospective, and blinded trial. Gut 2004;53:634–40.
[31] Dawsey SM, Fleischer DE, Wang GQ, Zhou B, Kidwell JA, Lu N, et al. Mucosal iodine staining improves endoscopic visualization of squamous dysplasia and squamous cell carcinoma of the esophagus in Linxian, China. Cancer 1998;83:220–31.
[32] Soetikno RM, Gotoda T, Nakanishi Y, Soehendra N. Endoscopic mucosal resection [review]. Gastrointest Endosc 2003;57:567–79.
[33] Uno Y, Munakata A. The non-lifting sign of invasive colon cancer. Gastrointest Endosc 1994;40:485–9.
[34] Kato H, Haga S, Endo S, Hashimoto M, Katsube T, Oi I, et al. Lifting of lesions during endoscopic mucosal resection (EMR) of early colorectal cancer: implications for the assessment of resectability. Endoscopy 2001;33:568–73.
[35] Ishiguro A, Uno Y, Ishiguro Y, Munakata A, Morita T. Correlation of lifting versus non-lifting and microscopic depth of invasion in early colorectal cancer. Gastrointest Endosc 1999;50:329–33.
[36] Yamamoto H, Kawata H, Sunada K, Satoh K, Kaneko Y, Ido K, et al. Success rate of curative endoscopic mucosal resection with circumferential mucosal incision assisted by submucosal injection of sodium hyaluronate. Gastrointest Endosc 2002;56: 507–12.
[37] Yamamoto H, Sekine Y, Higashizawa T, Kihira K, Kaneko Y, Hosoya Y, et al. Successful en bloc resection of a large superficial gastric cancer by using sodium hyaluronate and electrocautery incision forceps. Gastrointest Endosc 2001;54:629–32.
[38] May A, Gossner L, Behrens A, Kohnen R, Vieth M, Stolte M, et al. A prospective randomized trial of two different endoscopic resection techniques for early stage cancer of the esophagus. Gastrointest Endosc 2003;58:167–75.
[39] Seewald S, Akaraviputh T, Seitz U, Brand B, Groth S, Mendoza G, et al. Circumferential EMR and complete removal of Barrett's epithelium: a new approach to management of Barrett's esophagus containing high-grade intraepithelial neoplasia and intramucosal carcinoma. Gastrointest Endosc 2003;57:854–9.
[40] Ohkuwa M, Hosokawa K, Boku N, Ohtu A, Tajiri H, Yoshida S. New endoscopic treatment for intramucosal gastric tumors using an insulated-tip diathermic knife. Endoscopy 2001; 33(3):221–6.
[41] Hosokawa K, Yoshida S. Recent advances in endoscopic mucosal resection for early gastric cancer. Japanese Journal of Cancer and Chemotherapy 1998;25:483.
[42] Miyata M, Yokoyama Y, Okoyama N, Joh T, Seno K, Sasaki M, et al. What are the appropriate indications for endoscopic mucosal resection for early gastric cancer? Analysis of 256 endoscopically resected lesions. Endoscopy 2000;32:773–8.
[43] Matsushita M, Hajiro K, Okazaki K, Takakuwa H. Endoscopic mucosal resection of gastric tumors located in the lesser curvature of the upper third of the stomach. Gastrointest Endosc 1997;45:512–5.
[44] Lee TH, Hsueh PR, Yeh WC, Wang HP, Wang TH, Lin JT. Low frequency of bacteremia after endoscopic mucosal resection. Gastrointest Endosc 2000;52:223–5.
[45] Lambert R. Treatment of esophagogastric tumors [review]. Endoscopy 2003;35:118–26.

[46] Japanese Gastric Cancer Association. Japanese classification of gastric carcinoma: second English edition. Gastric Cancer 1998;1:10–24.
[47] Nijhawan PK, Wang KK. Endoscopic mucosal resection for lesions with endoscopic features suggestive of malignancy and high-grade dysplasia within Barrett's esophagus. Gastrointest Endosc 2000;52:328–32.
[48] Kodama M, Kakegawa T. Treatment of superficial cancer of the esophagus: a summary of responses to a questionnaire on superficial cancer of the esophagus in Japan. Surgery 1998; 123:432–9.
[49] Takeshita K, Tani M, Inoue H, Saeki I, Hayashi S, Honda T, et al. Endoscopic treatment of early oesophageal or gastric cancer. Gut 1997;40:123–7.
[50] Inoue H, Fukami N, Yoshida T, Kudo SE. Endoscopic mucosal resection for esophageal and gastric cancers [review]. J Gastroenterol Hepatol 2002;17:382–8.
[51] Narahara H, Iishi H, Tatsuta M, Uedo N, Sakai N, Yano H, et al. Effectiveness of endoscopic mucosal resection with submucosal saline injection technique for superficial squamous carcinomas of the esophagus. Gastrointest Endosc 2000;52:730–4.
[52] Shimizu Y, Tukagoshi H, Fujita M, Hosokawa M, Kato M, Asaka M. Metachronous squamous cell carcinoma of the esophagus arising after endoscopic mucosal resection. Gastrointest Endosc 2001;54:190–4.
[53] Nomura T, Boku N, Ohtsu A, Muto M, Matsumoto S, Tajiri H, et al. Recurrence after endoscopic mucosal resection for superficial esophageal cancer. Endoscopy 2000;32:277–80.
[54] Pech O, Gossner L, May A, Vieth M, Stolte M, Ell C. Endoscopic resection of superficial esophageal squamous-cell carcinomas: western experience. Am J Gastroenterol 2004;99: 1226–32.
[55] Shimizu Y, Tsukagoshi H, Fujita M, Hosokawa M, Kato M, Asaka M. Long-term outcome after endoscopic mucosal resection in patients with esophageal squamous cell carcinoma invading the muscularis mucosae or deeper. Gastrointest Endosc 2002;56:387–90.
[56] Hameeteman W, Tytgat GN, Houthoff HJ, van den Tweel JG. Barrett's esophagus: development of dysplasia and adenocarcinoma. Gastroenterology 1989;96(5 Pt 1):1249–56.
[57] Nigro JJ, Hagen JA, DeMeester TR, De Meester SR, Theisen J, Peters JH, et al. Occult esophageal adenocarcinoma: extent of disease and implications for effective therapy. Ann Surg 1999;230:433–8.
[58] May A, Gossner L, Pech O, Fritz A, Gunter E, Mayer G, et al. Local endoscopic therapy for intraepithelial high-grade neoplasia and early adenocarcinoma in Barrett's oesophagus: acute-phase and intermediate results of a new treatment approach. Eur J Gastroenterol Hepatol 2002;14:1085–91.
[59] Hirota WK, Loughney TM, Lazas DJ, Maydonovitch CL, Rholl V, Wong RK. Specialized intestinal metaplasia, dysplasia, and cancer of the esophagus and esophagogastric junction: prevalence and clinical data. Gastroenterology 1999;116:277–85.
[60] Inoue H, Endo M. Endoscopic esophageal mucosal resection using a transparent tube. Surg Endosc 1990;4:198–201.
[61] May A, Gossner L, Pech O, Muller H, Vieth M, Stolte M, et al. Intraepithelial high-grade neoplasia and early adenocarcinoma in short-segment Barrett's esophagus (SSBE): curative treatment using local endoscopic treatment techniques. Endoscopy 2002;34:604–10.
[62] Kaneko S, Yoshimura T. Time trend analysis of gastric cancer incidence in Japan by histological types, 1975–1989. Br J Cancer 2001;84:400–5.
[63] Moreto M. Diagnosis of esophagogastric tumors [review]. Endoscopy 2003;35:36–42.
[64] Yamada H, Ikegami M, Shimoda T, Takagi N, Maruyama M. Long-term follow-up study of gastric adenoma/dysplasia. Endoscopy 2004;36:390–6.
[65] Shimada S, Yagi Y, Shiomori K, Honmyo U, Hayashi N, Matsuo A, et al. Characterization of early gastric cancer and proposal of the optimal therapeutic strategy. Surgery 2001;129: 714–9.
[66] Inoue H. Endoscopic mucosal resection for esophageal and gastric mucosal cancers [review]. Can J Gastroenterol 1998;12:355–9.

[67] Inoue H, Fukami N, Yoshida T, Kudo SE. Endoscopic mucosal resection for esophageal and gastric cancers. J Gastroenterol Hepatol 2002;17:382–8.
[68] Amano Y, Ishihara S, Amano K, Hirakawa K, Adachi K, Fukuda R, et al. An assessment of local curability of endoscopic surgery in early gastric cancer without satisfaction of current therapeutic indications. Endoscopy 1998;30:548–52.
[69] Yamao T, Shirao K, Ono H, Kondo H, Saito D, Yamaguchi H, et al. Risk factors for lymph node metastasis from intramucosal gastric carcinoma. Cancer 1996;77:602–6.
[70] Miyamoto S, Muto M, Hamamoto Y, Boku N, Ohtsu A, Baba S, et al. A new technique for endoscopic mucosal resection with an insulated-tip electrosurgical knife improves the completeness of resection of intramucosal gastric neoplasms. Gastrointest Endosc 2002;55: 576–81.
[71] Akahoshi K, Chijiiwa Y, Hamada S, Sasaki I, Maruoka A, Kabemura T, et al. Endoscopic ultrasonography: a promising method for assessing the prospects of endoscopic mucosal resection in early gastric cancer. Endoscopy 1997;29:614–9.
[72] Overholt BF, Lightdale CJ, Wang K, et al. International multicenter partially blinded randomised study of the efficacy of photodynamic therapy using porfimer sodium for the ablation of high-grade dysplasia in Barrett's esophagus: results of 24 month follow-up. Gastroenterology 2003;124:151.
[73] Overholt BF, Panjehpour M, Halberg DL. Photodynamic therapy for Barrett's esophagus with dysplasia and/or early stage carcinoma: long-term results. Gastrointest Endosc 2003;58: 183–8.
[74] Franchimont D, Van Laethem JL, Deviere J. Argon plasma coagulation in Barrett's esophagus. Gastrointest Endosc Clin N Am 2003;13:457–66.
[75] Van Laethem JL, Jagodzinski R, Peny MO, Cremer M, Deviere J. Argon plasma coagulation in the treatment of Barrett's high-grade dysplasia and in situ adenocarcinoma. Endoscopy 2001;33:257–61.
[76] Gossner L, May A, Stolte M, Seitz G, Hahn EG, Ell C. KTP laser destruction of dysplasia and early cancer in columnar-lined Barrett's esophagus. Gastrointest Endosc 1999;49:8–12.
[77] Isshi K, Tajiri H, Fujisaki J, Mochizuki K, Matsuda K, Nakamura Y, et al. The effectiveness of a new multibending scope for endoscopic mucosal resection. Endoscopy 2004;36:294–7.
[78] Salameh FS. A new device for endoscopic mucosal resection. Endoscopy 2004;36:667.

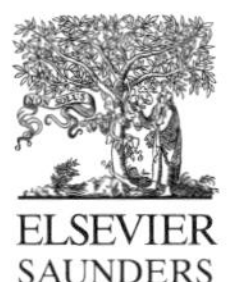

ELSEVIER
SAUNDERS

Med Clin N Am 89 (2005) 187–209

THE MEDICAL CLINICS OF NORTH AMERICA

# Laparoscopic surgery for the prevention, palliation, and cure of gastrointestinal malignancies

Jose E. Torres, MD, George Tsoulfas, MD[1], Kareem Hamdy, MD, Carol E.H. Scott-Conner, MD, PhD*

*Department of Surgery, Roy J. and Lucille C. Carver College of Medicine, University of Iowa, 200 Hawkins Drive, Iowa City, IA 52240, USA*

Medicine is a dynamic field, and physicians are constantly required to evaluate and re-evaluate treatment modalities. Diseases, such as pneumonia, trauma, cancer, and appendicitis, have been part of human existence since the beginning of civilization, and their treatment has undergone constant evolution. The pace of change has recently accelerated. For example, the development of first the sulfonamides and then penicillin revolutionized the treatment of infectious diseases. Standard therapy for peptic ulcer disease has evolved from bed rest with a diet of milk and antacids, to vagotomy, to histamine-2 antagonists, and finally to proton pump inhibitors and therapy for *Helicobacter pylori*. Just as these pharmaceutical advances revolutionized medical therapies, technologic innovations and instrument improvement have revolutionized the surgical management of many diseases.

Laparoscopy is a prime example of such a technologic revolution. The development of surgical laparoscopic techniques has revolutionized the way surgeons approach many diseases, including cancer. This article briefly discusses the historical development of surgical laparoscopy; describes laparoscopic surgical techniques, with a focus on techniques for common intra-abdominal malignancies; and reviews laparoscopic management of common gastrointestinal malignancies.

[1] Present address: Department of Surgery, Massachusetts General Hospital, Boston, Massachusetts.

* Corresponding author.

*E-mail address:* carol-scott-conner@uiowa.edu (C.E.H. Scott-Conner).



doi:10.1016/j.mcna.2004.08.012

## History of laparoscopic gastrointestinal surgery

Semm performed the first laparoscopic appendectomy in 1983, Muhe performed the first laparoscopic cholecystectomy in 1985, and Geagea performed the first laparoscopic fundoplication in 1991. In 1992, a Consensus Conference convened by the National Institutes of Health concluded that laparoscopic cholecystectomy was superior to the traditional open cholecystectomy. This is now the standard surgical procedure for symptomatic cholelithiasis.

Since that first laparoscopic cholecystectomy, progressive improvements in laparoscopic instrumentation and techniques have enabled surgeons to apply minimally invasive surgery as an alternative to traditional open surgical procedures. Some laparoscopic procedures, such as laparoscopic esophagomyotomy for achalasia and laparoscopic fundoplication for gastroesophageal reflux disease, have become the surgical procedures of choice. As laparoscopic techniques evolved, surgeons naturally began to apply them to treat cancer. Laparoscopy is now used, in conjunction with other modalities, for diagnosis and staging, and laparoscopic resection is increasingly being used for palliation or cure.

## Principles of surgical oncology

The objectives in cancer surgery are the same for laparoscopic or open surgery. They include cancer prevention, cancer diagnosis and staging, cure, tumor debulking, symptom palliation, and patient rehabilitation [1]. One or more of these objectives may dominate in a particular clinical situation. For example, cancer prevention is the objective in the surgical removal of organs at high risk of malignancy because of genetic predisposition or underlying pathologic disorders. Prophylactic proctocolectomy for ulcerative colitis with significant dysplasia, thyroidectomy for a patient with a multiple endocrine neoplasia syndrome, or esophageal surgery for refractory gastroesophageal reflux with Barrett's esophagus are applications of this objective.

The objective of diagnosis and staging requires procuring adequate tissue for a definitive pathologic diagnosis by histologic examination. This may require special stains or special studies, such as flow cytometry. Sufficient material for a pathologic diagnosis may be obtained by needle aspiration or by brushing for cytology, or may require tissue from a biopsy specimen. In staging, the extent of a gastrointestinal cancer is determined, including lesion size; depth of penetration; invasion into adjacent organs; involvement of regional lymph nodes; and the presence or absence of metastatic disease in the liver, on the peritoneal surfaces, or elsewhere. Laparoscopy is particularly useful to visualize the peritoneal surfaces and detect small peritoneal nodules, which can be biopsied under direct vision.

The objective of tumor removal for cure requires that the malignancy not be violated during surgical manipulation to avoid tumor spillage and remote implantation. Tumors should be removed en bloc with adjacent or adherent tissue. Adequate surgical margins, as defined for each malignancy, should be attained, and draining regional lymph nodes should be removed. Laparoscopic surgery must fulfill these requirements when performed for cure. This is particularly important because chemotherapy and radiation have limited efficacy for most gastrointestinal adenocarcinomas; properly performed surgical resection is the primary potentially curative therapy.

## Laparoscopic equipment and general techniques

Surgical laparoscopy is performed under general anesthesia, which provides muscle relaxation, airway control, and a stable and immobile operative field, except for the periodic rhythm of the diaphragm because of the ventilator. Surgeons access the operative field through small skin incisions, ranging from 3 to 5 mm in length for diagnostic laparoscopy to 10 to 12 mm for therapeutic laparoscopy. Air-tight cannulas, or ports, are placed through these skin incisions to permit instrument passage. The first port is usually periumbilical. Carbon dioxide gas is then insufflated, to a working pressure of about 13 to 15 mm Hg, to open the potential space between the anterior abdominal wall and the viscera. The same effect can be created by abdominal wall devices. For thoracoscopic surgery, the ribcage provides the necessary elevation once the lungs have been deflated.

After establishing the operative field, a rigid laparoscope is inserted into the port and the abdomen is inspected. The laparoscope illuminates the field and transmits visual images using rod-lens optics. A miniature video camera is attached to the rod and the visual image is transmitted electronically to an external video monitor. The video monitor provides powerful magnification and unparalleled resolution, but affords a limited field of view, loss of three-dimensional vision, and diminished tactile feedback.

After abdominal inspection, the surgeon selects the correct equipment for surgery, such as scissors, dissectors, graspers, biopsy forceps, stapling devices, clip applicators, cautery devices or their equivalents, retractors, suction-irrigators, and intracorporeal suturing devices. They are introduced through secondary ports placed around the periphery of the operative field. Standard laparoscopic instruments are 5 to 10 mm in diameter. Smaller, less than 3 mm wide instruments offer a slight advantage in terms of less postoperative pain, but have not yet been proved adequate for manipulation of thick tissue and are prone to break.

Laparoscopic surgery can be performed in any standard operating room. The instruments can be brought into the room. Specialized minimally invasive surgical suites have video monitors and laparoscopic surgical equipment mounted to the ceiling on moveable beams, decreasing the clutter and crowding around the operative field. They are increasingly being built.

## Benefits and risks

The benefits of laparoscopic surgery include shorter postoperative stay, improved cosmesis, decreased pain, decreased wound complications including fewer wound infections, less frequent pneumonia, and faster return of normal bowel function. The risks of laparoscopic surgery include risks from the carbon dioxide pneumoperitoneum, hernia formation at the trocar sites, and injury to adjacent viscera because of retraction or trocar placement. Major complications occur in less than 1% of laparoscopic surgeries [2]. Complications unique to laparoscopic surgery include complications from the pneumoperitoneum and injuries from trocar placement.

Carbon dioxide is chosen for insufflation to decrease the risk of gas emboli, if the insufflating gas should gain access to the venous system. Carbon dioxide is more rapidly absorbed than room air, but a large bolus of carbon dioxide, like an air embolus, can cause cardiac arrest. The increased intra-abdominal pressure caused by the pneumoperitoneum elevates the diaphragm and decreases venous return to the heart. The anesthesiologist must compensate for the consequent decrease in pulmonary compliance and for the hemodynamic alterations. Carbon dioxide is absorbed from the peritoneal surfaces and must be eliminated by the lungs. With good anesthesia support, most patients tolerate the pneumoperitoneum well. When it is tolerated poorly, lowering the insufflation pressure may alleviate the problem. Rarely, pneumoperitoneum is not tolerated and the procedure must be aborted or converted to an open operation.

Trocar injuries may be vascular, intestinal, or urologic. Laparoscopic surgery requires several small incisions to access the abdominal cavity. Most trocar injuries occur during the initial intra-abdominal entry, because the entry is performed blindly or with limited visualization. A special spring-loaded needle, called a Veress needle, is used to make the initial puncture and blind intra-abdominal entry. Tests are done to confirm access into the free peritoneal cavity. A trocar is placed after the pneumoperitoneum has physically separated the anterior abdominal wall from the underlying viscera. Newer trocars allow visualization of the layers of the abdominal wall as the first trocar is placed, but the visualization is limited. The Veress needle or the trocar may puncture viscera, blood vessels, or bladder. Recognition of the injury may be immediate or delayed.

Because of the hazards of blind trocar entry, an open technique with direct visualization and division of the fascial layers and peritoneum before placement of a blunt-tipped trocar (the Hasson cannula) has been advocated by some. This open technique provides very limited visualization and can cause bowel injury about as frequently as with the blind insertion [3]. Many surgeons routinely use the Veress needle technique, and reserve the Hasson cannula for patients who had previous abdominal surgery, are pregnant, or have other risk factors for trocar injury.

Vascular complications occur in 0.05% to 0.3% of cases [4]. The aorta, inferior vena cava, and iliac arteries or veins are most commonly injured and the injuries usually occur during trocar placement at the start of the surgery. Most of these injuries are identified when they occur, but they may sometimes be recognized only when hypotension occurs during surgery. A mortality of 15% has been reported [5].

Unlike vascular injuries, bowel injuries may not be identified until several days after surgery, sometimes after hospital discharge when the patient is readmitted with peritonitis. The incidence is similar to that of vascular complications [4]. About half involve the small intestine. Like vascular complications, most are believed to occur during trocar placement, with the remaining injuries caused by electrocautery burns or trauma during grasping or dissection.

The bladder and ureters are rarely injured. Unlike vascular and bowel injuries, most of these injuries occur not at the initiation of surgery but during subsequent dissection.

## Port site metastases

The most controversial complication of laparoscopic oncologic surgery is the development of tumor nodules at the sites of trocar placement, termed "port site metastases." In 1978, Dabronte et al [6] described port site metastasis 2 weeks after diagnostic laparoscopy for malignancy. Surgeons and gynecologists have subsequently reported numerous cases of this phenomenon.

Hypotheses to explain the pathophysiology of these metastases include hematogenous spread, the chimney effect of escaping insufflating gas, aerosolization of tumor cells, direct wound implantation, excessive surgical manipulation of the tumor, and the immunosuppressive effect of carbon dioxide pneumoperitoneum [7,8]. The risk of these metastases may be greater with certain cancers, such as gallbladder cancer, and laparoscopic surgery is not currently advocated for this cancer.

Port site metastases were initially believed to occur more frequently than wound recurrences after traditional open laparotomy. The incidence of port site metastasis is currently estimated at 0.71% [9], which is similar to the incidence of 0.6% for incisional recurrence following open colectomy for colorectal cancer [10]. In both surgeries, implantation usually occurs in patients with advanced cancer.

Several techniques may lower the risk of port site metastasis from laparoscopic surgery for malignancy. The surgeon must strictly adhere to the aforementioned guidelines of careful manipulation of the specimen to prevent rupture and intraperitoneal spillage of malignant cells. The surgeon may use a specimen retrieval bag to extract the specimen (avoiding contact with the incision); excise the trocar wounds at the end of the procedure; or irrigate port sites with chemotherapeutic agents, such as 5-fluorouracil [11,12].

## Training of laparoscopic and minimally invasive surgeons

Surgical residency programs currently provide training in basic surgical laparoscopy including laparoscopic cholecystectomy, appendectomy, and fundoplication. Skills learned in performing these procedures are transferable to other laparoscopic procedures. Surgeons in practice learn new laparoscopic techniques by attending short courses and by preceptorship by experienced surgeons. Surgical residency programs continue to introduce new techniques into their curriculums. Surgical residents are taught how to evaluate whether patients are suitable candidates for laparoscopic procedures. Surgeons must be taught during residency the pathophysiology of the malignancy being treated, alternative treatments, contraindications to laparoscopic surgery, and the indications for converting a laparoscopic procedure to a traditional open approach [13]. The surgeon in practice must, likewise, attain competency in these areas.

The Society of American Gastrointestinal Endoscopic Surgeons has established guidelines for training and credentialing surgeons for laparoscopic surgery. Teaching programs now provide training in operating rooms, animal laboratories, skills laboratories with laparoscopic trainers, and virtual reality simulators. Advanced laparoscopic surgical fellowships provide additional training after surgical residency, creating a highly competent cadre of practicing laparoscopic surgeons who will continue to develop new techniques and help train the next generation.

## Future of laparoscopic surgery

Recent advances have led to the development of laparoscopic endoluminal surgery, hand-assisted laparoscopic surgery (HALS), and robotic surgery. Laparoscopic endoluminal surgery involves the deliberate insertion of a trocar within the lumen of an organ by a small incision, without damaging the integrity or architecture of the organ. Laparoscopic endoluminal surgery has been applied to treat early gastric cancer, gastric leiomyoma, and pancreatic pseudocysts, and to remove giant cecal polyps [14,15]. Laparoscopic endoluminal surgery is currently limited because of the large size of the current surgical instruments and the technical difficulty of the procedures, but continued research and development may make laparoscopic endoluminal surgery very effective in the treatment of small and large bowel diseases.

In HALS, a variation of laparoscopic surgery, the surgeon creates a minilaparotomy and places a hand within the abdominal cavity. Special inserts through the incision allow the pneumoperitoneum to be maintained while the surgeon manipulates the surgical specimen and retracts under laparoscopic guidance. This facilitates traction, retraction, and exposure, and the removal of large specimens. HALS has been used for many surgical procedures, including transhiatal esophagectomy, gastroplasty, gastric bypass, repair of paraesophageal hernias, splenectomy, and living donor nephrectomy [16,17]. Preliminary studies demonstrate that HALS is effective in the surgical treatment of gastrointestinal tumors. Although HALS preserves the benefits of laparoscopic surgery in the treatment of colorectal disease, long-term prospective trials comparing HALS with traditional laparoscopic and open surgery are required.

Robotic surgery has developed recently, especially in neurosurgery, obstetrics and gynecology, and urology. Robotics has allowed surgeons to overcome some of the limitations associated with laparoscopic surgery, including lack of depth perception, lack of dexterity at the instrument tip, and hand discomfort. The da Vinci Robotic Surgical System (Intuitive Surgical, Mountain View, CA) allows the surgeon to be seated at a console looking at a three-dimensional imaging system. The surgeon controls the robotic camera and instruments by manipulating controls, which produce the same range of motion as the human wrist with no hand tremor. Robotic surgery is still in its infancy. Further improvements in instrumentation and surgical technique must be made to decrease the high cost and long time required for robotic surgery for it to become a practical alternative to the standard open or laparoscopic techniques.

Current laparoscopic and minimally invasive approaches to specific gastrointestinal malignancies are presently reviewed.

## Esophageal cancer

Minimally invasive esophageal resection began almost one century ago. Denk, in 1913, performed a transhiatal esophagectomy in animals and cadavers using a vein stripper, and Oshawa, in 1933, performed the first distal transhiatal esophagectomy in a human subject. Recognizing that the traditional transthoracic incision contributed greatly to the morbidity and mortality of esophagectomy for benign and malignant esophageal disease, Orringer and Sloan reported in 1978 a "blunt esophagectomy without thoracotomy" as a potentially safer and better tolerated alternative. This subsequently became known as "transhiatal esophagectomy." Although transhiatal esophagectomy avoids thoracotomy and reduces the pulmonary complications, it does not permit wide mediastinal lymphadenectomy, which has been shown to improve long-term outcomes by some investigators.

With the expansion of interest and experience in laparoscopic techniques in the late 1980s and 1990s, new approaches toward minimally invasive esophageal surgery were developed, including thoracoscopic esophagectomy combined with standard upper midline laparotomy and cervical anastomosis, and laparoscopic transhiatal resection. Several surgeons subsequently demonstrated the feasibility and safety of total minimally invasive esophagectomy combining a laparoscopic transhiatal technique with thoracoscopy.

Because of the aggressive natural history and poor prognosis of esophageal carcinoma, surgery often becomes palliative, despite an initially curative intent. Short-term outcomes and time for recovery are particularly important for palliative surgery. Nguyen et al [18,19] in a retrospective comparison of minimally invasive esophagectomy with transthoracic and transhiatal esophagectomy demonstrated significantly shorter operative times, less blood loss, fewer blood transfusions, and shortened intensive care unit and hospital stays with minimally invasive surgery.

Up to 30% of patients explored by the open technique for a curative resection had too advanced or too widespread cancer at surgery to undergo resection. Such patients incurred the morbidity of an open thoracotomy without benefit. Krasna et al [20] found that 14% of patients undergoing laparoscopy or thoracoscopy had a nonresectable primary tumor. These patients were then spared the morbidity of an unnecessary open thoracotomy. This is a decided benefit of minimally invasive curative resection. Moreover, thoracoscopy, compared with the open approach, seems to enhance the inspection of proximal and middle third esophageal cancers for signs of invasion.

Akiashi et al [21] studied the change in pulmonary function after a combined thoracoscopic esophagectomy and upper abdominal laparotomy in 39 patients. They demonstrated relative preservation of forced expiratory volume in 1 second and vital capacity, and a rapid return of pulmonary function tests to baseline. They hypothesized that total minimally invasive surgery could even better preserve pulmonary function; with a lower risk of pulmonary complications more individuals with compromised pulmonary function might become eligible for curative resection.

Significant advances in nonoperative palliation have rendered surgical options for palliation less attractive because of the greater morbidity and mortality of surgery. Accordingly, the preoperative evaluation focuses on identifying patients who are candidates for curative resection. Patients with distant metastases, distal lymph node involvement, or advanced local disease with involvement of the bronchi, the great vessels, or the recurrent laryngeal nerve are not candidates for curative resection.

Preoperative evaluation typically includes a chest radiograph, which helps demonstrate correlates of advanced disease, such as metastatic nodules or malignant effusions. A barium esophagogram is generally performed during the initial evaluation of patients with dysphagia to identify conditions that contraindicate or mandate caution with esophagoscopy. Depth of invasion, the primary measure of the extent of local disease in the staging system for esophageal carcinoma, correlates poorly with length of the lesion. Barium esophagogram has limited use in staging esophageal carcinoma. It does, however, provide important anatomic information regarding the location and length of the lesion, and associated pathologies, which could help guide the subsequent esophagoscopy and surgical approach.

Flexible esophagoscopy with a combination of punch biopsy and brush cytology is about 95% accurate in making a tissue diagnosis. Esophagoscopy also has a role in the diagnosis of early carcinoma in high-risk asymptomatic patients, such as those with a history of corrosive ingestion or Barrett's esophagus. The American College of Gastroenterology recommends that patients with Barrett's esophagus undergo regular endoscopic surveillance. Although retrospective studies have shown that endoscopic surveillance can sometimes detect early, curable neoplasms in patients with Barrett's esophagus, it is unclear whether routine esophagoscopic screening and periodic surveillance decreases mortality from esophageal cancer (see later discussion).

Several imaging modalities are used preoperatively to evaluate local and distant spread. Endoscopic ultrasound is the most useful and accurate imaging study to determine the local extent of the primary tumor. It also assesses regional lymph node involvement with excellent sensitivity and specificity. Tissue sampling through endoscopic ultrasound–guided fine-needle aspiration adds significantly to the accuracy and positive predictive value of this test. Endoscopic ultrasound–guided fine-needle aspiration can be useful when the tumor is inaccessible to esophagoscopic biopsy.

CT is most useful in evaluating the primary tumor when contiguous structures are clearly involved in a T4 lesion. Its principle role in the preoperative evaluation is to determine regional and distant nodal involvement, and the presence and extent of extranodal metastatic disease. CT determines nodal invasion primarily by size and this approach is somewhat inaccurate. CT is quite accurate in detecting distant metastases that are greater than 1 cm in diameter. MRI offers little advantage over CT. Fluorodeoxyglucose positron emission tomography is more sensitive in detecting smaller lesions.

Laparoscopy and thoracoscopy with biopsies are primarily used to assess regional nodes and detect distant metastases. T4 primaries, however, have been frequently diagnosed by these procedures [20]. These procedures are not without morbidity and can interfere with subsequent thoracoscopic procedures. They are accordingly indicated when the obtained information is decisive for selecting surgery (eg, determine the nature of inconclusive nodules that seem to be possibly metastatic on other imaging studies) (Figs. 1–3).

The preoperative evaluation should also identify patients at high risk for surgical intervention. In the Western Hemisphere, patients with esophageal squamous cell cancer have a high incidence of smoking tobacco and alcohol abuse, which correlates with other tumors and decreased cardiopulmonary reserve. The patient's cardiopulmonary reserve is assessed. This typically entails pulmonary function testing and a cardiac evaluation, including a cardiac stress test. Reversible conditions, such as bronchospastic disease, or surgically correctible coronary artery disease are identified and treated, and the patient's fitness for surgical intervention is reassessed thereafter. Screening of other organ systems, such as the liver for hepatic dysfunction, is performed as indicated by the patient history, physical examination, and routine laboratory test results.

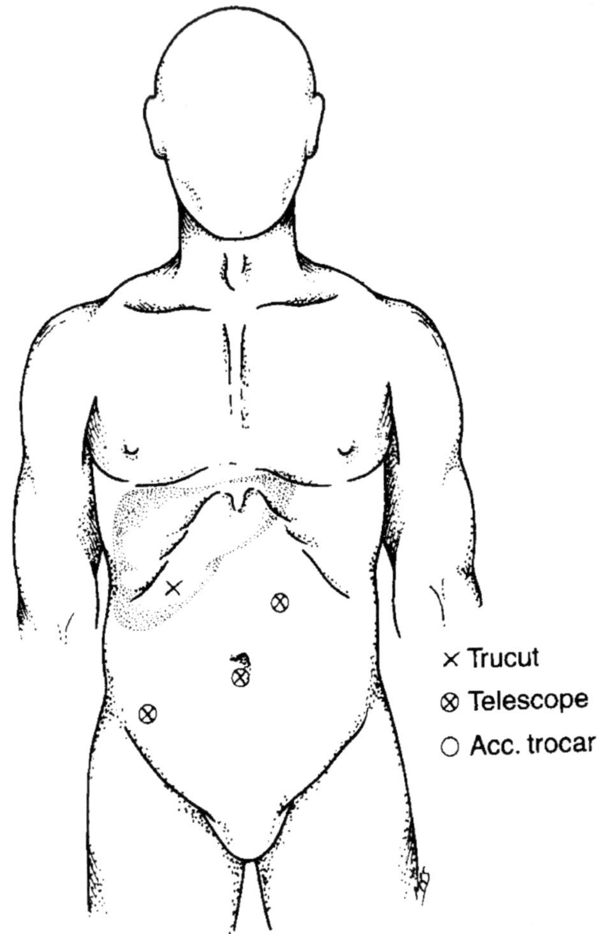


Fig. 1. Trocar sites for initial exploration including liver biopsy. (*From* Scott-Conner CEH, editor. The SAGES manual: fundamentals of laparoscopy and GI endoscopy. New York: Springer-Verlag; 1999. p. 117; with permission.)

A total videoscopic approach to esophagectomy for malignancy involves thoracoscopic mobilization of the esophagus, resection of paraesophageal and mediastinal lymph nodes, laparoscopic mobilization of the greater curvature, creation of a gastric conduit, and placement of a feeding jejunostomy. The procedure is completed by a small cervical incision through which the cervical esophagus is mobilized and the resected thoracic and abdominal portions are pulled through, along with the attached gastric conduit. The esophagogastric anastomosis is performed by this incision, thereby dramatically reducing the morbidity of an anastomotic leak. Other described techniques include a combined thoracoscopic and laparoscopic approach with an intrathoracic esophagogastric anastomosis and a solely

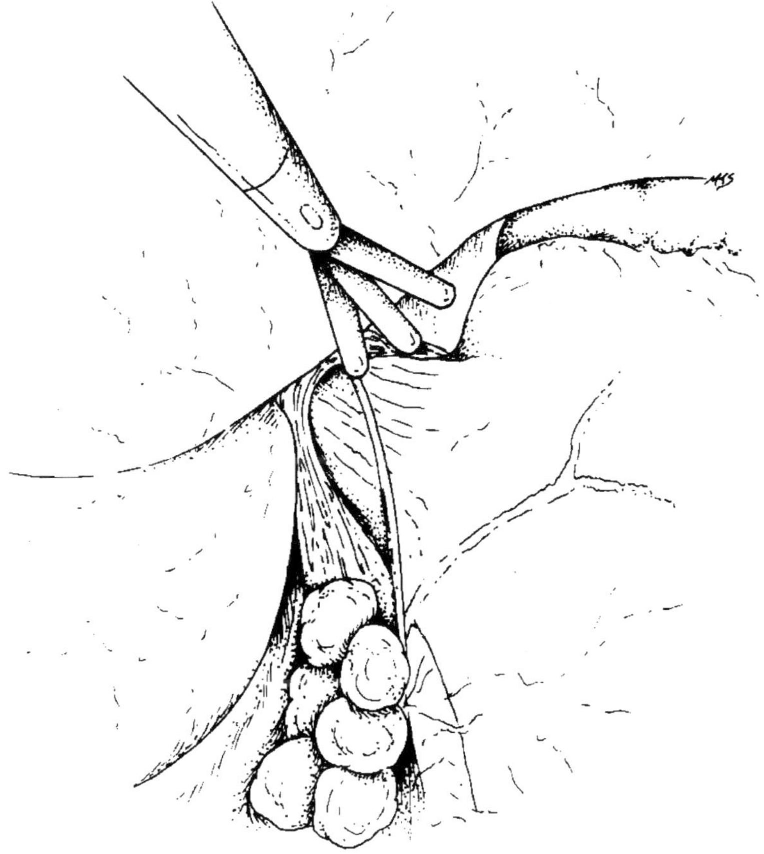

Fig. 2. Exposure of esophageal hiatus and nodes along lesser curvature of stomach. (*From* Scott-Conner CEH, editor. The SAGES manual: fundamentals of laparoscopy and GI endoscopy. New York: Springer-Verlag; 1999. p. 342; with permission.)

abdominal laparoscopic transhiatal resection. Choice of technique is guided by tumor location and the ability to obtain wide proximal and distal margins.

Immediate postoperative extubation, pain control, and initiation of jejunostomy feedings on the first or second postoperative days are important. A barium swallow is performed on day 3 to 6 and if an anastomotic leak is excluded, the nasogastric tube and the perianastomotic drain are pulled, and oral intake is resumed. The jejunostomy tube is pulled after adequate oral intake is established, several weeks postoperatively.

The mortality from thoracoscopic esophagectomy ranges from 0% to 11%, with most series reporting less than 5% mortality [22]. Pulmonary complications range from 0% to 36%, with most series reporting a 0% to 18% complication rate. Intraoperative bleeding occurs in less than 5% of

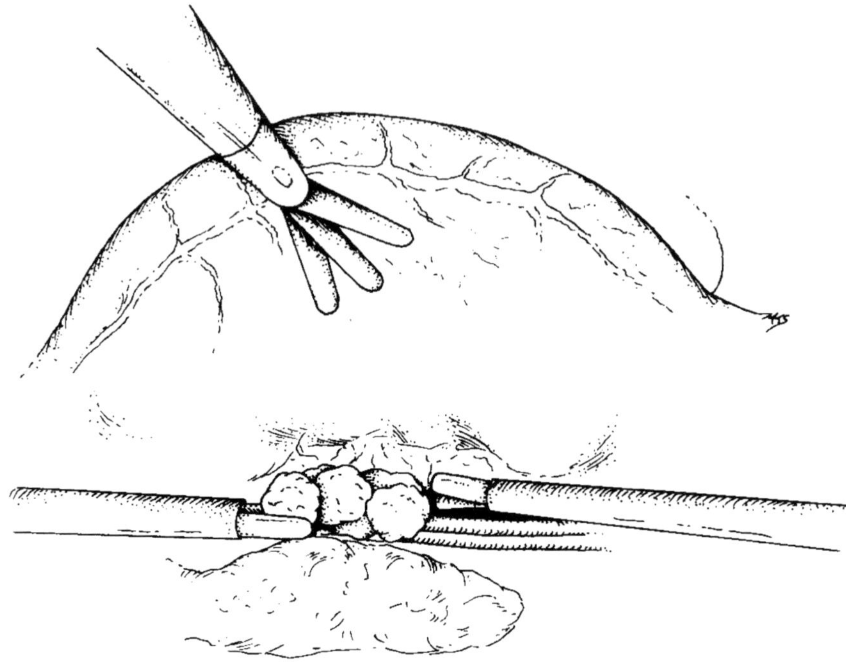

Fig. 3. Exposure of nodes around celiac axis. Stomach has been reflected cephalad and laparoscope inserted into lesser sac. (*From* Scott-Conner CEH, editor. The SAGES manual: fundamentals of laparoscopy and GI endoscopy. New York: Springer-Verlag; 1999. p. 343; with permission.)

cases. They are related to injury of the intercostal vessels, the azygos vein, or the aorta. The rate of conversion to an open procedure ranged from 0% to 27%, with most series reporting an 11% or less rate of conversion to an open procedure. The incidence of temporary recurrent laryngeal nerve palsy is about 15% [22]. Other complications, listed in Box 1, occur infrequently [22].

Early reports showed no advantage for the minimally invasive approach over traditional surgery. Some investigators attributed this to the small number of patients enrolled in these early studies. There is a strong learning curve effect for this surgery. Osugi et al [23] studied the outcome of 80 patients undergoing thoracoscopic esophagectomy and extensive mediastinal lymphadenectomy. The risk of pulmonary complications in their first 34 patients of 25% was equivalent to that of open esophagectomy. In their subsequent 46 patients, the operative time, blood loss, and rate of pulmonary complications (7%) decreased significantly. Akiashi et al [21] reported a reduction of pulmonary complications from 30% to 20% and a reduction of right laryngeal nerve palsy from 80% to 15% in laparoscopic as compared with open esophagectomy. The superior outcome was

**Box 1. Reported complications of minimally invasive esophagectomy for carcinoma**

- Pulmonary complications
  - Pneumonia
  - Air leak
  - Tracheal injury
  - Pleural effusion
  - Chylothorax
  - Pulmonary embolism
- Recurrent nerve paresis (right, left, bilateral)
- Anastomotic leak
- Mediastinal abscess
- Port site recurrence
- Wound dehiscence
- Delayed gastric emptying
- Anastomotic stricture
- Conversion to open
- Myocardial infarction

attributed to their prior experience in performing the thoracoscopic procedure on 20 pigs.

A concern regarding the minimally invasive approach is the completeness of mediastinal lymphadenectomy and its potential impact on long-term survival. Many investigators have addressed the completeness of the lymphadenectomy [17–24]. Both Akiashi et al [21] and Osugi et al [23] demonstrated that after sufficient experience the extent of mediastinal lymph node resection is at least equivalent to that with the open approach. Nguyen et al [18,19] demonstrated 3-year survival in 38 patients undergoing minimally invasive curative resection was comparable with the previously reported rate of 57% for open esophagectomy.

Laparoscopic antireflux surgery may help prevent cancer in patients with chronic gastroesophageal reflux disease [25,26], but a decrease in the incidence of carcinoma following the procedure has not been consistently demonstrated. Evidence in support of a decreased risk is largely inferential, including the demonstration of a decrease in bile reflux or a decrease in the incidence of new metaplasia. Barrett's metaplasia generally does not regress following the procedure and progression of Barrett's metaplasia to adenocarcinoma is a concern. The same concern occurs with medical management. Routine surveillance esophagoscopy and biopsy are still indicated after successful surgical or medical control of reflux disease.

The lack of an effective medical or surgical cure for Barrett's metaplasia, the persistent risk of malignant degeneration, and the subsequent need for regular endoscopic surveillance and biopsy has generated interest in minimally invasive interventions for this condition, specifically endoscopic ablation of the metaplastic epithelial lining of the esophagus, using argon plasma coagulation, photodynamic therapy, laser therapy, and endoscopic mucosal resection. The goal is to preserve the underlying layers of the esophagus during ablation while medically or surgically controlling the acid reflux, to permit squamous re-epithlialization of the columnar-lined esophagus.

Promising data are currently being compiled about prevention of malignant degeneration of Barrett's metaplasia with these techniques. If validated, a single session of ablative therapy, with minimal or no side effects, may sufficiently reduce the cancer risk to eliminate the need for long-term endoscopic surveillance.

## Gastric cancer

Although the incidence of gastric cancer has significantly decreased, the prognosis remains poor, with a 5-year survival of 10% to 20% [27]. In the United States, the median age of patients diagnosed with gastric cancer is 65 years, with 60% of cases occurring in men.

If distal esophageal and gastric cancers are identified early, they are curable by surgical resection. Unfortunately, widespread metastasis usually has occurred at diagnosis. Survival is optimized by extended lymphadenectomy in patients with negative peritoneal cytology, clear surgical margins, and apparently complete primary disease resection [28]. Extended lymphadenectomy is inadvisable in patients with a highly advanced primary tumor to avoid excessive morbidity [28].

Laparoscopy is an excellent tool for staging extent of disease before definitive therapy. CT scanning and ultrasonography are poor predictors of resectability [29]. Adding laparoscopy to the staging armamentarium significantly improves resectability rates at laparotomy.

Resection can be accomplished laparoscopically. Azagra performed the first laparoscopic gastrectomy for gastric cancer in 1993. Since then, the Japanese and Europeans have refined laparoscopic surgery for gastric cancer. In Japan most gastric tumors are discovered early, because of an aggressive screening program, and laparoscopy has become a viable option in the treatment of early gastric cancers. In Europe laparoscopic surgery has been used in the treatment of moderately advanced gastric cancers (T2N2M0).

Laparoscopic gastrectomy for malignancy is a viable alternative to open gastrectomy. Success in the attainment of clear margins and adequate lymphadenectomy was identical to that for the open procedure, and short-term survival and rates of wound seeding or trocar metastasis were identical [30]. Similar results were achieved in 106 patients undergoing laparoscopic resection for gastric cancer located in the middle or lower third of the stomach [31].

## Cancer of the small intestine

Although the small intestine comprises more than 90% of the mucosal surface of the gastrointestinal tract, it is responsible for only 5% to 20% of neoplasms and only 2% of malignancies [32]. The mean age of onset of both benign and malignant neoplasms is 60 years. Malignancies account for 75% of symptomatic tumors. Leiomyomas and adenomas comprise the most common benign lesions, whereas adenocarcinoma and carcinoid tumors comprise the malignant lesions.

Benign lesions can present with vague and nonspecific symptoms, including anorexia, dull abdominal pain, and dyspepsia. Most benign lesions are asymptomatic and are discovered at autopsy. Treatment of symptomatic benign tumors is surgical resection with primary anastomosis because of the significant risk of complications, such as bleeding or intussusception with obstruction without surgery.

Malignant tumors produce symptoms, including pain and weight loss, in most patients, with obstruction occurring in 15% to 30% of cases because of tumor infiltration and adhesions. The treatment of malignant tumors of the small bowel is wide cancer resection with regional lymphadenectomy. Pancreaticoduodenectomy (see section on pancreatic cancer) may be indicated for cancers of the duodenum. When surgical cure is impossible, palliative bypass procedures may be performed.

Laparoscopic lysis of adhesions has been demonstrated to be safe and effective in selected patients with small bowel obstruction who fail medical therapy. This approach most frequently succeeds in patients with less than three previous abdominal operations; prior appendectomy alone; early hospitalization after onset of symptoms; short duration of preoperative hospitalization (less than 24 hours); and simple adhesive bands as the obstructing mechanism discovered intraoperatively [33].

Although laparoscopic small bowel resection has been performed to treat Meckel's diverticulum and specially selected individuals with Crohn's disease, laparoscopic surgery for small bowel malignancy has been described only rarely in the surgical literature [34]. Several case reports have described laparoscopy, including laparoscopic-assisted small bowel resection, for a bleeding leiomyoma [35]. At present, there have been no large studies comparing the risks, benefits, and efficacy of laparoscopic surgery with that of the traditional open procedure for the staging, diagnosis, and treatment of small bowel cancers.

## Colorectal malignancies

The indications for laparoscopic colorectal resection are the same as those for open procedures and include inflammatory bowel disease, refractory bleeding, infection, trauma, and the removal of precancerous and cancerous lesions. Contraindications to laparoscopy include extensive previous abdominal surgery and tumors extending to adjacent organs.

The technique includes four or five small incisions for placement of the laparoscope and dissecting instruments. Specimen dissection and isolation is performed laparoscopically with the use of the harmonic scalpel or cautery. The oncologic principles of adequate margins of resection and wide resection of the colonic mesentery for complete lymphadenectomy are the same for laparoscopic surgery as for open surgery. Special precautions during laparoscopic resection include early vascular ligation, a no-touch technique, use of a wound protectomy, and release of the pneumoperitoneum before specimen removal. The specimen is removed in an impermeable bag to prevent spillage of cancerous cells. The anastomosis is performed either intracorporeally, especially for left-sided lesions, or extracorporeally in the HALS procedure. In the latter case, a mini-laparotomy incision, usually less than 7 cm, is made to remove the specimen and create the anastomosis [36]. The complications are identical between laparoscopic colorectal resection (LCR) and open colorectal resection (OCR). The most serious complications include wound infections, anastomotic leaks, bleeding, small bowel obstruction, and disruption of the autonomic nerves during rectal resection leading to urinary or sexual dysfunction.

Advantages of LCR over OCR substantiated in several studies include improved colonic motility with earlier initiation of oral intake, decreased postoperative pain, decreased length of hospitalization, and earlier return to work [37–39]. Length of stay data should be interpreted cautiously because they are highly influenced by health insurance company policies and by physician practices in different countries. Some studies have shown that LCR leads to significantly decreased intraoperative blood loss, and decreased need for transfusions, when compared with OCR [40–42]. This helps avoid the potentially immunosuppressive effects of transfusion. The primary disadvantage of LCR is an increase in mean operative time and in operating room charges, which increases the overall hospital cost [43]. The operative time declines with increasing surgical experience, and the operative cost is often counterbalanced by earlier hospital discharge and earlier return to work. Finally, the rate of wound complications decreases, possibly because of less wound contamination, decreased intestinal manipulation, and smaller incisions [44,45]. The incidence of anastomotic leaks and reoperation does not differ significantly between the two surgical techniques [46,47].

Surgery is frequently curative for colon cancer; the critical question is how LCR versus OCR affects patient survival. Chapman et al [48] reviewed 52 clinical trials on LCR: only five were properly randomized and in two of these the intention-to-treat analysis was violated. The rest of the studies were controlled clinical trials, case series, or case reports, reflecting the inherent problems in evaluating systematically a relatively new surgical procedure. Several randomized trials have analyzed the oncologic effects of LCR. Lacy et al [49] randomized 219 patients with nonmetastatic colon cancer into LCR versus OCR during a 5-year study. They verified the advantages of laparoscopic versus open surgery regarding less intraoperative blood loss, shorter onset to oral intake, shorter hospital stay, and lower morbidity, and some of the disadvantages, such as longer operative times. Although overall survival was not significantly different between the two groups, cancer-related survival and freedom from recurrence were significantly improved in the LCR group [49]. This difference seemed to be caused by improved results in patients with advanced nonmetastatic disease (stage III). The mechanism by which LCR was associated with a lower cancer recurrence rate and longer survival is unclear; one hypothesis suggests that the laparoscopic procedure results in decreased physiologic stress with a consequently more robust immune system, as supported by studies analyzing parameters of the immune response [50,51].

Port site metastases are a concern with LCR. These were initially estimated to occur in between 0% and 21% of cases [52–54]. In a prospective randomized trial, no port site metastases occurred in 91 patients treated by LCR and the overall recurrence rate was similar between LCR and OCR [55]. It is unclear whether abdominal wall recurrence is underreported in studies of OCR.

Overall, LCR seems an attractive surgical option that offers patients all the advantages associated with laparoscopy. Short-term oncologic results seem similar to that for OCR. There is a significant learning curve. Long-term results are still being analyzed.

## Hepatic tumors

Laparoscopy is primarily used for staging and biopsy of hepatic malignancies. Laparoscopy can be performed with three trocars. The liver is mobilized by dividing its ligamentous attachments, followed by complete laparoscopic evaluation of the liver, and biopsy of the hepatic lesions using cutting biopsy needles or cup forceps [56]. Hepatic lesions can have various colors and variable vascularity. They are usually superficial, however, and amenable to laparoscopic biopsy. Deeper lesions can be identified with laparoscopic ultrasound. The advantages of laparoscopy in this setting include the avoidance of the morbidity associated with a large subcostal incision, especially in the setting of hepatic cirrhosis, which frequently occurs in association with hepatic malignancy. This is especially important in patients who are deemed unresectable because of multiple lesions or advanced cirrhosis.

Recent technology, such as radiofrequency ablation, may be applied laparoscopically. Several small studies have demonstrated that radiofrequency can be delivered safely to ablate a liver lesion as an adjunct to laparoscopic resection, even in patients with Child's B or C cirrhosis [57,58]. In the latter group, radiofrequency ablation was usually used as a temporizing measure, and it prolonged the survival in patients who subsequently underwent orthotopic liver transplantation. Its success without orthotopic liver transplantation is uncertain.

Some groups have used laparoscopic or HALS surgery for partial hepatectomies or segmental resections [59–61]. These procedures include the establishment of pneumoperitoneum and a 5 to 10 cm long incision through which a hand can be inserted to facilitate manipulation of the target lesion. Technology used includes endoarticulating staplers, the ultrasonic scalpel, and hemostatic or occlusive glue. In studies of this procedure, the mean procedure duration of approximately 2.5 hours and the length of post-operative stay of 3 to 7 days were comparable with the historical experience with open surgery. Malignant tumors were resected with adequate margins. The complications were similar to those reported from open surgery.

Laparoscopic surgery has a role in the management of hepatic neoplasms for staging and biopsy, and for radiofrequency ablation as a bridge to transplantation. Its role in liver resection for malignancy requires further study. Most of the available studies are small and nonrandomized, because the technology is new and the learning curve is steep. The potential is great; laparoscopic lobectomies could provide an impetus to live-donor hepatic donation, to save the lives of people waiting a long time for transplantation of a cadaver liver.

## Pancreatic neoplasms

Pancreatic islet cell tumors represent a diverse group of neuroendocrine lesions, with greatly variable behavior. Successful treatment depends on accurate localization and ability to resect. Laparoscopy has significantly impacted the treatment of these tumors, because it has allowed improved intraoperative location (by use of laparoscopic ultrasound) followed by a less invasive resection than provided by open surgery [62,63]. Although many of these lesions are ideally suited for laparoscopic enucleation because of their small size and encapsulation, the adequacy of laparoscopic resection is of concern. The shorter hospital stay with laparoscopic surgery becomes a marginal benefit if patients with complications, such as pancreatic leaks (similar incidence for laparoscopic and open surgery), are included [64].

When enucleation is inadequate therapy, distal pancreatectomy may be required. This procedure is ideally suited for laparoscopy, because laparoscopic ultrasound can be used for tumor localization and the pathology is usually benign. Conditions for which distal pancreatectomy is indicated include cystadenoma, neuroendocrine tumors, cysts, and carcinoma of the pancreatic tail. When the splenic vessels are uninvolved splenic preservation may be possible. The surgery begins with an exploration to exclude metastatic disease, followed by entry into the lesser sac, after dividing the gastrocolic omentum to visualize the pancreas. The posterior peritoneum at the inferior border of the pancreas is divided. The dissection proceeds with division of the ligamentous attachments of the spleen and entrance into a fairly avascular plane posterior to the pancreatic tail. Mobilization proceeds from lateral to medial until the desired margin is reached. Endoscopic vascular stapling devices are used to control the splenic vessels, if the spleen is to be removed, and for the pancreas [65]. Complications include bleeding, which may require conversion to an open procedure; abscess; and pancreatic leak, which is usually adequately controlled with drainage and possible stenting of the pancreatic duct by endoscopic retrograde cholangiopancreatography.

Laparoscopic staging is frequently used for pancreatic adenocarcinoma to detect peritoneal carcinomatosis and hepatic lesions that may have been missed by conventional imaging studies. After thorough abdominal exploration, particularly of the liver, the lesser sac is entered and the pancreas examined. Intraoperative ultrasound, peritoneal cytology, and needle biopsies of suspicious lesions are useful adjuncts. About 10% of patients are found to have unresectable disease and spared the morbidity of an unnecessary laparotomy [66]. Some, however, argue that the limited detection rate of laparoscopic staging, the marginal benefit over MRI, and the absence of a large gain between surgical and endoscopic palliation, suggest that the benefit is only marginal [67–69]. Considering that laparoscopic staging is not a time-consuming procedure in experienced hands, it seems to be useful in properly selected patients when the preoperative imaging studies are inconclusive.

About 80% of patients with pancreatic and periampullary malignancies present with locally advanced or metastatic disease. These patients frequently require gastric or biliary bypass for palliation. Minimally invasive techniques may provide safe and effective alternatives to open surgery [70–72]. Although the biliary bypass of choice is a hepaticojejunostomy, the ease and safety of cholecystojejunostomy render it an attractive alternative for laparoscopic surgery. Patency of the cystic duct must be verified. Endoscopic biliary stents may be placed with significantly less morbidity than for any surgical procedure, but have a shorter half-life.

The data from the limited experience with laparoscopic pancreaticoduodenectomy have been encouraging, but the advent of HALS techniques has led to new enthusiasm. Very early limited reports show the potential for this technique [73].

## Summary

Laparoscopy is being used effectively for the staging, resecting, palliating, and preventing of gastrointestinal cancers. Continual improvement in surgical instrumentation and technical innovation will increase the applications of laparoscopic surgery in the diagnosis, staging, and treatment of gastrointestinal malignancies. Applications should continue to expand as novel techniques become routine.

## References

[1] Donohoe JH. Principles of cancer surgery. In: Norton JA, Bollinger RR, Lowry SF, Chang AE, Mulvhill SJ, Pass HI, et al, editors. Surgery: basic science and clinical evidence. New York: Springer Verlag; 2000. p. 1577–96.

[2] Barkun JS, Barkun AN, Sampalis JS, Fried G, Taylor B, Wexler MJ, et al. Randomized control trial of laparoscopic versus mini cholecystectomy. The McGill treatment Group. Lancet 1992;340:1116–9.
[3] Chandler JG, Corson SL, Way LW. Three spectra of laparoscopic entry access injuries. J Am Coll Surg 2000;192:478–90.
[4] Phillips PA, Amaral JF. Abdominal access complications in laparoscopic surgery. J Am Coll Surg 2001;192:525–36.
[5] Nordestgaard AG, Bodily KC, Osborne RW Jr, Buttorff JD. Major vascular injuries during laparoscopic procedures. Am J Surg 1995;169:543–5.
[6] Dabronte Z, Wittmann T, Karacsony G. Rapid development of malignant metastasis in the abdominal wall after laparoscopy. Endoscopy 1978;10:127–30.
[7] Ramirez PT, Wolf JK, Levenback C. Laparoscopic port-site metastasis: etiology and prevention. Gynecol Oncol 2003;91:179–89.
[8] Pearlstone DB, Feig BW, Mansfield PP. Port site recurrences after laparoscopy for malignant disease. Semin Surg Oncol 1999;16:307–12.
[9] Ziprin P, Ridgway PF, Peck DH, Darzi AW. The theories and realities of port-site metastases: a critical appraisal. J Am Coll Surg 2002;195(3):395–408.
[10] Reilly WT, Nelson H, Schroeder G, Wieand HS, O'Connell MJ. Wound recurrence following conventional treatment of colorectal cancer: a rare but perhaps underestimated problem. Dis Colon Rectum 1996;39:200–7.
[11] Eshraghi N, Swanstrom LL, Bax T, Jobe B, Horvath K, Sheppard B, et al. Topical treatments of laparoscopic port sites can decrease the incidence of incision metastasis. Surg Endosc 1999;13:1121–4.
[12] Swanstrom LL, Bax TL, Jobe B, Horvath K, Sheppard BL, Deveney C. Topical treatments of laparoscopic port sites can decrease the incidence of incision metastases. Surg Endosc 1999;13:1121–4.
[13] Society of American Gastrointestinal Endoscopic Surgeons. Integrating advanced laparoscopy into surgical residency training. Surgical Ultrasound 1998;12:374–6.
[14] Spivak H, Hunter JG. Endoluminal surgery. Surg Endosc 1997;11:321–5.
[15] Martinez-Serna T, Filipi CJ. Endoluminal surgery. World J Surg 1999;23:368–77.
[16] Targarona EM, Gracia E, Rodriguez M, Cerdan G, Balague C, Garriga J, et al. Hand-assisted laparoscopic surgery. Arch Surg 2003;138:133–41.
[17] Meijer DW, Bannenberg JJG, Jakimowicz JJ. Hand-assisted laparoscopic surgery: an overview. Surg Endosc 2000;14:891–5.
[18] Nguyen NT, Roberts P, Follette DM, Rivers R, Wolfe BM. Thoracoscopic and laparoscopic esophagectomy for benign and malignant disease: lessons learned from 46 consecutive procedures. J Am Coll Surg 2003;197:902–13.
[19] Nguyen NT, Follette DM, Wolfe BM, Schneider PD, Roberts P, Goodnight JE. Comparison of minimally invasive esophagectomy with transthoracic and transhiatal esophagectomy. Arch Surg 2000;135:920–5.
[20] Krasna MJ. The role of thoracoscopic lymph node staging in esophageal cancer. Int Surg 1997;82:7–11.
[21] Akiashi T, Kaneda I, Higuchi N, Kuriya Y, Kuramoto J, Toyoda T, et al. Thoracoscopic en bloc total esophagectomy with radical mediastinal lymphadenectomy. J Thorac Cardiovasc Surg 1996;112:1533–41.
[22] Peracchia A, Rosati R, Fumagalli U, Bona S, Chella B. Thoracoscopic esophagectomy: are there benefits? Semin Surg Oncol 1997;13:259–62.
[23] Osugi H, Takemura M, Higashino M, Takada N, Lee S, Ueno M. Learning curve of video-assisted thoracoscopic esophagectomy and extensive lymphadenectomy for squamous cell cancer of the thoracic esophagus and results. Surg Endosc 2003;17:515–9.
[24] Akiyama H, Tsurumaru M, Udagawa H, Kajiyama Y. Radical lymph node dissection for cancer of the thoracic esophagus. Ann Surg 1994;220:364–72.

[25] Abbas AE, Deschamps C, Cassivi SD, Allen MS, Nichols FC III, Miller DL, et al. Barrett's esophagus: the role of laparoscopic fundoplication. Ann Thorac Surg 2004;77:393–6.
[26] Jamieson GG, France M, Watson DI. Results of laparoscopic antireflux operations in patients who have Barrett's esophagus. Chest Surg Clin N Am 2002;12:149–55.
[27] Bass BL. What's new in general surgery: gastrointestinal conditions. J Am Coll Surg 2002; 195:835–54.
[28] Yildrim EM, Celen O, Berberoglu U. The Turkish experience with curative gastrectomies for gastric carcinomas: is D2 dissection worthwhile? J Am Coll Surg 2001;192:25–37.
[29] Kriplani AK, Kapur BML. Laparoscopy for preoperative staging and assessment of operability in gastric carcinoma. Gastrointest Endosc 1991;37:441–3.
[30] Weber KJ, Leyes CD, Gagner M, Divino CM. Comparison of laparoscopic and open gastrectomy for malignant disease. Surg Endosc 2003;17:968–71.
[31] Tanimura S, Higashino M, Fukunaga Y, Osugi H. Laparoscopic distal gastrectomy with regional lymph node dissection for gastric cancer. Surg Endosc 2003;17:758–62.
[32] Blanchard DK, Budde JM, Hatch GF, Wertheimer-Hatch L, Hatch KF, Davis GB, et al. Tumors of the small intestine. World J Surg 2000;24:421–9.
[33] Levard H, Boudet M, Msika S, Molkhou J, Hay J, Laborde Y, et al. Laparoscopic treatment of acute small bowell obstruction: a multi-coated retrospective study. Aust N Z J Surg 2001; 71:641–6.
[34] Aleali M, Milson JW. Laparoscopic surgery in Crohn's disease. Surg Clin North Am 2001; 81:217–30.
[35] Kok KYY, Mathew VV, Yapp SKS. Laparoscopic-assisted small bowel resection for a bleeding leiomyoma. Surg Endosc 1998;12:995–6.
[36] Weiss EG, Wexner SD. Laparoscopic segmental colectomies, anterior resection, and abdominoperineal resection. In: Scott-Conner CEH, editor. The SAGES manual: fundamentals in laparoscopy and GI endoscopy. New York: Springer-Verlag; 1998 p. 286–305.
[37] Guller U, Jain N, Hervey S, Purves H, Pietrobon R. Laparoscopic vs open colectomy: outcomes comparison based on large nationwide databases. Arch Surg 2003;138: 1179–86.
[38] Kasparek MS, Muller MH, Glatzle J, Manncke K, Baecker HD, Zittel TI, et al. Postoperative colonic motility in patients following laparoscopic assisted and open sigmoid colectomy. J Gastrointest Surg 2003;7:1073–81.
[39] Schlachta CM, Mamazza J, Gregoire R, Burpee SE, Poulin EC. Could laparoscopic colon and rectal surgery become the standard of care? A review and experience with 750 procedures. Can J Surg 2003;46:432–40.
[40] Kiran RP, Delaney CP, Senagore AJ, Millward BL, Fazio VW. Operative blood loss and use of blood products after laparoscopic and conventional open colorectal operations. Arch Surg 2004;139:39–42.
[41] Senagore AJ, Luchtefeld MA, Mackeigan JM, Mazier WP. Open colectomy versus laparoscopic colectomy: are there differences? Am Surg 1993;59:549–54.
[42] Muckleroy SK, Ratzer ER, Fenoglio ME. Laparoscopic colon surgery for benign disease: a comparison to open surgery. Journal of Society of Laparoendoscopic Surgeons 1999;3: 33–7.
[43] Lezoche E, Feliciotti F, Guerrieri M, Paganini AM, De Sanctis A, Campagnacci R, et al. Laparoscopic versus open hemicolectomy. Minerva Chir 2003;58:491–507.
[44] Milsom JW, Hammerhofer KA, Bohm B, Marcello P, Elson P, Fazio VW. Prospective randomized trial comparing laparoscopic vs. conventional surgery for refractory ileocolic Crohn's disease. Dis Colon Rectum 2001;44:1–9.
[45] Liang JT, Shieh MJ, Chen CN, Cheng YM, Chang KJ, Wang SM. Prospective evaluation of laparoscopic-assisted colectomy versus laparotomy with resection for management of complex polyps of the sigmoid colon. World J Surg 2002;26:377–83.

[46] Braga M, Gianotti L, Vignali A, Di Carlo V. Preoperative oral arginine and n-3 fatty acid supplementation improves the immunometabolic host response and outcome after colorectal resection for cancer. Surgery 2002;132(5):805–14.
[47] Vignali A, Gianotti L, Braga M, Radaelli G, Malvezzi L, DiCarlo V. Microperfusion of the rectal stump as predictive index of anastomotic leak. Dis Colon Rectum 2000;43:76–82.
[48] Chapman AE, Levitt MD, Hewett P, Woods R, Sheiner H, Maddern GJ. Laparoscopic-assisted resection of colorectal malignancies: a systematic review. Ann Surg 2001;234: 590–606.
[49] Lacy AM, Garcia-Valdecasas JC, Delgado S, Castells A, Taura P, Pique JM, et al. Laparoscopy-assisted colectomy versus open colectomy for treatment of non-metastatic colon cancer: a randomized trial. Lancet 2002;359:2224–9.
[50] Braga M, Vignali A, Gianotti L, Zuliani W, Radaelli G, Gruarin P, et al. Laparoscopic versus open colorectal surgery: a randomized trial on short-term outcome. Ann Surg 2002; 236:759–67.
[51] Harmon GD, Senagore AJ, Killbride MJ, Warzynski MJ. Interleukin-6 response to laparoscopic and open colectomy. Dis Colon Rectum 1994;37:754–9.
[52] Lacy AM, Delgado S, Garcia-Valdecasas JC, Castells A, Pique JM, Grande L, et al. Port site metastases and recurrence after laparoscopic colectomy, a randomized trial. Surg Endosc 1998;12:1039–42.
[53] Franklin M, Rosenthal D, Dorman J, Glass J, Norem R, Diaz A. Prospective comparison of open vs laparoscopic colon surgery for carcinoma: five year results. Dis Colon Rectum 1996; 39:S35–46.
[54] Wexner S, Cohen S. Port site metastases after laparoscopic colorectal surgery for cure of malignancy. Br J Surg 1995;82:295–8.
[55] Whelan R, Sellars G, Allendorf J, Laird D, Bessler MD, Nowygrod R, et al. Trocar site recurrence is unlikely to result from aerosolization of tumor cells. Dis Colon Rectum 1996; 39:S7–13.
[56] Greene F. Elective diagnostic laparoscopy and cancer staging. In: Scott-Conner CEH, editor. The SAGES manual: fundamentals in laparoscopy and GI endoscopy. New York: Springer-Verlag; 1998. p. 121.
[57] Arch-Ferrer JE, Smith JK, Bynon S, Eckhoff DE, Sellers MT, Bland KI, et al. Radio-frequency ablation in cirrhotic patients with hepatocellular carcinoma. Am Surg 2003;69: 1067–71.
[58] Croce E, Olmi S, Bertolini A, Erba L, Magnone S. Laparoscopic liver resection with radiofrequency. Hepatogastroenterology 2003;50:2088–92.
[59] Huang MT, Lee WJ, Wang W, Wei PL, Chen RJ. Hand-assisted laparoscopic hepatectomy for solid tumor in the posterior portion of the right lobe: initial experience. Ann Surg 2003; 238:674–9.
[60] Buell JF, Doty T, Schneider C, Gersin K, Rudich SM, Merchen TM, et al. Initial experience and evolution of laparoscopic liver surgery [abstract ]. In: Programs and abstracts of the Central Surgical Association; 2004, in press.
[61] Linden BC, Humar A, Sielaff TD. Laparoscopic stapled left lateral segment liver resection-technique and results. J Gastrointest Surg 2003;7:777–82.
[62] Spitz JD, Lilly MC, Tetik C, Arregui ME. Ultrasound-guided laparoscopic resection of pancreatic islet cell tumors. Surg Laparosc Endosc Percutan Tech 2000;10:168–73.
[63] Gagner M, Pomp A, Herrera MF. Early experience with laparoscopic resections of islet cell tumors. Surgery 1996;120:1051–4.
[64] Jaroszewski DE, Schlinkert RT, Thompson GB, Schlinkert DK. Laparoscopic localization and resection of insulinomas. Arch Surg 2004;139:270–4.
[65] Salky B. Distal pancreatectomy. In: Scott-Conner CEH, editor. The SAGES manual: fundamentals in laparoscopy and GI endoscopy. New York: Springer-Verlag; 1998 p. 307–313.
[66] Brooks AD, Mallis MJ, Brennan MF, Conlon KC. J Gastrointest Surg 2002;6:139–45.

[67] Schneider AR, Adamek HE, Layer G, Riemann JF, Arnold JC. Staging of abdominal metastases in pancreatic carcinoma by diagnostic laparoscopy and magnetic resonance imaging. Z Gastroenterol 2003;41:697–702.

[68] Hennig R, Tempia-Caliera AA, Hartel M, Buchler MW, Friess H. Staging laparoscopy and its indications in pancreatic cancer patients. Dig Surg 2002;19:484–8.

[69] Nieveen van Dijkum EJM, Romijin MG, Terwee CB, de Wit LT, van der Meulen HJP, Lameris HS, et al. Laparoscopic staging and subsequent palliation in patients with peripancreatic carcinoma. Ann Surg 2003;237:66–73.

[70] Rhodes M, Nathanson L, Fielding G. Laparoscopic biliary and gastric bypass: a useful adjunct in the treatment of carcinoma of the pancreas. Gut 1995;36:778–80.

[71] Bergamaschi R, Marvik R, Thoresen JE, Ystgaard B, Johnsen G, Myrvold HE. Open versus laparoscopic gastrojejunostomy for palliation in advanced pancreatic cancer. Surg Laparosc Endosc 1998;8:92–6.

[72] Rothlin MA, Schob O, Weber M. Laparoscopic gastro- and hepaticojejunostomy for palliation of pancreatic cancer: a case controlled study. Surg Endosc 1999;13:1065–9.

[73] Gagner M, Gentileschi P. Hand-assisted laparoscopic pancreatic resection. Semin Laparosc Surg 2001;8:114–25.

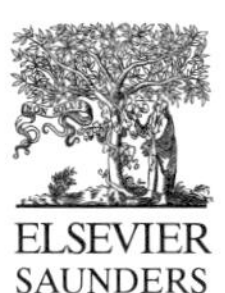

ELSEVIER
SAUNDERS

Med Clin N Am 89 (2005) 211–217

THE MEDICAL CLINICS OF NORTH AMERICA

# Index

*Note:* Page numbers of article titles are in **bold face** type.




doi:10.1016/S0025-7125(04)00168-3

## D



## E